PIVOTAL
MOMENTS
in Nursing

Leaders Who Changed the Path of a Profession

VOLUME II

BOOKS PUBLISHED BY THE HONOR SOCIETY OF NURSING, SIGMA THETA TAU INTERNATIONAL

Pivotal Moments in Nursing: Leaders Who Changed the Path of a Profession, Houser and Player, 2004 (Volume I) and 2007 (Volume II).

The W. K. Kellogg Foundation and the Nursing Profession: Shared Values, Shared Legacy, Lynaugh, Smith, Grace, Sena, de Villalobos, and Hlalele, 2007.

Daily Miracles: Stories and Practices of Humanity and Excellence in Health Care, Briskin and Boller, 2006.

A Daybook for Nurse Leaders and Mentors. Sigma Theta Tau International, 2006.

When Parents Say No: Religious and Cultural Influences on Pediatric Healthcare Treatment, Linnard-Palmer, 2006.

Healthy Places, Healthy People: A Handbook for Culturally Competent Community Nursing Practice, Dreher, Shapiro, and Asselin, 2006.

The HeART of Nursing: Expressions of Creative Art in Nursing, Second Edition, Wendler, 2005.

Reflecting on 30 Years of Nursing Leadership: 1975-2005, Donley, 2005.

nurseAdvance Collection. (Topic-specific collections of honor society published journal articles.) Topics offered are: Cultural Diversity in Nursing; Disaster, Trauma, and Emergency Nursing; Gerontological Nursing; Health Promotion in Nursing; Implementing Evidence-Based Nursing; Resources for Implementing Evidence-Based Nursing; Leadership and Mentoring in Nursing; Maternal Health Nursing; Oncology Nursing; Pediatric Nursing; Psychiatric-Mental Health Nursing; Public, Environmental, and Community Health Nursing; and Women's Health Nursing; 2006.

Technological Competency as Caring in Nursing, Locsin, 2005.

Making a Difference: Stories from the Point of Care, Volume I, Hudacek, 2005.

Making a Difference: Stories from the Point of Care, Volume II, Hudacek, 2004.

A Daybook for Nurses: Making a Difference Each Day, Hudacek, 2004.

Building and Managing a Career in Nursing: Strategies for Advancing Your Career, Miller, 2003.

Collaboration for the Promotion of Nursing, Briggs, Merk, and Mitchell, 2003.

Ordinary People, Extraordinary Lives: The Stories of Nurses, Smeltzer and Vlasses, 2003.

Stories of Family Caregiving: Reconsideration of Theory, Literature, and Life, Poirier and Ayres, 2002.

As We See Ourselves: Jewish Women in Nursing, Benson, 2001.

Cadet Nurse Stories: The Call for and Response of Women During World War II, Perry and Robinson, 2001.

Creating Responsive Solutions to Healthcare Change, McCullough, 2001.

Nurses' Moral Practice: Investing and Discounting Self, Kelly, 2000.

Nursing and Philanthropy: An Energizing Metaphor for the 21st Century, McBride, 2000.

Gerontological Nursing Issues for the 21st Century, Gueldner and Poon, 1999.

The Adventurous Years: Leaders in Action 1973-1999, Henderson, 1998.

Immigrant Women and Their Health: An Olive Paper, Ibrahim Meleis, Lipson, Muecke and Smith, 1998.

The Neuman Systems Model and Nursing Education: Teaching Strategies and Outcomes, Lowry, 1998.

The Image Editors: Mind, Spirit, and Voice, Hamilton, 1997.

The Language of Nursing Theory and Metatheory, King and Fawcett, 1997.

Virginia Avenel Henderson: Signature for Nursing, Hermann, 1997.

For more information and to order these books from the Honor Society of Nursing, Sigma Theta Tau International, visit the society's Web site at www.nursingsociety.org/publications, or go to www.nursingknowledge. org/stti/books, the Web site of Nursing Knowledge International, the honor society's sales and distribution division or, call 1.888.NKI.4.YOU (U.S. and Canada) or +1.317.634.8171 (Outside U.S. and Canada).

PIVOTAL MOMENTS
in Nursing

Leaders Who Changed the Path of a Profession

BETH P. HOUSER, RN, MS, FNP-C, DNSC
KATHY N. PLAYER, RN, EDD

VOLUME II

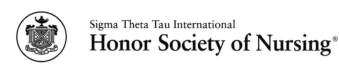

Sigma Theta Tau International
Honor Society of Nursing®

SIGMA THETA TAU INTERNATIONAL

Editor-in-Chief: Jeff Burnham
Acquisitions Editor: Fay L. Bower, DNSc, FAAN
Development Editor: Carla Hall
Copy Editor: Jane Palmer
Proofreader: Michelle Lilly

Cover Design by: Rebecca Harmon
Interior Design and Page Composition by: Rebecca Harmon

Printed in the United States of America
Printing and Binding by Printing Partners, Indianapolis, IN.

Sigma Theta Tau International
550 West North Street
Indianapolis, IN 46202

Visit our Web site at **www.nursingknowledge.org/STTI/books** for more information on our books.

ISBN-10: 1-930538-19-7
ISBN-13: 978-1-930538-19-1
Library of Congress Cataloging-in-Publication Data
Houser, Beth, 1957-
     Pivotal moments in nursing : leaders who changed the path of a profession / by Beth Houser and Kathy Player.
     p. ; cm.
Includes bibliographical references and index.
ISBN 1-930538-11-1
   1. Nurses—United States—Biography. 2. Nursing—United States—History.
[DNLM: 1. History of Nursing—United States. 2. Nurses—United States—Biography. 3. Leadership—United States—Biography. WZ 112.5.N8 H842p 2004]
I. Player, Kathy, 1962- II. Sigma Theta Tau International. III. Title.
RT34.H68 2004
610'.92'2—dc22
   2004005624

07   08   09   10   11   /   5   4   3   2   1

DEDICATION

"Imagine a world without nurses. Think of a world without persons who know what nurses know; who believe as nurses believe; who do what nurses do; who have the effect that nurses have on the health of individuals, families, and the nation; who enjoy the trust that nurses enjoy from the American people. Imagine a world like that, a world without nurses."

–Margretta Madden Styles
Presentation to the House of Delegates
American Association of Nurses annual meeting
Washington, DC, 2003

ACKNOWLEDGEMENTS

Beth P. Houser

I would like to acknowledge those who have helped me remain committed to my Daffodil Principle (see Introduction). First, I must thank my family for allowing me to pursue my dreams. Your patience and support have been appreciated and are the fuel that allows me to take one step at a time. Jessica, you have been there to care, and I thank you for your support. Rob, you have infinite leadership potential—go get life! Kevin, you have a grounded spirit and great vision—I look forward to watching you make your dreams become a reality. Bob, once again you have edited every word and applied your wisdom and intelligence. I couldn't have done it without you. Let me also thank Bill and Lorna Parsons (brother and sister in-law) and Sandy and Rich Hoch (sister and brother-in-law) for their unconditional love and support.

Lee Ford, RN, EdD, FAAN, has been a valued mentor and friend. She has carefully planted numerous seeds of vision. I recall a day when I burdened Lee with a *long* e-mail describing my cat-herding job. I expounded in great detail about my professional frustrations. The next day, she wrote back with a one-line reply that permanently changed my leadership perspective. She said, "Get some catnip, get in the middle of the circle, and make them come to you."

I must also give thanks to Sue Donaldson, RN, PhD, FAAN, who taught me how to write. I can hear Sue asking, "Is that the right word? Did you mean to say that? What is your point, and where are you taking the reader?" The sea of red ink on my work was your map for my growth. Thanks for continuing to apply pressure even when I resisted. I appreciate the energy you have invested. You helped me create a new understanding of my responsibility to scholarship. I also would like to thank my Scottsdale Healthcare colleagues: Peggy Reiley, RN, PhD, Kathi Zarubi, RN, MBA, Cathy Collette, and Doris Milton, RN, PhD, for proofreading many of the chapters and offering their insight into the final product. Last, but certainly not least, I would like to thank Nancy Queen, RN (John C. Lincoln —North Mountain) for always reminding me to reach further than comfortable and remain focused on what matters.

Lastly, I would like to thank Kathy Player, who is a consummate professional. She is a partner who is always on time! Thank heavens for Kathy. I admire her tireless commitment to our nursing profession. She has invested most of her career to enabling nurses to remain patient-focused and quality-minded through her work in professional organizations. Kathy is a master communicator and collaborator. It is a privilege to work with a colleague who is lives out the Daffodil Principle.

Dr. Kathy N. Player

I would like to thank Dr. Ken Blanchard and my colleagues in the Ken Blanchard College of Business at Grand Canyon University for their support in this undertaking. You each provided me with the encouragement needed to accomplish volume two and to now look to volume three. Thanks to Brent Richardson, CEO, for generously providing me the freedom to pursue my dreams. You allow me the opportunity to continuously impact nursing and healthcare through somewhat unconventional avenues.

Thanks go to my supportive friends and colleagues: Dr. Fran Roberts, dean of the College of Nursing at Grand Canyon University, you have a vision for what "can be" in nursing that is matched by few. Dr. Jody Summerford, dean of the College of Education, you are a true friend. Thank you both for always being just a phone call away.

As nurses, we are reminded daily of life's critical lessons, one of which is the importance of family. To my husband, who shares in the joy of my wins and provides encouragement through all life's challenges: Thanks for your devotion and love. Thanks to my mom and dad for being the strongest cheerleaders life offers. You both came to this country as immigrants and worked hard to provide a better life for your children. Any success I achieve along the way is my tribute to you both.

The initial concept for this book was Beth Houser's brainstorm, of which I accidentally got caught in the swirl. Interviewing these leaders, eating meals with them, meeting their families, and in some cases actually spending the night at their house to get the "whole story" will remain one of the most priceless moments in my nursing career. Thanks for all of it, Beth!

ABOUT THE AUTHORS

BETH P. HOUSER, RN, MS, FNP-C, DNSC

Beth Houser is director of Critical Care and Telemetry at Scottsdale Healthcare, Shea, and Osborn hospitals. Prior to this position, she was director of nursing research and Magnet projects for John C. Lincoln (JCL) Health Network in Phoenix, Arizona. She is also a Magnet appraiser for the American Nurses Credentialing Center and a Robert Wood Johnson Executive Nurse Fellow.

She graduated from the University of Arizona in 1978 with her Bachelor of Science in Nursing degree, and 20 years later completed her Master of Science degree from Arizona State University as a family nurse practitioner. In August 2004, Beth completed her doctoral dissertation, titled "Nursing Staffing Levels and Patient Outcomes," at Johns Hopkins University School of Nursing. The Hopkins Doctor of Nursing Science degree was devoted to educating nurses to utilize large databases to answer global healthcare questions, including the cost of implications. Her career interests include nurse-sensitive quality indicators and excellence in nursing practice.

Beth is adjunct faculty for Arizona State University and has spoken nationally on Magnet issues. She is an active member of the American Nurses Association, Sigma Theta Tau International, and the American Academy of Nurse Practitioners.

Beth is certified by the American Nurses Credentialing Center as a family nurse practitioner and remains active in clinical practice. She is the mother of three children, Jessica, Rob, and JJ, who have been the constant reminder to Beth of what really matters.

Kathy N. Player, RN, EdD

Dr. Kathy Player is dean of the Ken Blanchard College of Business and the College of Entrepreneurship at Grand Canyon University. She previously held the positions of chair of professional studies and director for the RN-BSN program. As dean, she oversees both the business division and professional studies division of the college. Kathy coordinated the development of an HLC-accredited Master of Science in Leadership program, which has been widely received by the healthcare community.

Kathy is the second vice-president for the American Nurses Association (2006-2008), serves on the boards of the American Nurses Credentialing Center (2006-2008) and Arizona Nurses Foundation (2006-2008), and is past president of the Arizona Nurses Association (2001-2005). She was awarded an RWJ Executive Nurse Fellowship in Leadership (2002-2005) and is an invited member of the Global Nursing Exchange. Kathy is the past vice president of Nu Upsilon Chapter of Sigma Theta Tau International and is a current member of Beta Mu Chapter.

Kathy co-authored volumes I and II of *Pivotal Moments in Nursing: Leaders Who Changed the Path of a Profession*. Other publications include: Entering a Community Dialog, *Nursing Administration Quarterly* (January, 2004); Retention: The Critical Challenge, *Nurse Leader* (July, 2003); and Take the Lead, *Reflections on Nursing Leadership* (May, 2003). She is also a contributing author for the chapter titled Legal Accountability and Responsibilities in the textbook *Nursing Fundamentals: Caring & Clinical Decision Making* (January, 2004).

Kathy has a global interest in improving the nursing profession and healthcare by providing nurses access to business, management, and leadership education. In 1999, Kathy traveled to Trang, Thailand, to work with Thai baccalaureate nursing students and faculty. In 2003, she participated in a healthcare leadership exchange in Cuba and met with directors and ministers of health to share U.S. and Cuban ideas and solutions for healthcare. In 2003 and 2004, Kathy went to Mexico as a participant in the Global Nursing Exchange.

Kathy lobbies actively at both local and national levels on behalf of nurses and nursing issues. She has worked on many successful healthcare proposition campaigns within Arizona, and she successfully coordinated efforts to receive a Leadership Initiative grant and a statewide Nursing Workforce Environment grant through the Arizona Nurses Association.

Kathy has an extensive background in healthcare. She graduated with her doctorate from the University of Sarasota in counseling psychology and holds a master's degree in counseling from Nova Southeastern University and a bachelor's degree in nursing from St. Joseph's College. She will graduate with both her MBA and MS-N in March 2007. She can be contacted via e-mail at kplayer@gcu.edu.

She lives in Phoenix, Arizona, with her husband, Ken. They enjoy traveling, skating, and photography.

TABLE OF CONTENTS

FOREWORD

Edge Runners, as described by Leland Kaiser, are individuals who combine knowledge, commitment, and will to push their ideas forward in the face of resistance. The ideas and the gathering of support for action often lead to necessary and permanent changes in systems and practices. The nurses profiled in this book are Edge Runners.* Each chapter describes the personal and professional journey to mastery and the impact of their work on the lives of others. Nurses and healthcare professionals around the world will be inspired by reading about the profiles in courage, leadership, and commitment as each of these leaders made the choices—sometimes very difficult ones—to effect change and to make a difference in the lives of others.

Readers will be engaged by the personal and professional stories of these exemplars of nursing excellence. The personal journey of each of these leaders often led to their choices to become nurses, to their perseverance, and to their lifelong commitment to making a difference in the lives of others. The stories of overcoming hardship, discrimination, and personal and professional struggles are profound. Readers should reflect on each story and how it fits into the mosaic of human caring pathways that exist within our profession. Each chapter presents a new pathway for us to examine and consider as we develop our own pathways.

Enjoy this book and allow the stories of these Edge Runners to inspire you in your personal journey.

—Linda Burnes Bolton, DrPH, RN, FAAN
Past President, American Academy of Nursing (2007)
Vice President and Chief Nursing Officer
Cedars-Sinai Medical Center, Los Angeles, CA
February 2007

*In November 2006, the American Academy of Nursing (AAN) launched the Raise the Voice campaign. For more information about this campaign or to nominate a nurse you know as an Edge Runner, visit www.aannet.org/raisethevoice/.

INTRODUCTION

As we wrote of the journeys of these exceptional leaders, those who changed the world through their tireless efforts, we were reminded of the story of the Daffodil Garden. In 1995, Jaroldeen Edwards wrote of the Daffodil Principle in her book *Celebration!* The story is of a daughter who knew of a magical place, a garden, planted by the hands of one woman named Gene Bauer who many years before had committed to change a small section of the world through her passion for daffodils. The daughter knew the wonder of Gene's efforts, but her mother couldn't see the need of visiting one more garden in her life, no matter how her daughter tried to convince her. What the mother missed in the message was that it wasn't only about the beauty of the Daffodil Garden; it was really about the possibility of changing the world in a sustaining way.

When the mother begrudgingly arrived at the Daffodil Garden, despite unpleasant weather, she was spellbound and rendered speechless by the beauty of Gene's 5 acres of the most astonishing colors and patterns displayed by the more than 50,000 bulbs planted by one woman, one bulb at a time, over nearly 40 years. The mother experienced the inspiration of the Daffodil Principle as:

- Moving toward a goal one step at a time.
- Loving the doing of one's goals.
- Understanding the power of accumulation over time.

When the awe and the enormity of that one woman's actions had washed over her, she was overcome by a deep sense of sadness and guilt that she hadn't committed to doing more with her own life's work. Her daughter, with a wisdom that exceeded her years, urged her mother to "start tomorrow." She reminded her mother not to fret about lost hours but instead to focus on how she might put the Daffodil Principle to use tomorrow.

The Daffodil Garden is located in the San Bernardino mountain range of southern California. In 1999, the Willow Fire destroyed Gene Bauer's A-frame home and most of the surrounding landscape. Miraculously, the daffodil bulbs beneath the ground survived and continue to bloom today. Gene's vision will long outlive her life. Her accomplishment will serve to inspire others to do something meaningful—no matter how large it seems or how long it will take.

We hope that as you read these remarkable leadership stories you will develop a sense of urgency around defining your professional "Daffodil Principle." We all have the opportunity to make a difference—one action at a time.

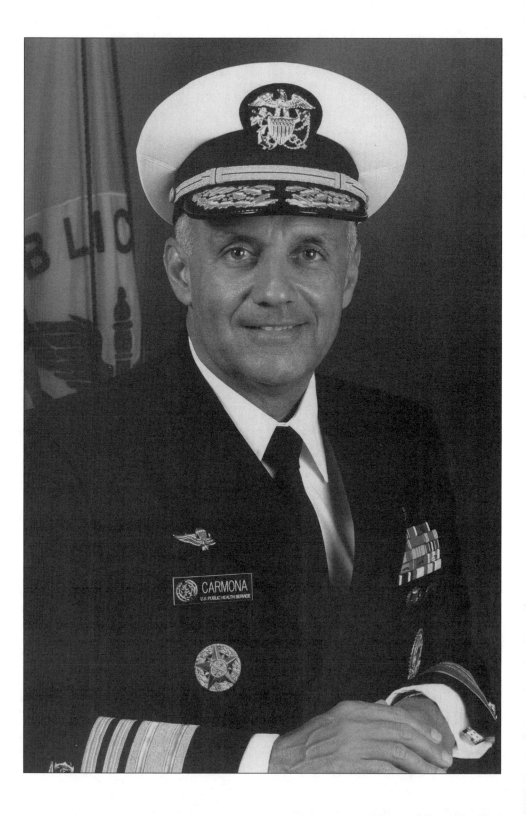

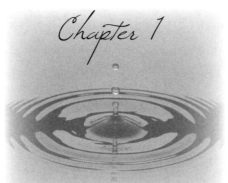

RICHARD HENRY CARMONA

"A recovering surgeon, always a nurse."
—Richard Carmona

On 5 August 2002, Richard Carmona, RN, MD, MPH, FACS, became the United States surgeon general, responsible for the health and well-being of almost 300 million U.S. citizens. In Rich Carmona, the president and Congress selected an accomplished medic; a combat-decorated, Vietnam veteran Army Green Beret; a nurse; a physician assistant; a physician; a police officer; a professor; a hospital administrator; and a public health officer. Rich's leadership brought credibility, trust, and integrity to the surgeon general's office because he prepared for the position by "living the experiences" that directly threaten public health today—high school dropout, poverty, addiction, homelessness, hunger, limited access to healthcare, family dysfunction, ethnic discrimination, and community chaos.

From very early in life, the decks were stacked against him. The irony is that he does not view himself as a victim. Rather, he views himself as a student of what life has offered him. For Rich, there were small windows in life that had a big impact in creating leadership opportunities. Rich credits his success to being more tenacious, wanting it more, and not being afraid to fail. He admits, "I have failed more times in my life than I have succeeded. The difference is I just continued to get up ... ultimately, I just got up one more time than the person who failed."

Rich describes himself as a recovering surgeon, but always a nurse. He believes he became a very good doctor because he was a very good nurse first. He insists that nursing's gift to his career is the holistic lens. He explains that physicians and nurses both care for patients, but each discipline approaches patient care from a different perspective. "Physicians see a problem on a body," he says. "Nurses see a person who happens to have something wrong, but they also see a family and an environment—nurses put the pieces of the puzzle together." Numerous influences have shaped his leadership style, but his strong sense of collaboration, communication, and compassion may be traced back to his nursing experience.

> *"I have failed more times in my life than I have succeeded. The difference is I just continued to get up. Ultimately, I just got up one more time than the person who failed."*

The leadership story of Rich Carmona is one of courage, commitment, and compassion. He is a global leader in public health policy for issues that lack geopolitical boundaries. He balances finite resources and infinite healthcare demands—an enormous responsibility that would appear daunting to most. Not, however, to Rich, whose passion is excellence and whose motto is "under-promise and over-deliver." He has created an exemplary record of success by understanding how to complete the mission. Rich is determined to improve, advance, and protect the health of the nation and the world. There is little doubt, given his leadership record, he will once again over-deliver.

Growing Up in Harlem

Rich was a first-generation American born 22 November 1949 in New York City (NYC). He was the oldest of four children (Rich, David, Phillip, and Susan) born to Lucy Martinez and Raoul Carmona. He was known most of his life as Richie or Rich to his family and friends. Both of his parents immigrated to the United States as young children and shared a common heritage of poverty; however, this tie is where the similarity started and ended. Lucy was an only child and Raoul was the youngest of 27 children, all of whom resided in a small apartment in a ghetto in Harlem. Lucy, although uneducated, was a scholar who spoke several languages. Raoul, a very nice man, was unfortunately a poor communicator even in his native tongue.

Rich's paternal grandmother, Maria Anglade Carmona, known to many as "Abuelita," emigrated from Puerto Rico without her husband to find a better life for her 27 children—nine of her own and 18 stepchildren. As a single mother, Abuelita was the family matriarch who ruled with an iron hand and a loving heart. She was the glue that held the family together through the good times and bad. Standing barely 5 feet tall and weighing less than 100 pounds soaking wet, Abuelita was a giant in Rich's eyes.

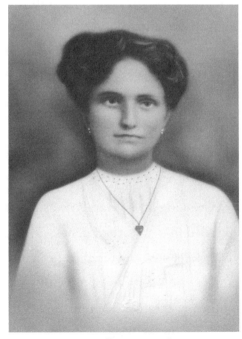

MARIA ANGLADE CARMONA, ABUELITA TO RICHARD CARMONA.

Abuelita was the neighborhood seamstress and the community ambassador. Every Sunday she would cook all day and open her home to those who needed food or support, and she welcomed newly immigrated families to the community. Abuelita taught Rich the lessons of cultural diversity and survival. Through her, he learned the value of the individual and the community, as well as the power of community service. Taking care of others was simply a way of life in the Carmona household.

It was no secret that Rich was Abuelita's favorite grandchild. As he struggled with delinquency and truancy through adolescence, Abuelita told anyone who would listen that "Richie is going to find himself and he will be fine," when no one else believed that—including Rich. Every Easter she would sew him a new suit. Rich would sit next to her and watch in amazement as she pumped the foot pedals of the old Singer sewing machine and magically produced handsome clothes that made him feel so proud. When she had Rich's attention, she was also sowing seeds of cultural heritage and responsibility. She forced Rich to speak Spanish, when it wasn't politically correct. Abuelita required that he listen to stories about Hispanic-American history so he knew and appreciated his roots. She earned respect from her family for her courage and integrity in dealing with whatever life sent her way. Rich admits that many of her early lessons were initially lost on him, but the seeds were planted. Decades later, it is not difficult to see that Abuelita's influence lived on in her favored grandchild. Rich was 14 years old when Abuelita died, and he was still "running the streets" of Harlem.

Growing up in Harlem was a test to the spirit. The neighborhood was engulfed in a culture of drugs, crime, and poverty. Street smarts and survival skills were required to fit in. Substance abuse was prominent in Rich's family. The "demons of alcohol" had overtaken his maternal grandmother, mother, and father. He remembers his maternal grandmother drinking and smoking all day long. As he watched her health decline, he was confused that someone that young could be so sick. Rich watched the devastation of poor lifestyle choices consume his grandmother's quality of life. His mother also chain smoked but reserved drinking alcohol for the evening hours. His father, a "good alcoholic," was frequently absent. His absences left a negative impression on his son, but Rich believes this helped him become a better leader, as he learned valuable lessons from the absence. Employment by any adult in the family was sporadic. Hunger was real and a daily worry. "It is hard to focus on homework or SAT exams when you are consumed with where the next meal will come from," he says. Surviving in the ghetto eclipsed vision or hope for the Carmonas.

Rich remembers returning from school one day to see the meager family belongings loaded in the back of a Salvation Army truck. At age 6, Rich and his parents and siblings were temporarily homeless and living in the streets. Abuelita took them in to her very small "projects" apartment. They stayed for about 18 months. Eventually, the family re-established residence in a Harlem tenement that was roach-infested. When the lights went out, the mice came out. In the winter, the apartment was too cold, and it was too hot in the summer. Whatever the season, there was rarely any hot water. His Abuelita would often bring food and basic comfort items. She was the family safety net—the safe port in the storm that often swirled around the Carmona household.

Despite the unstable lifestyle, Rich has very fond and vivid memories of his mother. He recalls in detail the dingy kitchen that had a little steel table and four uncomfortable steel chairs. It was here that his mother "would hold court." She would pontificate about "the power of education to set you free," and "there is life beyond poverty." Year after year, Lucy drilled into him that it was essential to think big and that he could be anything he

By the time Rich reached the sixth grade, the influence of poverty, addiction, ethnic disparity, family dysfunction, and community chaos had begun to negatively drive his choices.

wanted to be. For hours on end, while smoking and drinking, she would read to the children from encyclopedias and books borrowed from the library. Then she would quiz them on the new material, hoping to light the flame of inquiry and the quest for knowledge.

On a daily basis, Lucy would speak of world events and cultural differences. It was not unusual for her to vary her language among French, German, Spanish, and English to expand the children's vision of the world. She wanted them to know about the possibilities available to them. Rich describes his mother as a highly intelligent Renaissance woman who was born half a century too early. Lucy was also a talented, self-taught artist and musician. Perhaps the memory that sustained him through the years of instability was his mother's constant "hugs and kisses and telling us how much she cared about us."

His father was a man who had difficulty expressing himself. Rich cannot recall that his father ever told him he loved him, and he has no memory of spending time with his father. Rich describes him as a "guy I knew cared for me and was a very nice man, but someone I didn't see a lot." As a result, Rich became a surrogate parent for his younger siblings. Rich is careful not to criticize his father. As he says, "I didn't walk in those shoes." This wisdom has allowed him to see beyond injustice and helped prepare him for becoming a nondiscriminatory healthcare leader.

By the time Rich reached the sixth grade, the influence of poverty, addiction, ethnic disparity, family dysfunction, and community chaos had begun to negatively drive his choices. He developed truant behaviors that were episodic throughout his middle school years. His mother and Abuelita battled with him to attend class, but he simply wasn't interested in academics.

In the early 1960s, in an attempt to diversify the uptown schools, students were bused from Harlem to the Bronx. Rich found himself in a vastly different culture and also discovered that high school was a means to do something he was interested in—play team sports. The one glitch to team participation was the requirement of class attendance to make the team. Accommodating his interest in sports with the demands of school required some ingenuity on his part. Rich had to stay one step ahead of the coach and keep his real attendance record under cover. He did so by signing in each morning to homeroom class and then quietly taking the rest of the day off until it was time for team practice. Inevitably, Rich's truancy was discovered. He would pack up his sports gear and head to the school counselor's office.

Rich met the next set of positive influences on his life in the DeWitt Clinton High School counselor's office. Mr. Digrande and Mr. Blau both refused to give up on him. These counselors were committed to "saving me from myself" and repeatedly convinced a disbelieving principal that all Rich needed was one more chance. Digrande and Blau regularly shared with Rich that he was better than his choices; however, for him, life had so little structure that his choices seemingly had no value—positive or negative. By his senior year, Rich was an academic freshman. Graduation seemed hopeless, so he dropped out, like so many of his friends. Out of boredom, he began to regularly "run the streets" of Harlem with no particular purpose or passion.

The Compass and the Reality Check

During this period of personal turmoil and uncertainty, there were two influences that had huge life implications. The first was "the uptown girl" whom Rich calls "my compass for all things." Diane Theresa Sanchez lived a few blocks from his Abuelita's apartment. Rich noticed her for the first time at age 12. He managed to wrangle his way into a Catholic youth day trip so he could get to know Diane. She had a boyfriend, but this did not stop Rich from trying to spend time with her. He was fascinated by her nuclear family and found Diane easy to talk to. Everyone in the neighborhood knew not to mess with the Sanchez family, because most of the men in the family, including her father, were detectives in the New York City Police Department.

Three years passed before they became reacquainted when Rich coached Diane's younger brother's football team. Their first official date was 2 May 1965. He insinuated himself into her life, "even though she didn't want me there." Over time the friendship grew, and he recalls that she was the one constant in his life. He was amazed that Diane "liked me for who I was, and I didn't have much to offer."

He had no money, and it cost 70 cents to go uptown and visit Diane. The subway was 15 cents each way, and two slices of pizza and a soda to stave off the hunger consumed 40 cents more, when he had the money. Often Rich had only enough for the subway fare and could not eat. When he had no money, he would "sneak" on the subway to spend some time with Diane. He was too proud to let her pay for anything, so often their time together consisted of just walking and talking. The winter walks, with the bone-chilling wind and snow, were brutally cold. He owned only a plastic windbreaker jacket, but somehow these walks were some of the warmest and most comforting memories of his adolescence.

Diane's mother believed Rich was a good kid caught in difficult circumstances. She would invite him in for sandwiches, when Mr. Sanchez was not around, and took a motherly interest in him. This interest extended beyond food to another important motherly duty—laundry. One day Diane asked Rich if he did his own laundry, quickly adding her mother wanted to know. Confused and surprised, he confessed that when he had an extra dime, he would throw all his clothes into the washer at the local laundromat. Sorting the darks from the whites never occurred to him. Mrs. Sanchez had suspected this was the case and spent an entire day reclaiming the original bright white color to his clothes. Rich was overwhelmed by her kindness.

Vincent (Vinny) Sanchez, Diane's father, was a completely different story. He made it no secret that Rich was not good enough for Diane. Ironically, Rich agreed with Mr. Sanchez, which angered Diane. Vinny kept his hostility mostly to himself, until Diane announced that Rich was to escort her to her senior prom.

He recalls borrowing money to rent a tuxedo, buy a corsage, and arrange for transportation. Wearing a tux on the subway "guaranteed a mugging," so he was forced to spend $2 for cab fare, which ruled out the possibility of dinner. Mrs. Sanchez met him at the door and hurried to help Diane finish getting ready. As he waited, Rich heard Mr. Sanchez's heavy footsteps marching down the hall. When Mr. Sanchez rounded the corner, he was eye to eye with Rich and carrying a box under his arm. Rich offered an unanswered "Hello sir" as the detective unpacked the box of pistols onto the kitchen table. Mr. Sanchez began to clean his guns one by one, never taking his gaze off Rich. Not a word was spoken, but the message was deafening.

Diane was the stabilizing factor in Rich's life. She was "the grounding … my compass" at a time when he was still engaging in a lot of questionable activities. His friends in Harlem and the Bronx were transient.

Sal became Rich's reality check when he asked, "What do you do kid? What kind of education do you have? Where are you going?"

He never lived beyond the moment, because life was all about getting through the day. Rich saw an entirely different way of life in the Sanchez family. For the first time, he saw the results of stable relationships.

By age 17, Rich was still struggling to find a direction in life. He had no education and limited possibilities until he met Sal Hasson at a local candy store. Sal was dressed in an impressive Green Beret Special Forces uniform and was sharing with the neighborhood kids stories of seeing the world and serving his country. Rich was so drawn to Sal's stories that he returned to the candy store 3 days in a row to hear more about the Army. Rich describes this as "a very small window in time that had a major lifelong impact on my future."

Sal became Rich's reality check when he asked, "What do you do kid? What kind of education do you have? Where are you going?" Sal was holding up the proverbial mirror, and Rich saw the pathetic reflection of weak excuses and vague answers that rang hollow even to his own ears.

In 1967, Rich found himself in the recruiter's office, "being pitched" that the Army experience could "make him all that he could be." It was years later that Rich came to understand the depth of this statement. He took the Army entrance exams and returned to the block telling the kids he had signed up for the Army, and he was going to become a general. Soon after, Private Carmona was headed to boot camp and an entirely new life.

THE PLATFORM FOR SUCCESS

Rich boarded the train headed to South Carolina as a free-spirited kid who had spent his entire life on the battlefield of Harlem, where there were few rules and numerous casualties. When he arrived at Fort Jackson, South Carolina, he encountered a drill instructor who intended to transform the batch of "stupid ugly kids" into disciplined soldiers who understood duty, honor, country, and responsibility. After boot camp, Rich moved on to infantry training and parachute school, and then he joined the Special Forces as a medical and weapons specialist. During his training, Rich earned a general equivalency diploma (GED) so that he qualified for the Special Forces. While training for the medical specialist role, he received his basic nursing training.

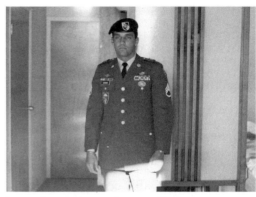

RICH CARMONA IN SPECIAL FORCES DRESS UNIFORM.

Moving through Army training provided Rich with a newfound maturity. During this 2-year period, he developed some skills and core competencies that he believes formed the platform for his success, both professionally and personally. He developed organizational and management skills, as well as an understanding of how to complete a mission. "You understand you have a mission to do; there are no excuses, and the guy above you is going to

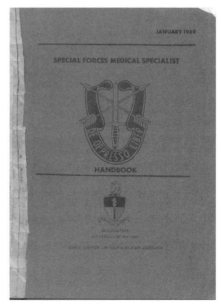

1969 SPECIAL FORCES MEDICAL SPECIALIST HANDBOOK.

hold you accountable," he says. Part of this understanding was to always have a Plan A, B, and C to accomplish the mission. He learned strategic planning, proactive thinking, risk taking, and action-based management.

During this period, Rich also learned that racial discrimination was alive and well in the southern part of the United States. In NYC, discrimination existed, but it was a much more subtle brand of discrimination. People were marginalized for their skin color or language by hiring decisions or by landlords refusing to rent apartments. In 1968, while training in Alabama, Rich encountered billboards recruiting for the Ku Klux Klan, an organization advocating "white" supremacy that was known to torture and kill non-Caucasians. Rich encountered segregated public drinking fountains, business entrances, and restaurant and public transportation seating. The racial tension had created palpable community chaos. Individuals of color became targeted victims of public violence as the South struggled with equality. Rich had not know that discrimination of this magnitude was possible. The power of oppression was a major lesson learned—and one not forgotten.

The instructor had only read about most of these organisms, while Rich had seen villages overcome by them.

VIETNAM—AN ERA OF EMANCIPATION

In 1969, Rich was deployed to the remote jungles of Vietnam. As a medical specialist, he and other team members were responsible for the healthcare of his "A" team of 12 Americans and thousands of Vietnamese civilians, with few resources. At 19 years of age, he found himself delivering babies without assistance. He was responsible for the treatment of burns, traumatic injuries from explosions, gunshot wounds requiring surgery, infectious diseases, parasitic diseases, malnutrition, and sanitation for the village.

Years later when Rich attended medical school and was studying microbiology and parasitology, the instructor was amazed that Rich knew how to diagnose, describe the sequela, and treat these rare diseases. The instructor had only read about most of these organisms, while Rich had seen villages overcome by them. Understandably, Rich views Vietnam as his training ground for understanding public and global health issues.

The Vietnam experience was not limited to medical care. As a sergeant in the Special Forces, he was also conducting combat operations as a weapons specialist. Generally, teams of two men, along with a group of indigenous forces, conducted reconnaissance or tactical missions. The missions, rotated among the team of 12 in the camp, were conducted in enemy territory and considered very dangerous. Because the medic was the most valuable person on the team, Rich frequently had to fight to take his assigned rotation on the combat missions. Everyone had combat skills, the argument went, but if anyone became sick or injured, only Rich, the medic, had the skills to save lives. Rich, however, would not allow his team members to take over his combat missions.

He was awarded the Bronze Star, two Purple Hearts, a Combat Medical Badge, the Vietnam Cross of Gallantry, and many other citations for his Vietnam service by the U.S. Army Special Forces division. He further earned leadership credibility as both a medic and weapons specialist by "never allowing others to do what I would not do myself."

Vietnam was also a time of lifelong relationships. Even today, he reflects on some of the lives that touched his. Rich was the medic in charge on a combat operation where there was significant gun and mortar fire. After the shooting stopped, the men conducted a bomb damage assessment by moving through the village looking for injuries. The team came across a young girl around 7 or 8 years old who had been caught in the cross-fire and wounded in the leg. After a team discussion on whether to leave her or take her to the camp for treatment, Rich assumed responsibility for the decision to take her back. She was a native child of the jungle or a "Montagnard girl," with no known age or family. Rich named her Linda, which means pretty in Spanish, and she became a part of the camp family. Linda would walk with Rich and the others to the gate when they left for a mission, and she would be waiting at the gate when they returned. She was like a daughter to the team. "Those guys would have died for her," Rich says. He wanted to adopt her but knew he was too young to assume this responsibility. He was just shy of his 21st birthday when he returned home and didn't have the stability in his own life to care for Linda. He still has a picture of her, though, and is grateful that some kindness evolved from the haze of destruction during the war.

Rich has another vivid memory of his Vietnam service. Diane sent him a letter every day he was away. She also sent him a birthday cake each year. Every holiday, he received a care package filled with items like toothpaste and cologne, things that only a loved one would remember. He didn't have the heart to tell Diane that the cologne was the joke of the camp, with the guys teasing him that the enemy would be able to smell him coming from miles away. When he received military rest and relaxation leave in Hawaii, Diane was there to meet him.

Two war zones—half a world apart, with vastly different causes yet remarkably similar outcomes—acted as reminders that Rich needed an education to escape the poverty jungle.

Reflecting back, he notes that he went to Vietnam expecting to see death and destruction. What he didn't expect was to return to NYC and discover that the war in Harlem, a place he called home, had also needlessly claimed many lives through drugs, violence, lifestyle choices, and poverty. Two war zones—

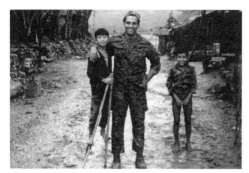

Rich Carmona, 1970, with "Montagnard" boys, in Ba To, Vietnam.

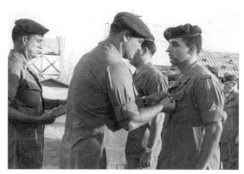

Rich Carmona, being presented with a Bronze Star and Purple Heart by Lt. Colonel Ronald Shackleton (pinning medal), Special Forces commander for I-Corp.

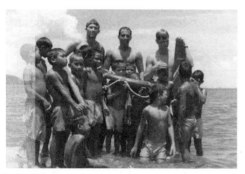

Rich Carmona (middle back row) with Special Forces team in the surf with combat-orphaned Montagnard kids, north of Danang, at China Beach, Vietnam.

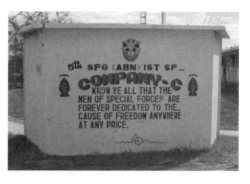

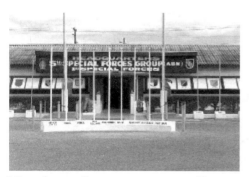

I-Corp Special Forces headquarters, Nha Trang, Vietnam, 1969.

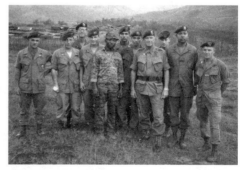

Carmona, far left, with his Special Forces team.

half a world apart, with vastly different causes yet remarkably similar outcomes—acted as reminders that Rich needed an education to escape the poverty jungle.

The Merging Disciplines

In 1970, after returning from Vietnam, Rich immediately started college with the eventual goal of applying to medical school. He worked part time as a lifeguard, a lifeguard instructor, and as a physician's assistant teaching emergency first responder courses while attending Bronx Community College. Rich and Diane married in NYC on 4 September 1971. On that day, Diane's father began talking to him. By February of 1974, Rich and Diane had grown weary of the cold New York winter and accepted an invitation to visit a Vietnam buddy in California. They fell in love with California, so Rich transferred to California State University at Long Beach to finish his baccalaureate. First, he had to immediately turn his attention to finding a job.

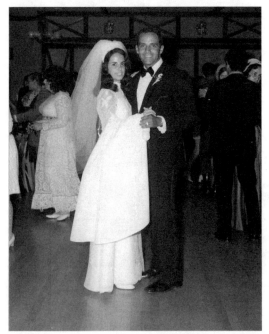

WEDDING DAY FOR RICH AND DIANE CARMONA.

The timing and location were right for Rich to take advantage of his medic training and become a nurse. In the early1970s, California offered medics the opportunity to take the state registered nursing exam based on the Special Forces curriculum. In mid-1974, Rich took the California nursing exam and began his career as an emergency department (ED) nurse while continuing full-time pre-med studies. It did not bother Rich in the least that he was sometimes the only male nurse in the entire hospital. As he says, "the gender difference was a bi-directional learning experience that improved all players."

Rich's medic background was invaluable to his ED experience. Emergency medicine didn't evolve as a specialty until the late 1970s. When Rich began working the ED, it was not uncommon for the moonlighting ED physician to be a dermatologist, radiologist, ophthalmologist, pathologist, or internist with little or no emergency experience. The good news was that many of the physicians had military backgrounds and enjoyed working with Rich because he had such a range of knowledge that could be used to help triage ED patients. He was able to utilize his medic skills while acquiring a new skill set—nursing. Nurses taught Rich the meaning of holistic care, collaboration, and interdisciplinary teamwork. He became a nurse and was proud of it.

In 1976, Rich began medical school at the University of California, San Francisco (UCSF). He received admission letters from several medical schools but chose UCSF, because it was diverse and the environment had the "right feel" for him. Sandy, Maria, and Rich were the three registered nurses in his medical school class, and they became kindred spirits. They knew that medical students went 2 years without patient contact, and when the time finally arrived, the students were often terrified and clumsy. The threesome convinced the UCSF nursing school to collaborate with the medical school to provide the first-ever "nursing skills lab" for medical students. The medical students learned vital signs, charting, and basic nursing skills. The students were taught how to write, flag, read, and take off orders. The importance of legible handwriting became obvious as they attempted to decipher the hieroglyphics masquerading as physician orders.

Rich watched as his fellow students had their eyes opened to how difficult, rewarding, and essential nursing is for the continuum of patient care. These physicians in training became indoctrinated into the life of a nurse, something Rich is very proud of. This collaborative nursing skills lab model was so successful that it continued on. Lesson learned? There is no substitute for the experience in the trenches and for walking in the shoes of another.

> *He acknowledges that he was not the smartest or most gifted student—he simply wanted it more, was willing to work for it, and was the most disciplined.*

Rich excelled in medical school. He was so happy to be in medical school and was one who never complained. "I didn't care where you sent me, because I thought this was the greatest thing in the world." Rich volunteered for extra rotations and even took his young daughter, Carolyn, on rounds with him. He graduated a year early, in 1979, and was number one in his class, receiving the coveted "Gold Headed Cane." He acknowledges that he was not the smartest or most gifted student—he simply wanted it more, was willing to work for it, and was the most disciplined.

With graduation nearing, Rich called his mother, who used to say that all she wanted was to see one of her kids graduate from high school, and offered to fly her to San Francisco for the ceremony. Rich also called his father with the same offer. Neither parent would commit to coming, but Rich sent them a ticket anyway, even though money was scarce. He really wanted to thank them in person and show them that he had turned out just fine, despite the rough start. Rich discovered just before graduation day that he had been selected as valedictorian and would be giving the commencement speech. He remembers looking down as he addressed the crowd and seeing the two empty, front-row seats reserved for his parents. He was struck by the fact that so much had changed, and yet so much had stayed the same. He tried in vain for many years to convince his parents to move from the ghetto, but it was home, no matter how bad it was. This was something Rich struggled to understand, but eventually came to accept.

He knows that a warm hug, handshake, hand holding, or eye-to-eye contact are methods to communicate human caring beyond the provision of healthcare.

During his surgical residency, Rich remembers a very famous attending surgeon telling him that he should have been a pediatrician because he spent so much time with the patients. At the time, Rich was upset by the implication that he wasn't surgeon material, but it did not take long for him to realize that this was really a great compliment. He believes that patients open their heart and soul during the physician/patient encounter, and "your goal is to make every patient feel they are the only patient in your practice for that encounter." He is firm that the encounter should not be distracted by the phone, note taking, or clock watching. Rich believes that this very "dignified encounter is an unquantifiable part of healing." He knows that a warm hug, handshake, hand holding, or eye-to-eye contact are methods to communicate human caring beyond the provision of healthcare. The power of relationships became an important component of success as Rich developed as a healthcare leader.

As a surgical attending, Rich would inform all new residents that it was wise to befriend the nurses. He would preach that the nurses would educate and protect them. He reminded them that "you are at the patient bedside 5-10 minutes each day and the nurses are there 24/7—nurses are the true caregivers and physicians only provide episodic care." Rich emphasized that "your patients will do better and your night will be smoother if you consider yourself a partner with the nurses" and show them their due respect. It took very little time for the residents to learn how right he was.

As Rich merged his nursing and medicine backgrounds, it became clear to him that inherent differences existed between the two professions. Nurses are taught collaboration from day one; physicians are trained to be independent thinkers. Nurses are holistic; physicians are focused on a diagnosis. Nurses cast the net to capture the family and environment; physicians drill down to a body part. The two professions approach patient care from opposite directions, but they need each other to create quality patient care. Rich contends that nurses are the drivers of the process. He states that "when a physician writes a discharge order, it is not magic. It is the nurse who gets the social worker, the administration, the clinic follow-up appointment; speaks to the caregivers; and manages every other detail to pull the whole thing together so that the patient is ready for discharge." Rich identifies the nurse as the collaborator and integrator of healthcare delivery.

In 1985, Rich completed his residency and a fellowship at UCSF in trauma, burns, and critical care. He also became a faculty member on staff. At the time, these were emerging specialty areas of practice. Across the country, joint trauma and emergency medical services (EMS) programs were being created that were supported by research evidence that patient and community outcomes would improve based upon these programs. In mid-1985, Rich accepted a similar trauma directorship at Tucson Medical Center and the University of Arizona Medical School. He became involved in community programs such as Safe Kids, Native American and Hispanic programs, school retention, and emergency preparedness. He became a nationally acclaimed preparedness and bioterrorism specialist and was instrumental in forming Arizona's first disaster medical assistance team. This same team now coordinates the state's efforts in bioterrorism prevention and emergency preparedness.

Rich recognized that to achieve his larger goals of injury prevention, he would benefit from further education. He enrolled in a master of public health and policy administration program (graduated 1998) at the University of Arizona. Along with other colleagues, Rich led seat belt, bike helmet, and pool safety awareness initiatives in an effort to proactively manage public health issues. His community involve-

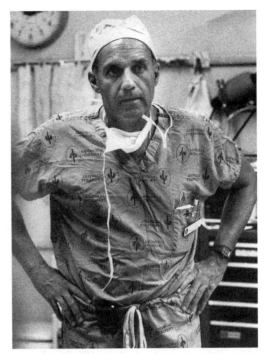

RICH CARMONA, DIRECTOR OF TRAUMA SERVICES AT TUCSON MEDICAL CENTER, AROUND 1988 AFTER A MAJOR TRAUMA RESUSCITATION.

ment placed him in contention for the position of chief medical officer and chief executive officer (CEO) at Kino County Hospital in Tucson, Arizona. Rich never intended to leave his clinical practice, but his record of community activism, educational and professional preparation, and public policy success made him a respected and coveted candidate. Rich accepted the position of chief medical officer and hospital CEO, once again acquiring an additional skill set in the delivery of healthcare.

A few years later, Kino County Hospital and health system experienced a financial crisis. The hospital was a provider of indigent healthcare for Arizona's poor. Kino County also served many patients who had illegally crossed the border from Mexico in desperate need of medical attention.

Some board members perceived that money spent to serve the indigent and the underserved was money "lost."

In 1998, Rich's reputation as Kino County's chief medical officer and CEO positioned him to become the new CEO of the county healthcare system. His biggest challenge as CEO was to work with the County Board of Supervisors to define and operationalize their mission statement. Rich acknowledged monies were being lost to system inefficiencies, which could be improved; however, he asked the leaders to make a decision if serving the underserved and indigent population was the hospital's mission. If not, then Rich suggested that they tell the poor and uninsured to find another hospital to take care of their needs. If the answer was yes, then it was important to budget sufficient funds to take care of this population and not view the care of this population as a financial loss, but rather as a commitment of services congruent with the mission. In 2 years as CEO, Rich influenced the board to change their well-entrenched fiscal outlook. Changing the cultural perception within an organization is a tremendous endeavor, and one that clearly shows the strength of Rich's character and his visionary leadership.

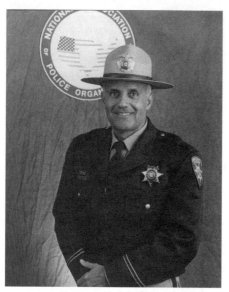

RICH CARMONA, DEPUTY SHERIFF OF PIMA COUNTY, ARIZONA.

Rich developed his career as a nurse, physician, public policy expert, community bioterrorism specialist, and hospital administrator, and in his spare time he had a parallel career track in law enforcement for most of his adult life. He was director of the Arizona Department of Public Safety Air

Rescue Unit, Pima County deputy sheriff, and S.W.A.T. team leader. He was involved in several harrowing shootouts and was wounded more than once while serving as a peace officer. He was awarded a Medal of Honor, Medal of Valor, Medal of Merit, two Purple Hearts, and many other commendations for his deputy sheriff and S.W.A.T. team leader service in Arizona. In 2000, Rich was selected as the nation's "Top Cop" and received the medical society "Top Doctor" Award.

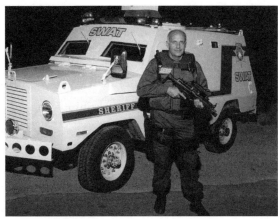

RICH CARMONA, PIMA COUNTY, ARIZONA, S.W.A.T. TEAM LEADER AND DEPUTY SHERIFF.

WEARING OF THE SHOES

Rich's leadership definitions, beliefs, and vision were influenced by a collage of experiences that have shaped his life. His leadership acumen, which took him decades to acquire, carries tremendous credibility with the people he leads, because he "has been there and done that" in just about every aspect of public health imaginable. Rich has walked in the shoes of many of the disciplines and individuals he interfaces with and offered guidance as the U.S. surgeon general. He can speak the professional language and has lived the challenges of nurses, physicians, police officers, public health officials, educators, hospital CEOs, emergency first responders, military personnel, the homeless, high school dropouts, addicts, victims of racism and inner city violence, and parents. With each experience, Rich has become wiser and more committed to make a difference.

Rich defines leadership "in its simplest form" as responsibility for the destiny of others. He states that as a Special Forces medic, he held the lives of others in his hands by his decision to move left, right, or withdraw. Leadership is the same whether you are a four-star general or a young sergeant—it is not about rank, but the responsibility to protect those you lead. As the U.S. surgeon general, Rich understood that "everything I say and everything I do has the potential to impact somebody." Rich laughs as he remembers a trip to a fast-food restaurant in Tucson, Arizona, shortly after being confirmed as U.S. surgeon general. The publicity surrounding the appointment had been intense, and everyone in the community knew of Rich's new role. That day, when he reached for one of his son's french fries, he turned to see that most of the restaurant was watching his lifestyle choice. He dropped the french fry and jokingly told his son, "Dad has a new job, so we'll have to do this french fry thing covertly!" While he made light of the situation, he really understood that as a role model for healthy living, this was an opportunity to lead by example.

Further, he believes that leaders must lead with integrity. For him, the definition of integrity is doing the right thing when nobody is watching.

Further, he believes that leaders must lead with integrity. For him, the definition of integrity is doing the right thing when nobody is watching. He is clear that leadership and integrity "go hand in hand." This symbiotic relationship between leadership and integrity requires subordinating one's own interests as the leader to the greater good of the organization or group. Rich adds, "I think true leaders think about what it means to be a leader; they don't just take it for granted. Leading is a privilege that is earned."

Leadership, he contends, is distinctly different from one's substantive area of expertise or rank and requires core competencies. Being a good nurse or good doctor or good officer doesn't make one the best leader for all situations. By way of example, Rich recalls that high-ranking officers would occasionally ask to participate in combat missions. However, it was understood that the team leader was the ranking member on the mission, because he had earned the leadership credibility within the group—the ranking officer would subordinate to the sergeant leading the mission. Great leaders have the wisdom to know when to subordinate to the more competent team member. More importantly, the leader recognizes that by doing so, his choice increases rather than marginalizes his leadership credibility.

"Leadership is best attained through credibility over your actions and your integrity over time. It is not only talking the talk, but walking the walk," Rich says. "The best leaders are those who are empowered by the people they lead." There is a bond of trust and the leader inspires confidence in the group. Attaining this level of leadership capability is initially difficult. A leader can assume a high level title or rank, but there is no means for the group to know if it should trust or second guess the decisions and direction of the new leader. According to Rich, the new leader will encounter non-believers, hidden agendas, and, worst of all, complacency. He explains that inspired leadership can come to a screeching halt by the "if it ain't broken, don't fix it" mentality.

Rich's leadership style to deal with barriers is to use the group to define appropriate behavior. He invests his leadership energy in the motivated majority to effect the change. When the nonbeliever's behavior becomes more and more removed from the majority, peer pressure becomes the driver for the minority change. These leadership lessons have been learned in the streets of Harlem, the jungles of Vietnam, wood-paneled boardrooms, and in Washington, DC, but the dynamics are always the same—leadership is leadership, regardless of the forum.

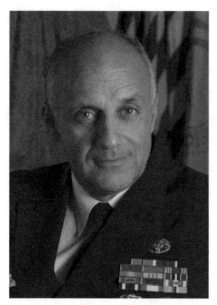

FORMER SURGEON GENERAL OF THE
UNITED STATES, RICHARD CARMONA.

Colleagues and friends describe Rich's leadership as visionary. Rich sees the problem from a different altitude, and he is not distracted by the surrounding chaos. As the U.S. surgeon general, he quickly understood that the most important aspect of his job was not just to safeguard the public health, but also to protect the integrity and dignity of the office. The holder of the position must stay above the political fray and "keep clean on the issues." He understood that when evaluating public policy, his job was to embrace evidence-based practice and quality data, which sometimes meant telling people what they didn't want to hear. Rich is firm in his proclamation that the office of the U.S. surgeon general should never be politicized, or future surgeon generals will never be successful, because national trust will be lost. Many polls show that the public views the surgeon general position as the most credible position in the U.S. government.

An important element of organizational vision is succession planning. Rich believes the first thing leaders should do in their new role is to determine who to prepare to fill the position in the future. What will they need to assume that responsibility of higher leadership? Rich believes that the leader is really the parent of the organization. His direct reports are like his children and he wants to "nurture them, inspire them, instill confidence in them, and have them appreciate their fullest potential because when the individuals grow, so does the organization."

He has had the good fortune of being mentored by some remarkable professionals and friends. Mentors will create a path of success through their experiences and lifelong lessons learned. In the Army, Richard Webber, his Special Forces squad leader, taught Rich leadership early in his life. During medical school and residency, Drs. Don Trunkey and Bob Lim left an indelible mark for attaining excellence. Don demanded that the residents remember they are first a physician and second a surgeon. The surgical residents did not order medical consults while on Don's service unless absolutely necessary. The residents should be able and willing to provide primary patient care. Rich describes Bob as one of the most dignified and humble surgeons he has ever known. Bob was a fine surgeon and extraordinary human being who taught Rich the immense responsibility of becoming a surgeon. Sheriff Clarence Dupnik (Pima County, Arizona) has been Rich's mentor and friend for 20 years. Clarence taught Rich about politics and the unique authority and power one has as a police officer. He taught Rich how to fairly use this authority for the good of the people. Clarence was a role model for leadership strength while maintaining great compassion and kindness. Lastly, Rich has been mentored by the small and unique fraternity of living U.S. surgeon generals—Richmond, Koop, Novello, Elders, and Satcher—who have imparted the dignity associated with the office and have made themselves available for counsel at any time.

The leadership role that may have taught Rich the most is parenting. Rich and Diane have four children—Carolyn (age 32), Jason (age 25), Robert (age 22), and Julianne (age 13)—who have been the center of meaning for his life. Carolyn is married to Robert Guillot and works as an ED/ICU registered nurse in Phoenix. Rich has been instrumental in Carolyn's career trajectory by teaching her to achieve maximum credibility and leadership in her role before moving on. He tells her, "You can't just punch your card.

The career stop is more than a stepping stone—it is a leadership opportunity, so get the most of it." Jason works in Tucson for Pima County and is in the Army National Guard. Robert is a college student in Maryland taking basic requirements as he develops his plan for life. And last but not least, Julianne is in high school. Rich is quick to identify that family is the most important thing in his life, and his children "have given to me, probably more than I have given to them—they have allowed me to be whole."

THE HUMBLE LEADER

One day, Rich received a phone message from the White House inquiring if he would consider the position of the U.S. surgeon general. He was sure that his buddies were attempting to set him up for a practical joke. What perplexed him was the caller ID box indicated the White House had called. How did they manage this? When Rich confirmed the call was real, he was sure the White House had mixed him up with another Richard Carmona. Rich became intrigued and decided there was no harm in beginning the interview process. When he discovered there were "hundreds and hundreds" of very qualified and politically connected candidates, he realized once again that this was a joke, but one worth entertaining. Rich sought guidance from an Arizona congressman that he had worked with for many years. Rich was so "embarrassed" that he was unable to say the words "U.S. surgeon general" until the congressman asked him directly what he was being considered for. When Rich told him, the congressman laughed and asked if he was kidding. He then asked if Rich knew the president or vice president or had any other political power cards. After several dead-end answers, Rich was advised to play the lottery, because he had better odds of collecting the jackpot than being selected as U.S. surgeon general.

As the process went on, Rich wondered if his misguided youth would eliminate him from contention. He was proud of his accomplishments, but realized he would be the first high school dropout and only the second Hispanic to hold the position. As the field of candidates for the U.S. surgeon general narrowed to a select few, Rich was simply grateful for the experience, regardless of the outcome. He recognized that being selected wasn't nearly as important as being considered a qualified candidate. He had memorized his rejection speech but had not written an acceptance speech. No one was more surprised by the selection than he was, but then again no one was more qualified. He had lived the American dream and spent a lifetime preparing for this global leadership role.

> *"When you take the elevator to the top floor, send it down for somebody else."*

SUMMARY

Rich's leadership journey had been guided by a few powerful messages to which he has remained committed. The first came from his mother, who would often say "to thine own self be true." It was many years into his adulthood before he understood that he had to be true to his values, principles, and ideals regardless of the choices of others. The second came from his Abuelita, who spoke and lived the message of the Golden Rule: Do unto others as you would have them do unto you. She was a role model for this character choice. Lastly, he learned from Susan, a social worker in southern California, that "when you take the elevator to the top floor, send it down for somebody else." Susan coached him to believe in himself and be comfortable with his past. Like his Abuelita, she knew his future would be bright. Living all three messages, Rich has "tracked as a leader, tracked as a mentor, and tracked as a role model to empower kids to see there is life after poverty and stress." Rich has devoted himself to local communities.

He has also openly communicated that there is life after failure—if you are willing to work hard. He believes anything is possible in this country and holds himself up as living proof. In June 2004, Rich visited his high school in the Bronx and was awarded his diploma 37 years later than expected. He accepted it with the excitement of a teenager.

With each leadership step he took, Rich remembered his roots and took his nursing experience of collaboration, communication, and compassion with him.

In August 2002, Rich and his family stood in the Oval Office taking pictures and having casual conversation with President George W. Bush as they prepared to enter the Green Room to announce to the world his nomination as the nation's 17th U.S. surgeon general. The administration had selected a man whose passion is excellence, whose motto is under-promise and over-deliver, whose priority is family, and whose commitment is to serve and protect the health of the nation. He describes his leadership legacy as: "Leave this very valuable position in a better condition than it was given to me. This means I must demonstrate that I have improved, advanced, and protected the health of the nation and world that I am part of." Rich is a warrior who has always finished his mission, with no excuses.

Rich had the courage to recreate himself numerous times as life presented the opportunities. He knew that each time he took on a new career path,

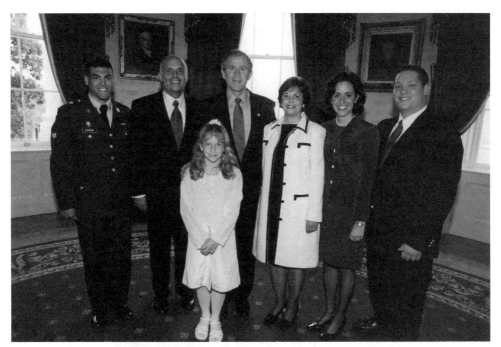

RICH AND DIANE CARMONA FLANK PRESIDENT GEORGE W. BUSH AND ARE
SURROUNDED BY THEIR CHILDREN. L-R: JASON CARMONA, RICH, PRESIDENT BUSH,
DIANE, CAROLYN CARMONA, ROBERT CARMONA, AND JULIANNE CARMONA, IN FRONT.

he had to do more than punch his card—Rich had to build leadership credibility. With each leadership step he took, Rich remembered his roots and
took his nursing experience of collaboration, communication, and compassion with him. As he would say, "A recovering surgeon, always a nurse."

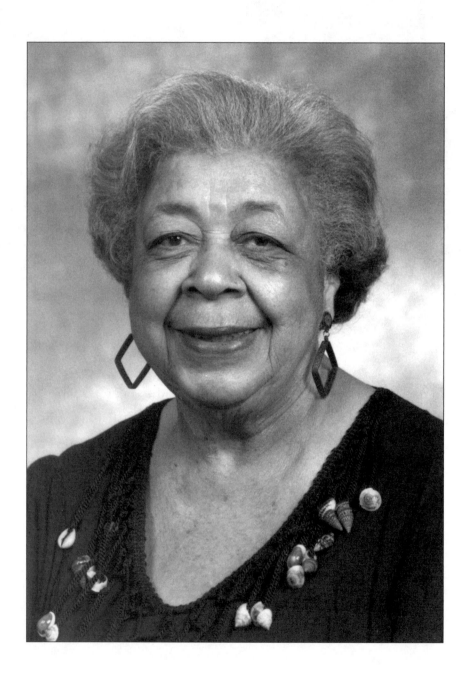

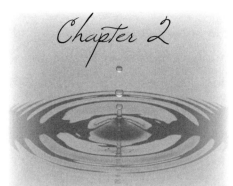

Chapter 2

MARY ELIZABETH CARNEGIE

"Times and people do change."
—M. Elizabeth Carnegie

Mary Elizabeth Carnegie, DPA, RN, FAAN, was born in Baltimore, Maryland, on 19 April 1916, to John Oliver and Adeline Beatrice Lancaster. Elizabeth, as she was called, was the fourth child in the family. She had one brother who died shortly after birth and two sisters. When Elizabeth was 2 years old, her parents divorced. Her mother struggled to meet the demands of raising three children as a single parent. To assist her mother in the responsibilities, Mary Elizabeth was "adopted" by her maternal aunt and uncle. At the age of 3, she went to live with Aunt Rosa and Uncle Thomas Robinson in Washington, DC.

This shift in living arrangements allowed Elizabeth to be nurtured and reared as an only child, since her aunt's daughter was grown and living independently. Elizabeth was raised in a strict household with firm rules to follow, but all within a loving environment.

During this time in history, growing up Black had its challenges. Except for public transportation, everything in Washington was segregated, including the school system, department stores, and neighborhoods. The era in which Elizabeth grew up influenced her passions and dedication throughout her nursing career. She always strove to see that minorities were treated equally and pushed to ensure that African American nurses were recognized. As a young child, Elizabeth could not imagine going to college because of the expense. As a professional nurse, she initiated the first baccalaureate nursing program in Virginia at Hampton University, an historically Black university, and forged impressive paths for nursing's minorities.

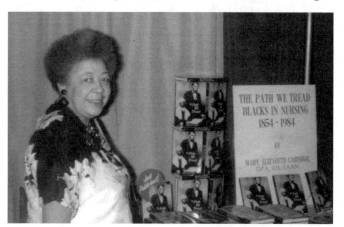

ELIZABETH CARNEGIE AT A BOOK SIGNING FOR HER BOOK *THE PATH WE TREAD: BLACKS IN NURSING 1854-1984* AT THE NATIONAL BLACK NURSES ASSOCIATION CONVENTION IN HOUSTON, TEXAS, 1986.

THE EARLY YEARS

Elizabeth was reared by her aunt, but her biological mother and sisters lived only 40 miles away in Baltimore. She continued to see them during holidays and family gatherings, so she never felt abandoned, and she adjusted quite well to her new surroundings. Perhaps these early changes in her life nurtured the flexible, tenacious qualities that she later displayed as a nursing leader. Her aunt valued education and instilled in her a tremendous drive to succeed and get ahead, even in the face of barriers most people will never encounter during their lifetime.

Under her cousin's instructions, she was taught to read and speak a second language—French. She entered kindergarten at age 4, but when the year was up and the other children advanced to first grade, she was told she could not move forward, because of a law that stated a child had to be 6 years old to enter first grade. Her aunt went to the school principal to protest the matter, and the following day Elizabeth attended class with her peers.

"I never knew what my aunt said to change the situation, but she was determined to see me enter first grade like the rest of the children," Elizabeth said. In those days, birth certificates were not required for school attendance, so Elizabeth imagined her aunt had told authorities that she was indeed of age to attend. Elizabeth enjoyed school and remembers at the end of some weeks, she would gather chalk and play school with her young friends. She, of course, was the teacher.

By the time Elizabeth lived with her aunt for 5 years, her mother's financial position had improved to the extent that she could support all three children. So at age 8, Elizabeth went home to Baltimore to live with her mother and siblings. She accepted this change in life events and felt no particular trauma leaving her aunt's home and school and starting over. She transferred into the fourth grade in Baltimore and did marvelously, until age 10. Only 2 years after being reunited with her family, Elizabeth was informed that her mother was gravely ill and could not take care of herself.

Aunt Rosa moved the two older sisters into an apartment in Washington, DC. Elizabeth and her mother lived with Aunt Rosa. It was a year before her mother's health improved to the point where the family could live on its own again.

Not only did Elizabeth's mother regain her health, but she was introduced to a gentleman by the name of Edward Davis. He would change the course of Elizabeth's life by marrying her mother. Elizabeth was excited about the positive turn of events and welcomed her new father into the family. Not long after her mother's marriage, Elizabeth was informed that her mother was going to have a baby. She was delighted and felt things could not get any better. However, the reality was that her good fortune, as she had recently come to know it, was about to end. Her mother died only 3 months after her baby brother, Roland, was born. Once again, her extended family stepped in to help take care of the children.

This was one of the most difficult times in her life, but Elizabeth used her strong Christian faith to guide her through this unhappy time. She was reared Catholic and had remained very involved in her church. She participated in the choir and played the church organ. Because she attended public school, it was required that she attend catechism classes on Saturdays. These classes were taught by the Sisters of Providence, an all-Black order. They had a deep influence on her, and she remembers, "I idolized these beautiful nuns and wanted to be one of them when I finished high school."

Elizabeth maintained good grades while in high school, even though she also worked to contribute to the family's finances. This time frame spanned the height of the Great Depression, and her Uncle Thomas had difficulty finding work. Elizabeth made money on the weekends and in the evenings preparing fruits and vegetables for a local cafeteria that served only Whites. Elizabeth worked hard to juggle both her job and school studies to the point where she was able to graduate while only 16 years old. By then, her original plan of becoming a nun had changed. She knew she wanted a professional career but was not sure what she should study. Her family did not have the money to send her to college, so Elizabeth had to earn her own way.

NURSING SCHOOL

Elizabeth asked her aunt's permission to live with cousins in New York, with the hope of furthering her education. Her aunt agreed to the plan and helped Elizabeth move her belongings. Once in New York, Elizabeth learned that one of the cousins had attended Lincoln School for Nurses, one of the two schools of nursing for Blacks in New York City. Her cousin suggested that she consider nursing as a profession, and the idea sounded like a good fit for her. However, just as when she was in kindergarten, Elizabeth found she was too young; she had to be 18 to attend nursing school.

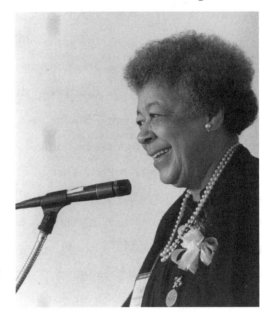

An earlier life lesson came back to her. She remembered her Aunt Rosa had been successful in getting her into first grade when she was younger than 6, so she was determined to fill out the application. When Elizabeth applied, she put down her age as 18. She proceeded to take the entrance exam and was notified a few weeks later by Lincoln School for Nurses that she had been accepted into the program.

Elizabeth came to enjoy nursing, partly because she had new and unaccustomed freedoms. "While at school, there were evenings when a group of us might stay out a bit late, until 10 p.m. or so, and that would not have been allowed under my Aunt Rosa's roof," she said. She also became very active in sports, playing tennis and basketball, swimming, ice skating, and riding horses.

Even though Lincoln was a Black nursing school, the instructors and director of the program were all White. During one particular class, a guest by the name of Mabel K. Staupers, executive secretary of the National Association of Colored Graduate Nurses (NACGN), was invited as a guest lecturer. NACGN had been established in 1908 to fight discrimination against Blacks in education, employment, and organized nursing. Lincoln School for Nurses was established by a board of directors comprised solely of White females. "As Black students in a Black school founded in 1898 by White philanthropists, we found that Mrs. Stauper's message had real meaning for the class," Elizabeth said.

Elizabeth looks back at the White nursing instructors and realizes that, as Black nursing students, they had very few role models in the classroom setting.

Elizabeth was learning for the first time how African American nurses were discriminated against not only in the South, but all over the United States. "When I was in New York at Lincoln, I did not know about discrimination outside my small city world," she said. "When Mrs. Stauper came to speak to my nursing class, it was at this moment I made a pledge to myself that I would do everything within my power to fight segregation and discrimination in the nursing profession. I planned then to take a leadership role in the fight against discrimination in my profession."

Elizabeth looks back at the White nursing instructors and realizes that, as Black nursing students, they had very few role models in the classroom setting. "As we were being taught the history of nursing, for example, we were not taught anything about other Black schools or Black nurse leaders; history was taught from a narrow perspective," she said.

More interestingly, Elizabeth did not even take care of African American patients while in school. "All our patients were from the Jewish neighborhood where the hospital was located, so I don't remember seeing any Black patients." She remembers working long hours while at school but enjoyed what she was doing.

During the 1930s, there were only two government hospitals that accepted Black nurses: Freedman's Hospital in Washington, DC, and Tuskegee Veterans Hospital in Alabama.

BEING A NURSE

Following nursing school, Elizabeth took her state board exams and was hired by Lincoln Hospital as a medical-surgical nurse. In addition, she took the civil service examination for nursing positions in government hospitals. During the 1930s, there were only two government hospitals that accepted Black nurses: Freedman's Hospital in Washington, DC, and Tuskegee Veterans Hospital in Alabama. Elizabeth passed her civil service exam and accepted a position at the Veterans (VA) Hospital in Tuskegee. She wanted to be placed at Freedman's Hospital, but a 1-year probationary period at Tuskegee was required before transferring. She set her mind on the long-term goal of completing her 1-year work commitment and then being transferred to a position at Freedman's Hospital.

At the VA hospital in Tuskegee, Elizabeth was working with other Black nurses and taking care of Black patients. As unremarkable as these two events sound in today's world, this was a novelty to Elizabeth at the time. Living and working in Tuskegee presented no racial problems during her year of employment.

True to her word, she went on to Freedman's after her year at Tuskegee. While working full time on the night shift at Freedman's, she took two courses during the day at Howard University, a Black school. Her eventual

It was my philosophy that we could not control what the Whites said to us, but we could control what we said.

goal was to earn her bachelor's degree. An offer from West Virginia State College came along that allowed her to work part time as a school nurse and go to school full time, so she took advantage of it. Again, as this was an all-Black school, she did not have to contend with racial problems.

Upon graduating with her bachelor's degree in sociology and minor in psychology, she was offered a faculty position at St. Philip Hospital School of Nursing, which was the Black school at the Medical College of Virginia in Richmond. The system was set up as a dual system—a school for Whites and a school for Blacks under the aegis of one institution that was run by Whites. "This is where I really faced racial discrimination among my colleagues," she said.

Working among both White and Black faculty members, Elizabeth noticed that "all the Black nursing instructors had academic degrees, but not all the White instructors."

One of the first major racial issues Elizabeth faced was in regard to her title. Nursing instructors were typically given the title of Miss or Mrs., but the Black instructors were not allowed this same courtesy.

"If you were Black, they would just call you nurse Lancaster, not Miss Lancaster," Elizabeth said. "It was my philosophy that we could not control what the Whites said to us, but we could control what we said." Thus, the Black faculty taught students to address themselves and Black instructors as Miss or Mrs. This issue did not get resolved until 1943, when a new nursing director was brought to St. Philip's.

"Even though she was White, she agreed with us that our nursing faculty and students should have the title of Miss or Mrs. It was a matter of self-respect and respect for each other," Elizabeth said.

CREATING THE FIRST BACCALAUREATE NURSING PROGRAM IN VIRGINIA

During the 1930s and 1940s, not many nurses of any race held a bachelor's degree, so when the first Black nurse—Estelle Riddle Osborne—was awarded a master's degree in 1931, it was cause for celebration. Estelle became a strong mentor in Elizabeth's life. "She saw the potential for leadership in me and suggested that I go to Hampton University and be groomed for the role of dean," Elizabeth said. It was Estelle who was able to get Elizabeth released from her position at St. Philip's so she could pursue advanced nursing roles. During World War II, jobs were frozen, so moving from job to job often wasn't possible, let alone feasible.

Even though Elizabeth's title was assistant dean, her charge was to start the first baccalaureate nursing program in the state of Virginia—until, that is, a nurse with a master's degree could be found for the position.

In 1943, however, Elizabeth was allowed to accept the new position of assistant dean at Hampton University. Her role was to be an apprentice of sorts for advancement into a dean's position. Even though Elizabeth's title was assistant dean, her charge was to start the first baccalaureate nursing program in the state of Virginia—until, that is, a nurse with a master's degree could be found for the position.

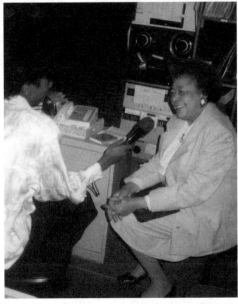

RADIO INTERVIEW WITH ELIZABETH CARNEGIE.

Many years later, Elizabeth went back to Hampton and taught research in its master's program in nursing.

Elizabeth enjoyed her tenure at Hampton University, but had a strong desire to go back to school and earn her master's degree. With the aid of a Rockefeller Foundation Fellowship, she was able to attend the University of Toronto in Canada and study nursing school administration, which led to a certificate of completion.

While in Toronto, she met and married Eric Carnegie, the brother of one of her students at St. Philip's in Richmond, VA. Her "long-distance" marriage lasted only 10 years, because Elizabeth refused to move to Canada and Eric refused to move to the United States.

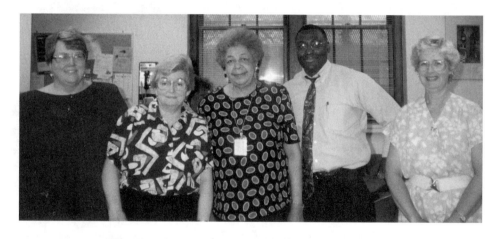

During this same time, Florida A&M University had applied to the General Education Board of the Rockefeller Foundation for funding to build a hospital to replace the old 40-bed frame building. The Rockefeller Foundation agreed to fund the project because the hospital served as a laboratory for students. It was stipulated that the school of nursing be re-organized under the supervision of a nursing dean, instead of the hospital medical director. As Elizabeth had just been educated with foundation dollars, she was the likely candidate with the proper credentials. Florida A&M agreed to accept her nursing school administration certificate as equivalent to a master's degree. Even though Florida A&M accepted the certificate as equivalent, Elizabeth could not. "I would not have been allowed to put on a master's gown as dean for the graduation ceremony, so my students and I would have been wearing the same gown. ... So, no, that was not okay with me," she said.

I walked into an organizational disaster and had numerous critical issues facing me, all needing attention immediately.

After a few years at Florida A&M, she went back to the Rockefeller Foundation and asked them for another educational grant, saying, "You have got to give me another scholarship to complete my master's degree before I can continue in this position at Florida A&M." The foundation agreed to fund her educational endeavors so she could attend Syracuse University's master of education program. It was a degree focused on the administration of higher education. She chose this route because a master's in nursing would have repeated the year of educational preparation she had had in Toronto. Syracuse gave her credit for the education she received in Toronto, so it was the logical choice at the time. While working on her master's, Elizabeth took an additional graduate course in nursing every semester, just to keep in touch with educational changes in the nursing profession. Once she completed her graduate education, she returned to the dean's position at Florida A&M College.

As one of only two schools for Blacks in Florida until 1950, it was also the only baccalaureate nursing program in the state. When she arrived at the school in 1945, she realized what would lie ahead for her. The hospital in which the students had their clinical experience was substandard. It was so inadequate that before students from Florida A&M could sit for their nursing state board exams, they had to go all the way to Baltimore and spend a year training at a larger hospital. "I walked into an organizational disaster and had numerous critical issues facing me, all needing attention immediately," Elizabeth said.

Now that Florida A&M had a nursing dean at the helm and not a physician, the General Education Board of the Rockefeller Foundation committed funds to build a hospital.

Dean of Florida A&M College

Elizabeth Carnegie did not need much time to assess that she had walked into a situation that could be described as more than difficult and challenging—it was "horrible," she said. She had to reorganize the school of nursing, seek national accreditation, and make the school an integral part of the college. Another opportunity that Elizabeth saw was the chance to help Black nurses gain the respect of the public in general and the respect of other nurses, regardless of race.

The list of issues Elizabeth faced was daunting. For example, nursing students were not selected by any particular criteria or standard. The registrar at the school would go into a full auditorium of new students and ask, "All of those who are interested in nursing, stand up!" Those students who stood were sent to the hospital. That was the admission process. There were no records or high school transcripts, no birth certificates, and no aptitude test scores.

This was the area Elizabeth first changed, by administering an aptitude test. "I got one of the national tests that used to be given before entrance into nursing school, and that exam cleared out half of the students. I told them that I was not putting them out of college, but I was putting them out of nursing." It took Elizabeth some time to institute changes, such as requiring birth certificates for potential student candidates, along with high school transcripts. Eventually, she did get the standards of the nursing school raised, but not without threatening to leave. She called the Rockefeller Foundation and told them she could not stay in these conditions any longer, but they wrote back to say they would see her in the spring of the next year—which meant she had to stay.

> *She was faced with the difficulties of going into hospital nursing programs led by White nursing directors, where not so much as a handshake would be shared.*

The second area that Elizabeth focused on was finding a different clinical site for her nursing students. As the hospital at Florida A&M had only 40 beds, with just 25 usually full, her students had to get most of their clinical experience elsewhere. For 10 years, they had been affiliating at Provident Hospital, a Black facility in Baltimore that was nearly 1,000 miles away. There was no excuse for the conditions in one area to be so poor that students had to transfer to a hospital in Baltimore to receive proper clinical experiences. As reality would have it, after one site visit to Baltimore, Elizabeth realized that conditions were not much better there. In 1946, she requested permission to visit larger facilities within the state of Florida.

Again, she was faced with the difficulties of going into hospital nursing programs led by White nursing directors, where not so much as a handshake would be shared. "My hand would be left dangling in every instance," Elizabeth said. If this was the discrimination she had to face, she felt students should not be subjected to those same conditions.

In planning meetings between the hospital and school, she was addressed with her proper title, Dean Carnegie, *but her students continued to face the issue of being called* nurse Smith *instead of* Miss Smith.

It was not until she consulted a friend that she received some helpful guidance in her quest. She was referred to the nursing director at Duval Medical Center in Jacksonville, FL, and Elizabeth gained the hope she needed for the future of her school. During the initial introductions with the White director of nursing, she was greeted with a handshake. Elizabeth felt hope not only for her school, but "for the human race." However, she would still have her work cut out for her. She received permission from Duval Medical Center for her students to receive clinical experience there, but was told they had no funds to house the students. That issue would rest with Florida A&M—more specifically, Elizabeth—to figure out. She made an appointment with the president of Florida A&M and convinced him that it was the school's responsibility to keep

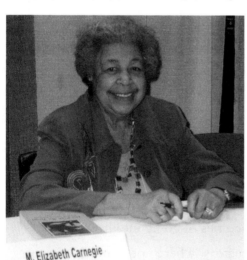

M. Elizabeth Carnegie

ELIZABETH CARNEGIE AT AN HONOR SOCIETY OF NURSING, SIGMA THETA TAU INTERNATIONAL BOOK SIGNING, OCTOBER, 2001.

control of the nursing program and provide housing and faculty. Again, funds were requested and received from the Rockefeller Foundation to purchase a house in Jacksonville, near the hospital, that was large enough to accommodate 12 to 16 students. In addition, the monies from the grant enabled the school to employ faculty members, a dietitian, a cook, office furniture for empty space within the hospital that had been set aside, a small library of books, and a furnished classroom. The contract was signed and the partnership sealed.

Elizabeth continued to help Blacks gain respect within White society. In planning meetings between the hospital and school, she was addressed with her proper title, *Dean* Carnegie, but her students continued to face the issue of being called *nurse* Smith instead of *Miss* Smith. Elizabeth felt that with a new start, she was not going to accept this indignity. She attempted to explain that her nursing students should be referred to as *Miss*, but was informed that the southern custom was being followed, and students would be referred to as *nurse*. Elizabeth had learned much along her journey, so she thought she might be able to turn the tables in the conversation with the hospital director by arguing that the students could not be called *nurse* because they were not yet nurses. The director thought about it and replied, "That's true, so what should we call them?" Elizabeth responded, "Why not *Miss*?" She pushed by saying the students had been taught to respect themselves and others, and the students expected the same in return. Elizabeth told the director that she should set the example for her staff to follow, and it worked. From that point forward, nursing students at Florida A&M were referred to as *Miss*. What seems like a small win was a major victory for her at the time.

However, the challenges created by discrimination did not stop with this one victory. Just one week before students were scheduled to start their clinical rotation, Elizabeth remembers the Jacksonville newspaper reporting that White nurses were threatening to walk out of Duval Medical Center if Black students were placed there. The newspaper article made the students nervous, but Elizabeth assured them the contract allowed them to go to school. There was no strike, and the students conducted themselves with dignity and fortitude. The first year of the contract, however, students were allowed to staff only the wards where all the patients were Black. Within the year, though, that portion of the contract was dropped and "the entire hospital was made available to our students," Elizabeth said.

Elizabeth started to turn an inadequate employment situation around. She was able to hire additional faculty and start a public health program, all because she had the cooperation and support of the Florida A&M administration. "They supported me because I had the Rockefeller Foundation behind me, and money talks. I did not fail to remind the administration of that either, so they did not play with me."

Even though Elizabeth's students had a new clinical setting in which to learn, her long-term plans were for the Florida A&M campus to have its own hospital. Again, she had the support of the administration. President William H. Gray of Florida A&M appealed to the Rockefeller Foundation again to fund this undertaking. The school was awarded $50,000 for construction, but had to conduct a fund-raising campaign to acquire the rest of the money. It only took a few years before the groundbreaking event took place and a modern hospital was erected.

She received praise after presenting her clinical rotation plan at a meeting of the Florida State Board of Nurse Examiners, which was held at a White hotel. When lunch was served following the presentation, Elizabeth was relegated to a table in a far corner of the room, where she ate alone.

Elizabeth's hard work and achievements did not come easy. Besides focusing on completing work for the nursing school, she had to persevere through discriminatory remarks and acts of unkindness. As an example, she received praise after presenting her clinical rotation plan at a meeting of the Florida State Board of Nurse Examiners, which was held at a White hotel. When lunch was served following the presentation, Elizabeth was relegated to a table in a far corner of the room, where she ate alone. "I wanted to walk right out the door, but I was afraid such an action would lead to sanctions against my program and my students," she said. She was humiliated by the experience and could not bring herself to join in the discussions that afternoon.

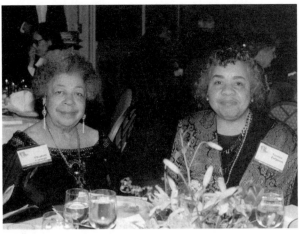

ELIZABETH CARNEGIE, LEFT, AND VERNICE FERGUSON, FORMER HONOR SOCIETY OF NURSING, SIGMA THETA TAU INTERNATIONAL PRESIDENT, AT A SIGMA THETA TAU INTERNATIONAL DINNER.

After 7 years with Florida A&M, she was able to achieve national accreditation by what today is known as the National League for Nursing. Florida A&M was the first nursing program in the state of Florida to receive this accreditation. Furthermore, it was the only Black school run by a Black dean in the state, which made it even more special to Elizabeth. At the time, Whites did not have a baccalaureate program within the state of Florida, only diploma programs.

By the early 1950s, the White state universities in Florida (University of Florida and Florida State University) established baccalaureate nursing programs. Elizabeth remembers when the University of Florida hosted its 25th anniversary celebration in 1981. "I was invited as a guest and was cited for having pioneered baccalaureate nursing education in the state of Florida. ... Times and people do change," she said.

ADVANCEMENT IN THE STATE NURSES ASSOCIATION

Prior to the early 1940s, Black nurses in the South were not allowed to join their state nurses association, which would have provided them membership in the American Nurses Association (ANA). An organization known as the Florida Association of Colored Graduate Nurses (FACGN), a constituent member organization of the National Association of Colored Graduate Nurses, had been started years earlier. Elizabeth wanted to bridge this gap in the profession's associations and create inclusion within the organizations.

Even after a 1942 vote allowed Black nurses to join the Florida State Nurses Association (FSNA), they still were not allowed voice or active participation. They were members only through their payment of dues. In 1946, when Elizabeth was attending the FACGN convention in Miami, she remembers that "we met in the basement of a Black church in the Black section of

Before the convention, it was rumored that if I spoke, the White nurses would walk out. I did speak, and no one walked out.

town; however, our president was invited to attend one program session of the Florida State Nurses Association convention. Our association, in turn, asked the president of FSNA to attend one of our sessions." Progress was slow in happening, but it was happening.

A year later in 1947, the same two organizations met in Daytona Beach, in separate sections of town. The FSNA had its meeting in a White hotel, while the FACGN held its meeting at the Black college. This time, all the Black nurses were invited to attend the joint program session of the FSNA convention, and the Florida State League of Nursing Education. This time, Black nurses were allowed a voice in the educational issues being presented. Since Elizabeth had a strong academic background in nursing education, she surfaced as a natural voice for Black nurses across the state. This was the year she was elected president of the Florida Association of Colored Graduate Nurses.

> *We pounced on every absurdity thrown at us until all efforts at segregation were eliminated.*

In 1948, Elizabeth was invited to keynote the convention of the Florida State Nurses Association. "Before the convention, it was rumored that if I spoke, the White nurses would walk out. I did speak, and no one walked out." In 1998, 50 years later, Elizabeth was again invited to keynote the convention of the Florida Nurses Association. The speech she gave in 1948 and the one she had given in 1998 were published together in FNA's official newsletter.

In 1949, at the National Association of Colored Graduate Nurses convention in Louisville, KY, the Black nurses voted for the association to cease operations, and it officially went out of business in 1951. In 1950, the Florida Association of Colored Graduate Nurses was dissolved. This was not an easy process, because there were issues such as dues and transfers of members to consider. "I remember one White nurse in the FSNA suggesting that there be a Black section," Elizabeth said. She responded, "If we do that, then a Chinese and other racial sections would have to be formed! We pounced on every absurdity thrown at us until all efforts at segregation were eliminated."

The year that FACGN voted to dissolve was also the year that Elizabeth was on the election ballot of the Florida State Nurses Association, running for a position on the board of directors. She was elected for 1 year and re-elected in 1950 for 3 years. She remained on the Florida State Nurses Association board of directors until 1953, when she moved to New York to accept a position as an editor at the *American Journal of Nursing*. This was Elizabeth's step from state leader to leader on the national level.

Elizabeth was the pioneer in forging integration within FNSA. "I think they got tired of my demands as president of the Black nurses association," she said. For example, when both associations met in Panama City one year, a guest speaker was brought in specifically for the Florida State Nurses Association. Elizabeth knew the guest speaker, and after the presentation, which was held in a White hotel, Elizabeth invited the guest speaker to give the same address on the Black side of town, where the Black nurses association was meeting.

Once it was agreed that Black nurses would have equal voice and vote in the FSNA, the next issue was finding a place where both races would be allowed to meet without violating state segregation laws. In Tallahassee, the meeting place would be right at the Leon County Courthouse. This was a location where it would be easy for all to attend. However, Elizabeth remembers the early games that were played between the two races. The first she remembers as "musical chairs." Initially, the White nurses

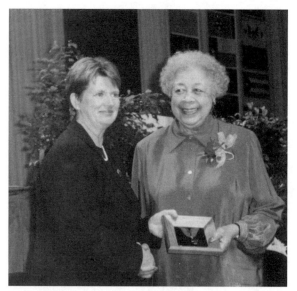

ELIZABETH CARNEGIE AT HER INDUCTION INTO THE AMERICAN NURSES ASSOCIATION (ANA) HALL OF FAME IN 2000. WITH HER IS MARY FOLEY, THEN PRESIDENT OF ANA.

would wait outside the courthouse for the Black nurses to arrive before assuming their seats. This way, if the Black nurses gathered more to the front or rear chairs, the White nurses would take the opposite seating. However, at the next meeting, the Black nurses arrived early and waited outside for the White nurses. "We could scatter in our seating and ensure integration in the seating arrangement, at the very least," Elizabeth said. The nurses did succeed in becoming an integrated community that addressed issues in a democratic fashion. Fortunately, the games did not last long before everyone settled down to do the real work of the association.

On Staff of the *American Journal of Nursing*

In 1953, Elizabeth moved into a national role when she accepted an editor position for the *American Journal of Nursing*. It was another step up the leadership ladder. She was now in a position to influence change and opinion through her position. However, relocating to New York was not without its challenges. Elizabeth faced the same blatant racial discrimination she had encountered in the South. For months, she attempted to rent an apartment near her office, only to be turned away by White landlords with the explanation that "We don't rent to coloreds." With financial help from a relative, Elizabeth purchased her own home in Queens, New York.

Elizabeth remembers her chief editor, Nell Beeby, being concerned about the consequences of sending Elizabeth on the road, traveling to southern states for the journal. "I assured her that I could take care of myself, and nothing could be worse than some of the situations I had already encountered," she said. Her career with the journal was fruitful. After 3 years, she was promoted to associate editor of *Nursing Outlook,* with educational content as her responsibility. By 1970, Elizabeth was senior editor for *Nursing Outlook*.

Through her various positions there, Elizabeth traveled nationally and internationally. She had the opportunity to attend the inauguration of William Tubman, president of Liberia in West Africa. Her charge was to write an article about nursing in Liberia, Ghana, and Nigeria. While in Africa, she visited and guest lectured at nursing schools. Five years went by before Elizabeth made her second trip to Africa. She served on the board of Women's Africa Committee of the African American Institute. Each year, a selected board member traveled to Africa to interview women finalists to come to the United States for leadership training, and some of these women were nurses.

During the late 1960s and early 1970s, Elizabeth felt it was time to go back to school and earn a doctoral degree. "It was not required for my job, but it was something I wanted to do for myself," she said. Elizabeth started her doctoral program at the Graduate School of Public Administration at New York University on a part-time basis, but she soon enrolled full time. She successfully completed the program and in 1973, published her dissertation with the National League for Nursing as a book, titled *Disadvantaged Students in RN Programs*.

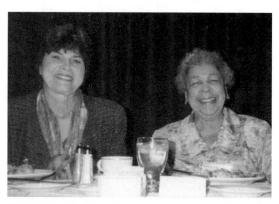

ELIZABETH CARNEGIE, RIGHT, WITH PAT MESSMER, THEN PRESIDENT OF THE SOUTHERN NURSING RESEARCH SOCIETY (SNRS) AT SNRS CONFERENCE APRIL 1997.

After graduating with her doctoral degree, Elizabeth accepted a position as chief editor of *Nursing Research*.

As a result of her first editorial in *Nursing Research,* she was able to influence change for minorities. "My first editorial was titled *ANF Directory Identifies Minorities with Doctoral Degrees in Nursing,*" she said. In this editorial, attention was drawn to the fact that there were few minorities in nursing who were prepared at the doctoral level. With national attention on this issue, the American Nurses Association applied for and received a grant to fund minority nurses seeking PhDs. The ANA board of directors appointed Elizabeth to the advisory committee for the minority program. In 1980, she chaired the committee that has funded the doctoral education of more than 200 minority nurses.

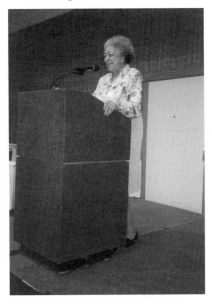

Elizabeth is passionate about ensuring that more minority nurses are provided with the opportunity for graduate education. Each year, through Nurses Educational Funds, an independent nonprofit organization that grants and administers scholarships to registered nurses for graduate study, she has earmarked funds for the Carnegie Scholarship, which aids a Black doctoral student. She also has an endowment fund in her name at the American Nurses Foundation to give financial assistance to Black nurses engaged in research. And, Howard University in Washington, DC, has an annual M. Elizabeth Carnegie Research Conference, which has become international in scope.

While Elizabeth was chief editor for *Nursing Research,* she was inducted into the American Academy of Nursing. She was soon elected to the position of treasurer on the academy's board of directors and was elected president in 1978.

THE RETIRED NURSE

Upon retiring after 25 years of service to the *American Journal of Nursing* family of publications, Elizabeth started her own consulting business. She continues to travel nationally, consulting with nursing schools, guest lecturing, conducting writing workshops, and working as a distinguished visiting professor. In all of Elizabeth's scholarly research, one area she felt was never addressed was that Black nurses had been left out of the history books of America, "with the exception of one or two sentences alluding to the first Black nurse, Mary Mahoney."

Elizabeth wrote a book titled *The Path We Tread: Blacks in Nursing.* However, even as a successful writer and editor, Elizabeth could not get publishers to accept her book. Lippincott [Lippincott Williams & Wilkins] told her that because it was about one group of nurses, it would not sell. Other publishers would not give her a reason for their rejection. Instead of giving up on her dream of publication, Elizabeth took her own innovative

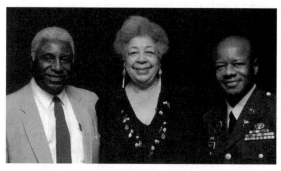

L-R, ERIC CARNEGIE, ELIZABETH CARNEGIE, AND LTC PATRICK A. WESLEY OF THE UNITED STATES ARMY NURSE CORPS.

advice published in an editorial, "Rejection Can Be a Challenge." She approached Lippincott a second time with $5,000, which was required for the publication of her book. She was then given a contract. Subsequently, the book has gone through second and third editions, published by the National League for Nursing. The third edition includes Black nurses in Africa and the Caribbean.

Elizabeth's book drew attention to the void of Blacks in history books. She has made television and radio appearances, fulfilled speaking engagements, and attended book signings all over the country. As a result, White authors often include more than one sentence about Black nurses. As new nursing textbooks are published, Elizabeth is frequently invited to contribute content on the history of Black nurses.

"My most cherished honor for the book came as a legislative resolution made May 22, 1986, by the New York State Senate," she said.

It reads:

> Resolved that this legislative body pause in its deliberations to honor Mary Elizabeth Carnegie for her contributions to the field of nursing as a nurse practitioner, educator, and author, and be it further resolved that this legislative body congratulate Mary Elizabeth Carnegie on her new book, *The Path We Tread: Blacks in Nursing*.

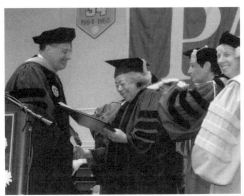 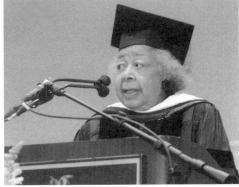

ELIZABETH CARNEGIE BEING AWARDED THE HONORARY DOCTOR OF HUMANE LETTERS BY PACE UNIVERSITY FOR HER SIGNIFICANT CONTRIBUTIONS TO THE DEVELOPMENT OF NURSING AS A PROFESSION, SCIENCE, AND DISCIPLINE. MAY 23, 2004.

Elizabeth realizes many Black nurses lived through the same history of discrimination she did and fought many of the same battles. "The times today are much improved from when I was growing up, but we still have further to go," she said.

Even retired, Elizabeth keeps a full calendar of engagements related to nursing. As long as hurdles remain in place for Black nurses, the profession can be sure Elizabeth will continue fighting the battle she is most passionate to win ... national equality for Black nurses.

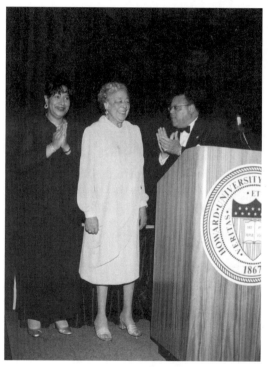

ELIZABETH CARNEGIE, CENTER, RECEIVING THE LEGACY OF LEADERSHIP AWARD, DISTINGUISHED HEALTHCARE EDUCATOR, FROM HOWARD UNIVERSITY, WASHINGTON, D.C., IN 2001. ON HER RIGHT IS DR. DOROTHY POWELL. H. PATRICK SWYGERT, PRESIDENT OF HOWARD UNIVERSITY, IS AT THE PODIUM.

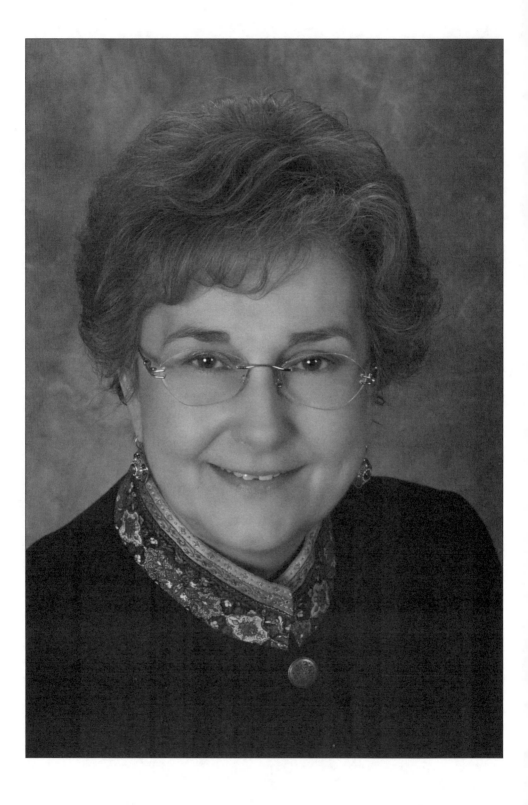

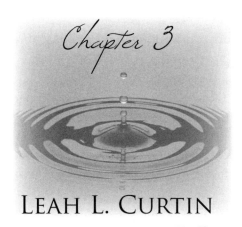

Chapter 3

LEAH L. CURTIN

When you draw a line in the sand about a principle or a stance, understand it is your line and your sand, and nobody else is going to defend that turf with you.

—Leah Curtin

Leah Curtin, RN, MS, MA, FAAN, is one of nursing's most provocative, compelling, and multifaceted leaders. She fought for societal causes and the rights of patients and nurses. Most know Leah as the "mother of nursing ethics," but her prolific writing career and her presentations on practice, leadership, and healthcare reform and restructuring touched nearly all aspects of healthcare and nursing. She is a philosopher, teacher, amateur paleontologist, author, editor, linguistic analyst, and international leader on ethics. Her love for nursing is the common thread throughout her work.

Describing Leah is like trying to catch a butterfly. Just when you think you have captured her essence, the story darts in another direction and reveals an entirely new aspect of her expertise and intelligence. In 1981, Leah's son Chris was assigned to write a school essay about the person he most admired. He chose his mother. Through the purity of a child's perspective, Chris wrote the following:

> Leah Curtin was a tomboy. She was also the strongest kid on
> the block. As she got older, she wanted to join the convent, and
> she did. She was in a missionary order and tried to help the poor
> overseas, but then she got sick and had to leave the convent.
> When she came home, her parents nursed her back to health. Leah
> still wanted to help people, so she decided to go to nursing school.
> After she got out of school, she married my dad and had four
> children. She worked for hospitals for a while. She also worked in
> public health. Because she wanted to help people more, she went
> back to college. She got a master's degree in health administration
> and one in philosophy. She won lots of awards. After years and
> years and years as a nurse, her name got around. After a while,
> she became quite good at her work. She was offered more than
> a few jobs, but she decided to be the editor of a nursing journal
> and a teacher of ethics (that means how to be good). She wrote
> two books about ethics. She gets to go everywhere telling speeches
> about how to be good. She was telling every person how wrong
> it is to kill. She mostly wants to tell people that the best thing is
> to love and serve each other. She got more than just a few laughs.
> But many believed her. Now she still does it, but she mostly makes
> speeches in other countries. The End.

It's a pretty complete story, and Chris succinctly captured Leah's leadership journey and her influential role in shaping the nursing profession, and he did it with love and devotion. What he left out—stories such as Leah being "poisoned" by her nursing-school colleagues; nearly being kicked out of nursing school; stopping abuses of power; and identifying unethical practice, societal neglect, and misdirection—is told in the pages to come.

As a result of Leah's leadership, the nursing profession plays a key role in healthcare ethics today. She reached beyond the world of ethics to push, pull, and coax other nurse leaders to individually and collectively engage in a more meaningful conversation about everything that affects patient care and the well-being of nursing staff. In whatever she does, she minces no words and selects them carefully to add the greatest possible clarity and power to her message.

EARLY INFLUENCES

Leah was born 8 March 1942 in Chicago, Illinois, to Jean Wilson Sutter (Bill) and Veronica Eloise Dunst Sutter. An electrical engineer, Bill moved the family to Cleveland, Ohio, for a career opportunity when Leah was 6 months old. Her father's early dreams were to attend medical school, but the Great Depression emptied the family savings account and took with it his dreams. Veronica (Vonnie) was a housewife who had more than a full-time job raising a family of four girls—Jeanne, Leah, Patty, and Louise. When the children were all in school, Vonnie went to work. Her most interesting job—as secretarial assistant to the Hamilton County coroner—put her right in the middle of a number of notorious murder cases in the Cincinnati area— where the family had settled. All of the girls, except Patty, would become nurses.

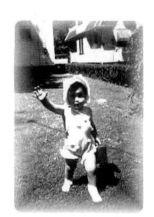

A TODDLING LEAH CURTIN

Dinnertime in the Sutter household was always busy and full of discussion—even arguments—about politics, religion, current events, the latest murder, educational needs, work issues, and almost anything imaginable. Often the discussions would end with one person or another pulling out an encyclopedia to prove a point. Having lived through the Great Depression, her parents had painful and hopeful memories that, in many ways, colored their approach to and attitude about work, life, and religion.

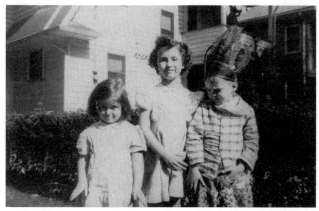

A young Leah, her sister Jeanne, and a neighbor boy. Leah and Jeanne are both Fellows of the American Academy of Nursing (FAAN). Sister FAANs are quite a rare event in the nursing profession.

Leah's paternal grandmother had an enormous influence on her when she was young. Every week, Grandma would send each grandchild a small gift through the mail—perhaps a package of lifesavers, a fancy straw, or a coloring book. Receiving mail from Grandma made the girls feel important and special. During the Great Depression, Grandma and Grandpa were among the lucky ones; he still had a job, and they "almost owned" the two-family house where they lived. The upstairs was rented to a nice young family whose rent paid her grandparents' mortgage.

Every day, people would come to Grandma's door looking for work. Grandma always found some work for them to do and paid them what little money she had. Because *everyone* was poor, no one—not even Grandma—could afford to give presents, even for special occasions. But she could and did give the gifts of compassion, love, and laughter. She would make and actually *wear* what can only be described as amazing hats full of feathers and flowers and fruit, always with a little veil that went to the tip of her nose. The harmless jokes she played on family members became the stuff of legends.

When their tenants couldn't pay the rent, her grandparents let them stay anyway. Finally, even Grandma and Grandpa lost their home when they couldn't keep up the mortgage payments. They were never able to buy another home, but Grandma kept her family, her friends, her life, and her soul intact. She never stopped giving.

She gave from her heart, and she never expected anything in return. She gave because she wanted to give: no *quid pro quo*, no owing or being owed. She gave of herself in good times and bad, even to strangers. Grandma's kindnesses were hugs, and they were as essential to life as clean water and good food. When Leah was 8 years old, Grandma was killed by a drunk driver, but her spirit lived on through stories and memories.

ALWAYS A REBEL

In the middle of her freshman year in high school, Leah's family moved from Cleveland to Cincinnati. There, Leah transferred to Mother of Mercy High School. The Catholic school would have a tremendous influence on her future thinking and direction.

Leah was reminded regularly of her disobedient behavior at Mother of Mercy High School, where "the sisters didn't really care if you liked the rules." She was popular with the other students and active in many extra-curricular activities. The sisters doted on her, even though she was often reprimanded for breaking rules that Leah thought "didn't make sense," such as talking in the halls. Leah remembers thinking, "How much trouble can you get into by talking in the halls?" She has come to believe that such rules served the purpose of allowing children to rebel. Rebellion, she believes, is fundamental to personal growth. "Every thinking person is going to rebel, especially against stupid rules, so it's better to break the rules when you are young, when the consequences are minimal compared to later in life," she says. During her teenage

Rebellion, she believes, is fundamental to personal growth.

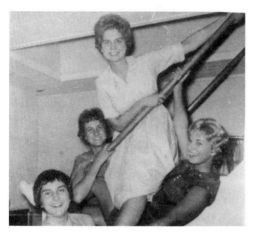

LEAH, ON THE FAR LEFT, WITH HER BEST FRIENDS AT HER HIGH SCHOOL GRADUATION PARTY.

years, Leah excelled at challenging authority and violating stupid rules. Along the way, this behavior helped her summon the courage to ask the hard questions.

Leah had not been raised Catholic. However, she became enculturated into the religion and decided to join a Catholic convent after high school. When Leah announced she was joining the Maryknoll Sisters of St. Dominic, Vonnie cried for days. This decision meant that Leah would never spend a single night under her parents' roof again. Leah was committed to learning how to be a religious sister and had high respect for the work the sisters were attempting to accomplish. She spent nearly 3 years at the Maryknoll convent before she realized it really was not a good fit. The obedience factor was looming once again.

Leah laughs and says: "I had no idea I didn't fit in. I thought I fit in just fine." While in the novitiate, Leah was directed to begin preparing herself to become a librarian. She was assigned to assist the librarian in various ways—including learning to classify books according to the Dewey Decimal System. Leah loved to read, and she loved books, which led to her downfall as a librarian; instead of classifying the books, she spent hours reading them.

Ironically, it was Leah's health that changed the course of her religious training. While living in the convent, Leah was diagnosed with an ulcer. The treatment for ulcers at the time was a "sippy diet" that consisted of milk and cream to neutralize stomach acids. Leah grew more and more symptomatic, and her weight dropped to a mere 90 pounds. Ultimately, she left the convent for health reasons. Later, she was diagnosed with cholelithiasis, which had significantly worsened because of the "therapeutic" sippy diet.

Leah returned home from the convent in December 1962 feeling derailed and disappointed. She decided to attend college to explore one of her life interests, paleontology. As a young girl in Cleveland, she had been an avid collector of rocks. She would bang the rocks together hoping the cracked interior would display a rare find of a fossil—and it did often enough to create quite a collection.

When her family moved to Cincinnati during her childhood, she discovered, much to her delight, the area was one of the world's centers for Ordovician fossils. As luck would have it, the transportation department was digging a cut through a hill to accommodate Interstate 75, and workers uncovered a bed of fossils. The fossils were 300-400 million years old, primarily sea creatures and invertebrates. Leah was in heaven. She kept a log of her fossil discoveries and managed to find some brachiopods that had never been catalogued. At 18, Leah received an Outstanding Scientific Achievement award from the Engineering Society of Cincinnati for developing a new theory for the evolution of the brachiopod Platystrophia. Between

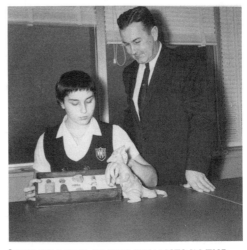

LEAH WAS ONE OF THE FINALISTS IN THE 1960 NATIONAL WESTINGHOUSE SCIENCE TALENT SEARCH, THE MOST PRESTIGIOUS RESEARCH-BASED SCIENCE COMPETITION IN THE UNITED STATES FOR HIGH SCHOOL STUDENTS. THIS PHOTO SHOWS LEAH WITH HER PROJECT AND HER FATHER.

1958 and 1960, Leah received 11 awards for outstanding achievement in earth science, paleontology, and science from The Ohio State University, University of Cincinnati, and Miami University for her work with fossils. In 1960 she also was one of the finalists in the National Westinghouse Science Talent Search, the most prestigious research-based science competition in the United States for high school students. (Today, Intel is the sponsor of the "Westinghouse Competition.") Prestigious colleges eagerly sought winners and finalists in the competition. American Telephone and Telegragh (AT&T), her father's employer, published an article about her accomplishments in their in-house journal. Leah was offered several scholarships but preferred entering the Maryknoll convent.

Now "back in the world" again, Leah spent a semester pursuing general and paleontology studies before deciding that it was time to settle on something more socially relevant than studying specimens that had been dead more than 300 million years. Leah's older sister, Jeanne, was already head nurse in charge of a psychiatric unit. Since Leah enjoyed science so much, she decided to become a nurse, as nursing offered a way to earn a living by helping other people.

MEMORABLE EXPERIENCES FROM NURSING SCHOOL

In 1963, Leah enrolled in the Good Samaritan Hospital School of Nursing in Cincinnati, OH, where she found her education to be far less challenging and entertaining than her experiences with fellow students. All student nurses were required to live in a dormitory and work long hours at the hospital, often managing an entire nursing unit with little assistance. They rotated day, evening, and night shifts, even if they had a full schedule of classes the next day.

This schedule played havoc on the students in more ways than stress and sleep deprivation. One night after Leah worked the night shift, she rushed back to the dorm to change clothes and get to her morning classes by 8:30. While running out the door, she grabbed a piece of pizza from the dorm refrigerator, little knowing that it had sat out all night. Leah began to feel ill. By the end of the first class, she was very sick with nausea and abdominal pain. She and her close friends huddled at break and decided that the pizza had caused food poisoning. Since they had just studied how to induce vomiting, they decided they should treat Leah in this way. The group concocted the soap and water brew from memory and encouraged Leah to gulp down the remedy. Just as she finished swallowing the emetic, one of her co-conspirators noticed they had accidentally added disinfectant rather than soap to the mix. At this point, panic and chaos began to grow at the same rapid rate as Leah's abdominal girth. Quickly, her co-conspirators ran to the infirmary for help and left Leah alone to manage the simultane-

ous waves of vomiting and diarrhea. By the time they returned with the aging infirmarian, Leah's pain had decreased substantially. The pizza and any other food or liquid had long since left her gastrointestinal tract. Hospitalized for observation, Leah was easy prey for Sister Andrew, the director of the nursing pro-

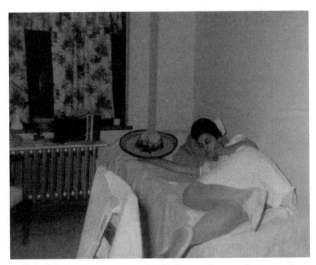

LEAH IN HER DORMITORY ROOM AT GOOD SAMARITAN HOSPITAL SCHOOL OF NURSING CATCHING A QUICK NAP BETWEEN WORKING THE NIGHT SHIFT AND PUTTING IN A FULL DAY OF CLASSES. 1964.

gram. Sister Andrew was furious and demanded that Leah receive a psychiatric evaluation. She was convinced Leah had done this to attract attention. Leah met with the psychiatrist, Maria Krocker, who listened intently and then laughed and told her the next time she wanted to vomit, "You tell me and I will write you a prescription, and you can avoid all this trouble." The only diagnosis Dr. Krocker arrived at about Leah was "terminal stupidity." Sister Andrew was not happy.

DEFINING MOMENTS

Two profound experiences during the pediatric rotation of Leah's final year of nursing school had a significant impact on how she perceived herself as a nurse and also on her understanding of the potential for nurses abusing one another. The first experience was a defining moment of responsibility. Just a few days into her pediatric rotation, Leah was assigned a young boy who was admitted for a high fever of undetermined origin. He had been in the hospital less than 24 hours and his parents had just gone home when he began to bleed from every orifice of his body. Leah asked the charge nurse to call a medical emergency. The charge nurse also kept trying to reach the parents. Leah stayed with the boy, carrying him quickly to the treatment room. The physicians worked frantically to save him, but he bled out. When his parents finally arrived, Leah covered the blood on her uniform with a patient gown and stayed with the parents to assure them their son had not died alone and afraid. She and the boy's parents cried together, and it comforted them to think a nurse cared enough about their son to cry with them.

Nurses are present at the most important times in people's lives—what they do, or fail to do, has enormous impact.

Later, Leah reflected on the enormous privilege of being a nurse. Nurses are present at the most important times in people's lives—what they do, or fail to do, has enormous impact. After this experience, Leah developed a deep and abiding respect for those who work with sick children. She also clearly realized that she wasn't cut out for pediatrics because she "wouldn't survive it." Not all nurses are a "fit" for all practices, she says, and it is okay to admit that.

The second pediatric experience created an understanding of the impact nurses have on one another, sometimes for the worse. Leah's pediatric instructor had categorized her as an older student—at the advanced age of 22—and sent the clear message to Leah that she would never be a favorite student. Much to Leah's delight, this instructor was on vacation at the beginning of her pediatric rotation. During this time, Leah noted that one of her infant patients was developing pressure wounds from his pre-surgical traction for repair of a congenital hip problem. She tried one thing after another to prevent further damage. Finally, she brought an idea to the attention of the head nurse and a physician. Leah's ingenious idea was immediately implemented with great results. She was pleased to have made a difference in patient care outcomes. The head nurse and physician, wanting to encourage creativity, asked her to demonstrate her "method" to LPN students and resident physicians, which she did. When her instructor returned and heard about Leah's project, she was furious. She called Leah into the classroom and harangued her for several hours about arrogance and insolence. Over and over again, she asked: "Who do you think you are? How could you possibly think about teaching anyone about anything?" The instructor failed Leah in pediatrics.

Leah was once again called to the director's office to meet with Sister Andrew. The conversation began along the lines of, "Do you realize that

> *Never abuse your authority, however small or great it may be.*

you have been given an F in pediatrics?" Sister Andrew showed Leah a list of deficiencies submitted by the instructor. For once in her life, Leah was diplomatic enough to say, "I think that I have a personality conflict with this instructor." Seeking resolution to the opposing stories, Sister Andrew turned her attention to the National League of Nursing test scores that had just arrived, thinking they would show Leah to be deficient in pediatrics and thus support the instructor's opinion. Instead, Sister Andrew discovered Leah had scored in the 99th percentile. The case was closed, but the story didn't end there.

A few years later, Leah's pediatric instructor returned to school seeking her master's degree. She was assigned to Leah's unit to complete necessary clinical work. The tables had turned: This time the charge nurse was none other than Leah. Leah gave her the most difficult patient assignments (commensurate with graduate education). When her previous instructor performed well, Leah resisted the temptation to seek revenge and gave her the high marks she deserved. The lesson learned is *never abuse your authority, however small or great it may be.* Moreover, nursing is a small world and you never know when you may be on the other side of the table. Professional and collegial behavior—or the lack of it—will almost certainly be remembered.

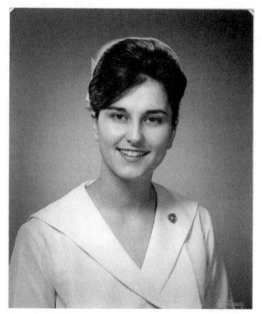

LEAH'S 1965 NURSING SCHOOL GRADUATION PHOTO.

THE COURAGE TO QUESTION

Today, the Institute of Medicine (IOM), the Agency for Health Research and Quality (AHRQ), the Joint Commission on Accreditation of Healthcare Organizations (JCAHO), and numerous other professional organizations mandate that hospitals create a work environment where questioning unsafe or unethical practices is accepted and welcomed. Additionally, the expectation is that hospitals will create systems of redundancy and checks to ensure safe practice. This was not the case in previous decades. In the 1960s, few nurses questioned physicians' orders, much less refused to follow them. Nonetheless, questioning a physician's orders was commonplace in the hospital program Leah attended. It was always done respectfully, with the hope of learning and understanding the medical regimen, but it was done—and it was expected. Thus, early in her career, Leah learned to question what she did not understand.

After completing nursing school in 1965, Leah was employed at a large teaching hospital. Initially, she worked in acute care, but transferred to a tuberculosis unit after a few months. Leah was a very new nurse—she had not yet taken her state boards—but had enough knowledge to be concerned about the practice of one of the medical interns who was ordering unusual medications at doses that far exceeded the limits found in the *Physician's Desk Reference*. Leah had numerous heated exchanges with the ordering intern and eventually reported her concerns to the chief of service. On several occasions, Leah refused to give the medications as ordered. The head nurse supported her—and either gave the doses herself or called the resident to give them himself. One day, Leah was caring for a patient who was receiving an experimental drug that listed respiratory failure as a possible side effect. All experimental medications were under lock and key, and the charge nurse carried the key. Leah became suspicious when the intern in question asked for two vials of the drug rather than the one that was ordered for him. The intern retorted that one vial was for the patient, and the second vial was to complete stability testing. Leah gave him the two vials but was not comfortable about it. Her shift ended at 3 p.m. that day, but she was scheduled back at 11:00 to work the night shift, at which time she planned to check on the patient again.

When Leah took report that night, she was told the patient had died from respiratory failure. The patient's diagnosis was scleroderma. He had been tolerating the drug very well, but there was the matter of the two vials Leah had given to the intern earlier that day. Moreover, even though it was almost midnight, the patient's chart was already gone, even though standard practice was for charts of patients who died to be processed by the ward clerk in the morning and then sent to medical records. Leah checked the medication cupboard: All vials (and their accompanying literature) were gone. Leah then checked the unit's experimental drug file, which provided information about the drugs and their side effects, but the information about this drug had been removed. Leah was in charge of 52 patients that night and had very little time to look into the details.

The next morning, the day nurse called in sick. Leah was required to work another shift—and the chief of service made rounds on the day shift. As part of the protocol, autopsies were performed on patients who died while taking experimental drugs. Leah asked the chief if she could attend this patient's autopsy, but she was informed that no autopsy would be performed. A bit later, Leah called the chief of pharmacy and asked for information on the experimental drug, but he refused to provide it.

When Leah was finally relieved for lunch, the chief nursing officer (CNO) sought her out. "What's with this?" Leah wondered. Shortly after that, the chief of medicine arrived and asked Leah if he could sit with them. Then, along came the chief of pharmacy as well as the hospital administrator. Leah now felt like a butterfly pinned to a board.

The "chiefs" said they knew that Leah was upset, and they wanted to know why. Mincing no words, Leah told the story of the extra vial, the patient death with no ordered autopsy, the information that was missing, and the history of the intern's overdoses, to which she had vigorously objected. She told them not to take her word for it but to read all the patient's charts for themselves. The written orders could speak for themselves.

After that fateful lunch, it seemed the hospital needed her services day and night. She worked 30 to 40 days in a row and often a double or even triple shift. Her schedule was changed nearly every day, making the quality of her life more miserable by the moment. It appeared the chiefs wanted her out of the organization. Though she was "slow on the uptake," Leah decided that it was time to change jobs. On her last day of work, her former boss from the acute unit met her in the parking lot and told her that she would be happy to provide Leah with a positive letter of reference. She also gave Leah her home address and advised her to have requests for references sent there rather than to the hospital. As for the intern, he was not seen in the hospital again. Rumor had it that he lost his license to practice medicine and was sent to a forensic institution. For sure, the students at the medical school heard a number of lectures on appropriate prescribing and the dangers of overdosing patients.

This experience taught Leah that she must have the courage to advocate for the safe care of her patients. It also taught her that in any job-related confrontation, no matter how right you might be, your colleagues are unlikely to come to your defense, and you have to forgive them for that. After all, Leah drew the line

"For better or for worse, nurses create nursing," she says. "We—you and me—are the profession ... and often the patient's last line of defense."

in the sand when she persisted in asking questions about the patient who died—and she could not expect others to risk their jobs, income, and security for her decision.

Abuse of power was a recurrent theme for Leah during her early nursing career. Her awareness of and concern for abuse of power permeated her future professional decision-making. She learned to "fly low" and hope that authority figures wouldn't even know her name. Years later, when addressing the National Council of State Boards of Nursing, Leah began her remarks by assuring them that she had *never* wanted to come to *their* attention.

Through it all, her passion for nursing was never dampened. Leah believes that nursing has everything to do with patients, and that nursing comes into existence when the nurse lays hands on the patient. "For better or for worse, nurses create nursing," she says. "We—you and me—are the profession ... and often the patient's last line of defense."

What she experienced in her early years as a nurse had everything to do with politics and agendas that were way outside her realm of knowledge and, of course, completely unrelated—often even contrary to—good patient care. The lesson she learned? Advocate for what you believe to be *right* for the patient. This was the beginning of her lifelong passion for ethics.

A LEADER OF RIGHTS—GETTING THINGS DONE

On 16 March 1966, Leah married Peter Curtin, a hospital finance director. Two years later, the first of their four children, Peter, was born, followed by Rose in 1970, Chris in 1971, and Joe in 1973. When she had been in high school, Leah learned to love oil painting. In fact, she even sold a few canvasses that she painted when she was a nursing student. But now, Leah painted pictures with a mission: to decorate the otherwise bare walls of the family home. She painted several still lifes and even some Disney characters that she hung in the children's rooms.

However, Leah's next "real" job after leaving the hospital was with the Visiting Nurses Association of Cincinnati (VNA), which covered several counties in Ohio and northern Kentucky. Her inner city district included a patient load of tens of thousands of people, and she filled in for other nurses too. She saw it all—from racial riots in the city to children dying in the hills of Kentucky because they couldn't get antibiotics. Leah was frustrated by the systemic barriers that prevented patients from receiving care for their illnesses or traumas. Thus was born her driving concern for reform—specifically justice in allocation of resources and access to care.

In early 1968, Leah recalls the dire circumstances of a patient who had been diagnosed with cervical cancer and treated with radiation implants. As a result, the patient suffered severe internal radiation burns that caused intractable pain. The final line of treatment was a chordotomy for pain control, with the trade-off of partial paralysis, and a colostomy. When the patient was finally discharged to home she "had nothing, absolutely nothing," Leah says, and didn't qualify for welfare because she had a paid-up $5,000 life insurance policy.

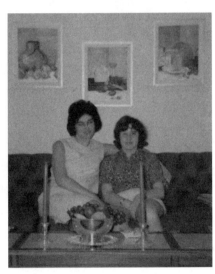

LEAH, LEFT, WITH HER SISTER LOUISE IN HER AND PETER'S FIRST APARTMENT IN 1966. BEHIND THEM ARE THREE OF LEAH'S PAINTINGS.

When Leah arrived at the patient's home, it was clear the patient had little to eat, a pressure ulcer exposing her coccyx, a dependent father who was a bilateral amputee, and no one to help her with activities of daily liv-

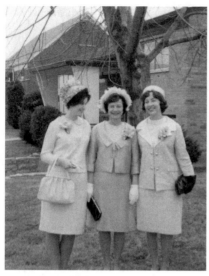

LEAH, LEFT, HER MOTHER, CENTER, AND HER SISTER PAT DRESSED FOR EASTER IN 1967.

ing. Setting priorities, Leah first found a resource for food. She went to the patient's neighbor and negotiated a deal: If the patient cooked supper for the all-male neighboring family with their food, she and her father could eat for free. This accomplished three things: The patient and her father ate, the patient was forced to be up on her walker and active, and most importantly, the patient felt useful and capable again. Meanwhile, the neighboring family—a widower and his sons—came home to a hot meal every night.

The next step was finding a way to get the rent paid. Leah attempted to meet with the hospital social service worker without success. Finally, she staged a one-woman sit-in outside the social worker's office. She arrived in full VNA uniform and sat there most of the day. When the social worker tried to go home, Leah stopped her and described the patient's desperate situation. The social worker found a way to put the patient on partial welfare—enough to cover the rent.

If you can't go through the front door, then find a side door or a window.

Two important things Leah learned at the VNA were:

1. If you ask, people are almost always willing to help.
2. If you can't go through the front door, then find a side door or a window.

To Leah, leadership means getting done what needs to be done. It does not mean a title of authority.

One example of Leah's ability to get things done was her leadership in protecting the integrity and conscience of nurses. In doing so, she became entangled in another career crossroads—legalized abortion. Veteran nurses had been taught to deal with two patients (mother and fetus), not just one. Thus, abortion required a huge paradigm shift in nursing practice for which many nurses were unprepared. Some nurses were forced to participate in abortion procedures or face loss of their jobs for insubordination. When a panel of three district court judges struck down Kentucky's institutional and individual conscience clause in *Wolfe v. Schoering*, 1976, Leah was among the leaders of the legal drive to reinstate it. Despite the fact that the Kentucky statute included a severability clause, the district court went further and invalidated Kentucky's individual conscience clause (that had not even been challenged). In the appeal from that decision, Leah was the force behind an *amicus curae* brief on behalf of Kentucky registered nurses that was entered in an attempt to save the individual conscience clause, even if the institutional conscience clause failed.

The U.S. Court of Appeals for the Sixth Circuit reversed the district court's decision in regard to both private institutions and private individuals but upheld the district court in regard to public institutions. Thus, nurses and other healthcare personnel had a clearly defined right to freedom of conscience—a right that soon was supported by conscience clause legislation in most states.

At the time of this court case, Leah was caring for four small children, working a part-time night shift at a local hospital, and also attending two graduate programs simultaneously—one for a master of arts in philosophy (Athenaeum of Ohio—1977) and the other for a master of science in health planning and administration (University of Cincinnati—1977). She was overextended, but someone needed to insist on a definitive legal opinion

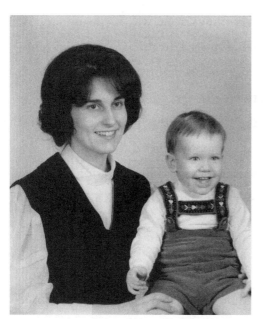

LEAH WITH HER FIRST CHILD, PETER, WHEN HE WAS 18 MONTHS OLD.

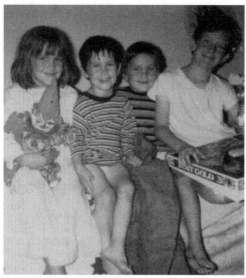

FROM LEFT TO RIGHT: ROSE, JOE, CHRIS, AND PETE CURTIN, 1976.

about nurses' freedom of conscience rights. Thus, she conferred with attorneys, gathered nurses in public and private sectors for a class action brief, and raised money to pay the legal defense. At one point, several of the nurses (all employed at the same hospital) withdrew from the case. A director of nursing from a Catholic hospital in Kentucky threatened the nurses with job loss if they went to court. Leah called this director to assure her that none of the nurses would be required to testify in court, thus none of them would be taking time away from their duties at the hospital. The goal of this suit was not to limit women's rights to abortion, but rather to address nurses' freedom of conscience rights. Having clearly informed the director about the nature of the case, Leah's call was transferred to the president of the hospital. Once connected with the president, she was put on hold for hours, after which the president's secretary informed her that he had to leave the office for another engage-ment. Frustrated, but not yet defeated, Leah called the U.S. papal nuncio, who quickly understood the situation and referred her to the order of sisters who owned the Kentucky Catholic hospital. After an extensive dis-cussion about the purpose of the lawsuit and its impact on the nursing pro-fession in particular and Catholic hospitals in general, this order's mother general promised to take action to protect the nurses, and she did.

The ultimate outcome of this case meant that nurses were no longer merely instruments of the order of others, but rather independent human beings with consciences who have responsibilities and also rights. This was a groundbreaking case for the rights of nurses. The long-term consequence of this case is that freedom of conscience was established. This right ex-tends well beyond abortion, as healthcare workers grapple with ethical and moral consequences of current and future technologies and procedures.

When asked what she learned from the experience, Leah replies with a wry smile, "Lawyers are darned expensive." Fortunately, no one knows better than Leah that it is impossible to put a price on professional freedom of conscience.

THE BEGINNING OF NURSING ETHICS

One of the first bioethics centers to emerge in the United States was the Hastings Center in Garrison, New York. Founded in 1969, the Hastings Center is a nonprofit, nonpartisan bioethics research institute that was founded to explore fundamental questions in healthcare. Leah was inter-ested in ethics in a variety of ways. She attended Hastings Center meetings soon after it was founded to gain a greater understanding and perspective of ethics.

At the time, nursing ethics did not exist as a discipline. Leah had noticed that many of the attendees at Hastings Center meetings and national ethics conferences were nurses, and yet nobody was talking about nursing's ethical practice issues. Mary Josephine Flaherty was among the outstanding people that Leah met. At that time, Mary was dean of the faculty of nursing at the University of Ottawa, and she became one of Leah's mentors. The Hastings Center discussions centered on medicine and various biological sciences, as though nursing practice was irrelevant to ethics discussions. Leah began to talk with other nurses about starting a nursing ethics center. While all agreed that it was a great idea, there was no time or money to operationalize a center for nursing ethics.

In the mid 1970s, Leah was a philosophy student at Anthenaeum of Ohio. She was asked to teach what might well have been the first interdisciplinary course in ethics actually held in a clinical setting—the Cincinnati Center for Developmental Disabilities (CCDD). She was a clinical intern in ethics at CCDD when Dr. Rubinstein, founder and head of the clinic, arranged for her to teach this controversial class. It undoubtedly was the first time many of the students discussed ethics at all—no less in an interdisciplinary "classroom"—and Leah struggled to get anyone to open up for discussion. She would say something "positively outrageous," in her words, to generate a response, and then she would wait for the controversy to begin.

As an intern with the CCDD, Leah became involved in issues surrounding the treatment of infants born with significant congenital defects. John Lorber, a British ethicist, had recently published an article proposing "criteria for humanhood." This discussion was particularly relevant to CCDD, because 80-85% of the children who came to the center were meningomyelocele patients.

At the 1975 National Spina Bifida Association meeting in Cincinnati, Barbara Engstron, director of nursing at CCDD and another of Leah's mentors, introduced her as the director of an organization that did not exist—the National Center for Nursing Ethics. Leah was stunned she had been appointed to direct a hoped-for, but as yet unrealized national center for nursing ethics. Barbara told her the center needed to be developed, and Leah had more time than anyone else. Making the announcement more or less forced the issue of whether or not the center should be established. Meanwhile, at this first meeting of the National Spina Bifida Association, Leah facilitated a multidisciplinary panel on treatment versus nontreatment of children born with spina bifida. She even spoke with the parents about this subject in a special breakout session. The panel included a neurosurgeon, neonatologist, pediatrician, clinical nurse specialist, social worker, intensive care nurse, parent, and clergyman. At the end of the debate, the panel was evenly split. The neurosurgeon, social worker, neonatologist, and intensive care nurse approved of euthanasia. The pediatrician, parent, clinical nurse specialist, and clergyman disapproved. Leah observed that the difference between the two groups was that those who favored nontreatment entered the child's life during episodes of crisis and saw only the trauma. Those who favored treatment saw the personality of the child emerge over time—and also saw the joy and triumph of both child and parents.

Almost immediately after the conference, Leah began receiving correspondence for the National Center for Nursing Ethics. During the first year, she received more than 1,500 letters and answered them from the center's headquarters—her kitchen table. Officially, the National Center for Nursing Ethics was formed in 1975, and the original board members included Barbara Engstrom, RN, MSN; M. Josephine Flaherty, RN, PhD; Helen Creighton, RN, JD; Anne Davis, RN, PhD, FAAN; Luther Christman,

RN, PhD, FAAN; Helen Eileen Ridgeway, RN, PhD; Gina Giavinco, RN, MPHN; and Sr. Eileen Kantz, RN, MSN.

The board set and accomplished several goals, including encouraging the development of a code of ethics for nurses, disseminating ethics information via mainstream nursing journal publications, and convincing the National League for Nursing to incorporate nursing ethics into the core curriculum for nursing education. Leah also became editor of *Update on Ethics* and *The Journal for Nursing Ethics*, both of which were published by the National Center for Nursing Ethics. The ethics ball was rolling, and Leah was at the center of the movement. She was engaging in high-level ethics dialogue and developing the practice of ethics with other national and international leaders. It was a rare time in practice development. Leah was in the right place at the right time with the perfect opportunity to lead not only nursing but also healthcare in the development of ethics.

When Leah began teaching ethics at Northern Kentucky University, she recalls being frustrated that she could not find an ethics textbook she liked. She contacted M. Josephine Flaherty, the principal nursing officer of Canada, and together they wrote *Nursing Ethics: Theories and Pragmatics*. The effort was one of the first of its kind and was recognized by the *American Journal of Nursing* as Book of the Year in 1982.

> *Leaving may mean nurses are left with no one at executive levels to advocate for patient care; staying may be seen as participating in an immoral system. Judging either is an exercise in arrogance."*

Leah was publishing, teaching, and making presentations on ethics around the country. As her son Chris wrote in his essay, Leah's name got around.

Ethics, Integrity, Principles, and Ego

Leah believes that one of the foundations of nursing practice is trust. Patients must trust that nurses will bring their knowledge, skill, and integrity to their practice when administering medications and providing hands-on care. Leah defines integrity as doing what one thinks is right.

According to Leah, the restructuring, redesigning, and re-engineering of hospitals in the 1990s and the reduction of RN-to-patient ratios were challenges to the integrity of nurse leaders. They suffered considerable angst, and many of the best nursing leaders left their jobs because they believed the changes would be damaging to patient-care outcomes. Others chose to stay and try to mitigate the harmful effects of economic pressures. Which leaders were right? "It is a true moral dilemma," Leah says. "Leaving may mean nurses are left with no one at executive levels to advocate for patient care; staying may be seen as participating in an immoral system. Judging either is an exercise in arrogance."

When drawing a line in the sand, Leah believes it is important to distinguish between what is ego and what is principle. Ego is associated with self-righteous or self-aggrandizing choices. Choices made on principle involve deeply held values and doing what one truly believes to be the right thing in a given situation.

Leah believes the most pervasive ethical problem for nurses is that they cannot practice nursing the way they believe it should be practiced. This is where the nurse executive has the greatest opportunity. Nurses in executive leadership roles have the power to influence the work environment, but they are not omnipotent. They cannot change the economic environment and its constraints. Nurse leaders have to work with chief executive officers, chief financial officers, and others to reduce costs, but they can use their influence judiciously to minimize negative impacts on patient care. Her advice is to "weigh carefully the good of leaving versus the good of staying," because nurse executives can do a lot of good in those roles even with limitations. Additionally, those leadership positions are few and far between. Nurse executives who leave their job may be unable to find another position where they have the privilege of influencing quality of patient care.

Leah warns that when nurses are considering action as a result of a threat to integrity, they should do so with the full knowledge that they may stand alone. Speaking from experience, Leah says: "When you draw a line in the sand about a principle or a stance, understand it is your line and your sand, and nobody else is going to defend that turf with you. You are on your own. No matter how 'right' you are and no matter how close your friendships, they may not support you." When drawing a line in the sand, Leah believes it is important to distinguish between what is ego and what is principle. Ego is associated with self-righteous or self-aggrandizing choices. Choices made on principle involve deeply held values and doing what one truly believes to be the right thing in a given situation.

As an example, Leah describes her friend Carolina Zurlage, a former high school teacher. Carolina was a brilliant woman who was truly an educator, not merely a teacher. In her youth, Carolina had been a Marine working in the historical archives at the Pentagon. At the time she was teaching, the national debate over the Vietnam war was spawning a rising number of protests that were escalating into violence. Some of her students refused to say the Pledge of Allegiance before class. To deal with the protests, Carolina asked the students to complete an assignment: Rewrite the Pledge of Allegiance in such a way that they could say it sincerely and in good conscience. She sent a letter home to the parents explaining the assignment and why it was to be undertaken. Someone informed the John

Birch Society, an organization founded to defend the United States against perceived threats to the Constitution, especially communist infiltration. The John Birch Society turned this student assignment into a media circus about "subversive" teachers, with Carolina being the subverter. Carolina was condemned in the press and accused of everything from being unpatriotic to being immoral. Eventually, the turmoil led to a public meeting of the board of education at which Carolina, though defended by many students and their parents, was required to defend herself.

Leah believes the biggest ethical challenge in most people's lives is trying to maintain integrity.

Shortly thereafter, her contract was up for renewal. The school offered her a 1-year contract. She resigned. Her administrator wanted to keep her, but offering her the standard 2-5 year contract wasn't advisable for him, given the high profile and political nature of the situation. He suggested a way for her to survive the controversy. She was fighting for principles—student rights and academic freedom. However, Carolina wouldn't accept any compromise, even one that did not involve her principles, but rather the circumstances of her employment. The administrator wanted to give the appearance of putting Carolina on probation while keeping her on staff. Carolina would have none of it. She reacted with her ego instead of her principles. Ultimately, the resignation made her bitter because she lost the ability to do something she loved, teaching, and her students lost a gifted educator.

Leah believes the biggest ethical challenge in most people's lives is trying to maintain integrity. Regardless of the position, "maintaining one's integrity is the hardest thing to do, because you can play such games with your own mind. You can lose little pieces of your soul until you don't even know who you are any more," Leah warns.

She tries to maintain her own integrity by never making excuses. Her motto is, "To thine own self be honest." Justifying poor, foolish, or self-serving choices is an exercise in self-delusion that leads to your own moral disintegration. Leah recommends that to stay grounded, healthcare leaders should stay in close contact with patients. "We go to work each day to give wonderful care to people," she says. Few healthcare providers would refute this statement. Thus, patient-centered decision-making should be foremost among the leadership priorities of nurses.

Medicine would not have advanced beyond bloodletting if lawyers made the decisions, she says, as they are "too legalistic at times to promote humanistic progress."

THE ROLE OF AN ETHICS COMMITTEE

Patient circumstances resulting in an ethics committee consult are daily occurrences in healthcare. Leah believes bioethics committees are very useful if they function properly. In her opinion, the committee should be multidisciplinary, but lawyers should be consultants rather than committee members, because their opinions are taken as "law" and often stop discussions. Medicine would not have advanced beyond bloodletting if lawyers made the decisions, she says, as they are "too legalistic at times to promote humanistic progress." Having lawyers advise the committee is necessary to assure that recommendations are legal, but the legal perspective must not dominate the thinking of the group.

Additionally, Leah thinks ethics committees should be able to set up subcommittees to deal with cases outside the expertise of the committee members. The foundation of ethical decision-making is accurate facts, and utilizing content experts at the subcommittee level is important to accurate discovery.

Leah asserts that the primary function of an ethics committee is two-fold: to assist the organization or institution in developing policy about how ethical issues should be handled, not necessarily what should be done in a specific case; and to educate people about ethics, including administrative practice as well as clinical practice. Only as a last resort should the ethics committee make decisions regarding a specific clinical case. Most people easily identify ethical issues related to clinical cases; however, less obvious are the situations involving the ethical accountability of hospital administrators for providing the infrastructure essential for good clinical outcomes.

Through this and other opportunities she made for herself, she learned that some of the most important and compelling conversations occur at the end of the conference, often in the bar.

Hospital administrators are responsible for providing leadership; up-to-date, accessible policies and procedures; professional development and education; supplies; technology; and adequate staffing. If administrative decisions focus on the bottom line, ethical dilemmas inevitably ensue.

THE POWER OF NETWORKING

Leah was in her late 20s when she was serendipitously thrust into a national leadership role for nursing ethics. She was debating and socializing with some of the nation's finest scholars while completing graduate studies. She remembers a weeklong, world-class conference on bioethics and the law that was held in her hometown, but she could not afford to attend it. Not to be denied, Leah contacted Father Della Pica, the program organizer, and volunteered to pick up guests from the airport, introduce speakers, hand out evaluations, and run any and all conference errands, just to get in the vicinity of the discussion and become a "sponge" for ideas. Through this and other opportunities she made for herself, she learned that some of the most important and compelling conversations occur at the end of the conference, often in the bar. Leah learned that "if you want to make friends on a dry campus, it helps to have good Scotch," so she always bought the best. The benefit of networking for new leaders is to broaden their perspectives through the wisdom of others. Leah learned a great deal in this way.

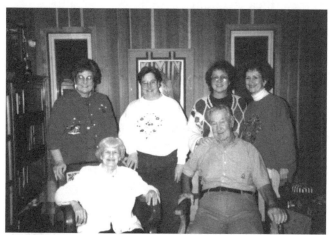

LEAH AND HER SISTERS WITH THEIR PARENTS IN 1998. SEATED ARE MOM AND DAD. STANDING, FROM LEFT TO RIGHT, ARE LEAH, LOUISE, PAT, AND JEANNE.

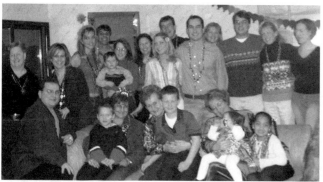

LEAH'S FAMILY AND FRIENDS GATHER FOR A SURPRISE 60TH BIRTHDAY PARTY FOR HER IN 2002.

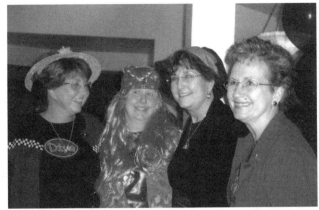

Nurse leaders such as Alice Clark, M. Josephine Flaherty, Grayce Sills, and Hildegard Peplau individually provided Leah with numerous professional opportunities and remarkable mentorship. Alice had been editor of *RN* magazine for years and was publisher of *Nursing Forum* and *Perspectives in Psychiatric Care* when she first met Leah at the Center for Nursing Ethics booth at an American Nurses Association (ANA) conference. They spoke at length about the future of nursing ethics, and Alice invited Leah to stay with her when Leah was invited to speak on the subject in New York and Connecticut. Alice also invited Leah to write articles for both *Nursing Forum* and *Perspectives in Psychiatric Care*. Furthermore, she introduced Leah to Mike Kelly, then associate publisher of the journal *Supervisor Nurse*. Alice knew that *Supervisor Nurse* needed an editor-in-chief and that Leah was a gifted writer. The match seemed perfect. Leah had never envisioned a career in writing, but she kept her mind and options open to this potential new career path.

> *I don't play games, and people are so shocked that I come out with what I think.*

She had never heard of the *Supervisor Nurse* journal, but her master's in health planning and administration had prepared her well. Leah admits that her interest in that master's degree was "an attempt to understand what the heck managers and administrators were thinking." After careful consideration, Leah accepted the position as editor-in-chief of *Supervisor Nurse* at age 35. The publisher of the journal, John Harling, asked her not to write about ethics in the journal, but he agreed that she could write about the topic in other journals. Leah then asked him to change the name of the journal. After 18 months of vigorous discussion, the journal's name was changed to *Nursing Management*. She wrote about leadership, practice, and relevant healthcare issues. Several years later, John asked Leah to write a monthly column on ethics. He believed in a strict separation between editorial and advertising and allowed her complete editorial freedom—a privilege she treasured and never abused. John became her friend as well as her publisher.

Her master's degree in philosophy, with a minor in linguistic analysis, helped Leah develop her new career path. She was educated to write and speak plainly. She communicates precisely what she means to convey, and every word is selected carefully toward this end. "I don't play games, and people are so shocked that I come out with what I think." She does not try to be shocking but simply tries to say what she interprets. The feedback she often receives is that readers are pleased they can understand what she is saying, even if they don't agree with the message.

Leah points out that criticism is finding fault, while critique is challenging, expanding, or changing the viewpoint to improve the outcome. Criticism can be demoralizing, while critique is elevating and necessary for professional growth.

When Leah's articles or editorials create a stir among readers, she always gets the message. She specifically recalls a letter of response from

Hildegard Peplau, a prominent leader in psychiatric nursing. Leah had come to know Hildegard well following an ANA meeting in Phoenix, AZ, when Hildegard and Grayce Sills invited Leah to join them for a post-conference trip to the Grand Canyon. Hildegard was well into her 70s, so hiking was out of the question. This meant there was time for hours of debate about everything imaginable, and a bond of mutual respect formed among the three nursing leaders. When Leah wrote a *Nursing Management* editorial titled *"The Bottom Line Be Damned"* in 1997, she received a letter from Hildegard that began, "Never did I think I would see such a word in a professional journal, not to mention on its front cover." The letter ended, "But if ever it was justified, and I am not saying it ever could be, *this* would be the case." Over the years, Hildegard mentored Leah primarily through letters in which she critiqued the content of Leah's articles and editorials. This gift of critique is something Leah treasured. She remembers that Hildegard would "cross mental swords" with the editorials and either agree, disagree, or ask for more information—but always with a purpose and explanation for her thinking. Leah explains that Hildegard would never come out and say, "You are wrong," but rather, "I got the message." Leah was a better writer and thinker thanks to this gift of critique.

Leah points out that criticism is finding fault, while critique is challenging, expanding, or changing the viewpoint to improve the outcome. Criticism can be demoralizing, while critique is elevating and necessary for professional growth. Nurses need to learn how to offer and embrace the gift of critique.

THE POWER OF THE PEN

For nearly 20 years, Leah educated, entertained, and expanded the vision of the nursing profession with *Nursing Management* editorials such as

"*Free the Hospice 6*" (July 1991), "*The Ghost of Jacob Marley*" (December 1994), "*Unsafe Patient Care: The Road to Abilene*" (April 1995), "*The Tsunami Effect*" (April 1994), "*Mirror, Mirror on the Wall*" (September 1992), and "*Nurses: Bimbos on the Boob Tube?*" (May 1990). Leah writes her editorials as if she is speaking directly to people. Readers can almost feel her elbow in their side as she whispers, "Hey, do you see what I mean? Isn't this obvious and worthy of further thought?"

Leah's editorials can make readers laugh out loud, hang their head in shame, or get angry, but she has the gift of making others *feel* her point—whether they agree or disagree with her. In 1983, Leah was elected a fellow of the American Academy of Nursing, and several years later her sister Jeanne Clement, RN, EdD, joined her as a fellow. They are one of only two sets of sisters elected to the academy.

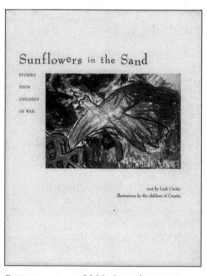

Sunflowers in the Sand

STORIES
FROM
CHILDREN
OF WAR

text by Leah Curtin
Illustrations by the children of Croatia

PUBLISHED IN 2000, LEAH'S BOOK,
SUNFLOWERS IN THE SAND,
TELLS THE POIGNANT STORIES OF
CHILDREN CAUGHT IN THE MIDST
OF THE BALKANS WAR OF THE 1990S.

Leah believes that some people are born with a unique ability to take the reader on a journey that is interesting and informative. Others struggle to make their point known at the most basic level. In either case, writing is a skill that improves with practice. Leah urges that professionals share what they have learned—for the benefit of the patient. The clinical discovery that has absorbed so many hours and so much talent and revealed such valuable findings deserves to be shared with the profession. Leah refused to "let the labor go to rack and ruin" and began to publish in graduate school.

In 1975, one of her health management professors was so taken with Leah's project on euthanasia that the professor nearly forced her to create and publish her first book, *The Mask of Euthanasia*. The professor helped her with all the illustrations and gave her the confidence to get her ideas out there for the world to see. In 1990, Leah was one of several nurses invited to have lunch with Laura Bush at the White House in honor of Nurses Day. In 1995, Springhouse Corporation collected her editorials and published them in a book, *Nursing into the 21st Century*, which is still in use today.

Leah encourages writers to publish for passion and not just profession. She is a strong advocate of, as she calls it, "doing what gives you life." In January 2000, Leah wrote a book titled *Sunflowers in the Sand: Stories from Children of War*. Sister Joanne Schuster and the Franciscan Sisters of the Poor Health System challenged her to break her traditional publication mold and write about the impact of war on the lives of children. The book tells poignant stories about the impact of war on the lives of children in the area formerly known as Yugoslavia. Many times Leah had to stop writing because she could no longer see through her tears. The book received a positive review in the *New York Times* Sunday Book Review section and has raised tens of thousands of dollars for the care and treatment of children affected by the war.

STATING THE OBVIOUS: THE WISDOM AND COURAGE OF LEADERSHIP

Leah spent 20 remarkable years leading *Nursing Management* through some of the most turbulent times in healthcare. She was given the freedom to chronicle those years as well as to hold the profession and healthcare accountable. She helped create the Nursing Management Congress more than 25 years ago as a forum to generate and disseminate new knowledge in the field. Leah survived the sale of the journal in 1995, and when she resigned from *Nursing Management* in 1998, it was with many lessons learned and a lifetime of career experiences.

She offers simple advice to all nurse executives: "Don't worry about contracts. Contracts only help the people who have enough money to enforce them, and if you don't have the money don't bother." She believes if you are not dealing with honorable people, a contract is not worth the paper it is written on, unless you are very wealthy. If you are dealing with honorable people, then you probably don't need a contract in the first place.

The real nurses are nurses who practice the profession. The rest of us live on their backs.

As a result of her position at *Nursing Management*, Leah was frequently invited to present the keynote speech at conferences. Through these and other opportunities, she was often provided with the opportunity to influence the thinking of a large number of professionals. Leah recalls being invited to be the closing speaker for a conference on nursing science and theory. She had attended the entire conference and took it all in with growing agitation. Leah went to the podium and began her presentation: "Let me remind you that nursing is a practice discipline not an academic discipline, and we should stay married to our practice. You are not nurse scientists. You are nurse researchers! And you are responsible for researching things that will improve the practice of nursing. If you do not work to improve the practice of nursing, then please stop taking our money." She went on to tell the audience that "the real nurses are those who practice the profession. The rest of us live on their backs."

The crowd was electrified by Leah's closing remarks. She received numerous questions and a standing ovation; however, she says with a chuckle,

"I was never invited back to speak at that conference again—can you imagine?" But the privilege of her position allowed her to take a similar message to the masses and put it permanently in print in an editorial titled *Real Nurses Don't Whine* (December 1992), which can be found in Leah's book *Nursing into the 21st Century,* a collection of her editorials.

Leah is still very busy professionally. Since leaving *Nursing Management,* she has founded (and closed) *The Journal of Clinical Systems Management* (*JCSM*) and has written 60 more editorials and more than 100 articles for *JCSM* as well as various other journals. She is the director of Cross Country Education's Nurse Manager Boot Camp, which provides rigorous preparation for future nurse managers. She is also clinical professor of nursing at the University of Cincinnati College of Nursing and Health, and she teaches online for Excelsior University and the University of Colorado at Denver. In addition, she is president of Metier Consultants, a columnist for several journals, and a consultant and speaker at events throughout the United States as well as overseas. Leah and Franklyn Shaffer, RN, PhD, are co-directors of the National Forum on Healthcare Leadership, and she still makes keynote addresses, gives workshops, and otherwise remains very busy. She is a member of the board of directors for Firefly Medical Inc. and serves on a number of nursing advisory boards. When asked if she will ever retire, Leah points out that she's far too young to even think about retiring—besides, there is still far too much to do. Her passion for ethics remains intact, only now she has broadened her horizons to include "leadership of the spirit."

> She points out that as a leader, "Chances are if you say anything at all, someone is going to disapprove," so prepare yourself for it and be comfortable with your message.

Leah believes bedside nurses are at times unduly criticized through assumptions made by others. She becomes incensed when she hears others refer to bedside nurses as "refrigerator nurses" or disparage nurses who choose to work for agencies. Leah remarks that if a "bedside nurse works because she or he needs to buy a refrigerator, then doesn't this thinking apply to everyone in some way? Does that make a nurse administrator a jewelry nurse or a Mercedes Benz nurse? Is it really any different? Is there any less commitment from the bedside nurse than the nurse administrator?" Additionally, Leah believes criticizing nurses who work for agencies is just plain wrong. Those nurses simply have chosen a different career path.

There are times that nursing leaders must state the obvious and call it as they see it, even if it creates controversy. Leah encourages nurse leaders to stand up for what they think is the right thing to do—for patients, for nursing, and for health service delivery. She points out that as a leader, "Chances are if you say anything at all, someone is going to disapprove," so prepare yourself for it and be comfortable with your message. Leah doesn't think that creating controversy makes a nurse a leader, but responding effectively to conflict situations will.

Regrets and Gratitude

Leah has always regretted that she didn't complete a baccalaureate of science in nursing (BSN) or finish her doctorate. She had devoted 5 years to earning a diploma in nursing and very much wanted to complete the requirements for her BSN. Leah approached the University of Cincinnati College of Nursing about attending its program in the early 1970s. She was told that in order to be "properly socialized," she would need to leave her husband and four children to live in the dormitory. Leah could not abandon her family to be "resocialized," and her hopes for earning a BSN vanished.

After earning two master's degrees, Leah was eager to pursue a doctoral degree. She began a program, but she never finished because neither her husband nor her parents supported the choice. She had been married to Peter for nearly 15 years. Many of those years, Leah had been in school or working on projects that consumed much of her attention. Peter couldn't understand her desire to pursue doctoral studies and wouldn't financially support the decision. Leah appealed to her parents for support, but her mother felt that Leah should be home with the children. Even today, she would like to return to school for doctoral studies, believing that "anytime you can learn it is a wonderful thing." Fortunately for Leah, two universities have conferred honorary doctorates on her for her work and for her humanitarian services. But as Leah says, "It isn't the same thing at all!"

Leah's career took off when she was in her mid 30s, and the travel commitments increased exponentially. She deeply regrets the impact her frequent absences had on her children, even though she cannot regret the work she did. Leah expressed some of this distress in a poem of sorts. It reads:

Rose Mary fell and cut her knee,
and I wasn't there to care.
Seventeen stitches to close her knee,
and I wasn't there to care.

Peter aced his S.A.T.s,
and I wasn't there to care.
He was the valedictorian of his class,
and I wasn't there to care.

Christopher hit a long home run,
and I wasn't there to care.
He was the hero of the day,
and I wasn't there to care.

> *Life has become so intensely goal-driven that people aren't even aware of what and who they are passing up along the way.*

Little Joseph's thumb was crushed,
and I wasn't there to care.
He ran to me for help,
but I wasn't there to care.

I was chairing a meeting, or giving a speech
Or consulting with influential folks
I loved the work—and did some good
But O! How I wish I'd been there to care.

She reminds us that "there is always a price to pay for any choice you make, so whenever possible, find a way to pay the price yourself—or at least to minimize the price others pay for your choices." Many nurse leaders board the next plane with great angst for what family experiences they are leaving behind while feeling the pressure of what business is awaiting them in the next city.

As her career unfolded, Leah wasn't always able to predict or control some professional demands. Nor was she cognizant of the professional legacy she would ultimately leave. This is the dual-edge sword of achievement. However, she feels blessed to have had a life and career filled with great opportunities.

Leah and Peter divorced in 1986, after 20 years of marriage. She is grateful for the family and life they built together, but "the marriage was not a good fit." Leah identifies her children as what she is most proud of, stating categorically, "They are good citizens and good people." She beams as she says, "Let met tell you about them."

- *Peter*, a lawyer, is married to Susan Grassman. They have two daughters, Katie Rose and Leah Paige.
- *Rose,* a fitness manager, is married to David Aleman. They have a son, David Kai.

- *Christopher,* an educational administrator, is married to Krista St. Claire. They have a son, Conner, and twins on the way.
- *Joseph*, a print analyst, is married to Melanie Kern. They have a daughter, Marina Louise.

There is no doubt that at this point in her life, she does not miss any opportunities to show her family that "she is there to care." Her home is filled with family photos, fossils from her many years of collecting, artwork from around the world, and her beloved pets—Buster and Zach. She has devoted a whole room to toys for her grandchildren.

Leah is also grateful for all the people she met as a nurse. She is profoundly thankful that she was given the opportunity to write, to influence, to talk to people, and to share ideas. She cautions others not to be so intensely goal-driven that they miss splendid people and other great opportunities on their way to the goal. Leah understands that short-term goals are necessary, but "serendipity may be the best long-term goal—let life come to you."

Summary

Leah Curtin is known to many nurses as the mother of nursing ethics, but her contributions far exceed the singular category of ethics. Leah has fought for nursing practice rights, advocated for administrative responsibility, publicly proclaimed the value of the bedside nurse, and published prolifically on most topics relevant to improving outcomes.

Leah is a nurses' nurse. She has reinvented her career a few times—bedside nurse, public health nurse, author, editor, educator, and consultant—but at the heart of every career choice is her devotion to high-quality patient care. She has been willing to publicly debate difficult and often unpopular topics on behalf of patients and nurses. She is a brilliant strategist who measures each word for its power and clarity. Her pen is her favorite weapon. Leah's direct style and bold message have opened the minds of many.

She says she never really saw herself as a leader; she just happened to have the right interests that meshed with the spirit of the time. Her numerous accomplishments and recognitions tell a very different story—she stands alone in her ability to create change and enhance vision around doing the right thing. Just ask her son Chris.

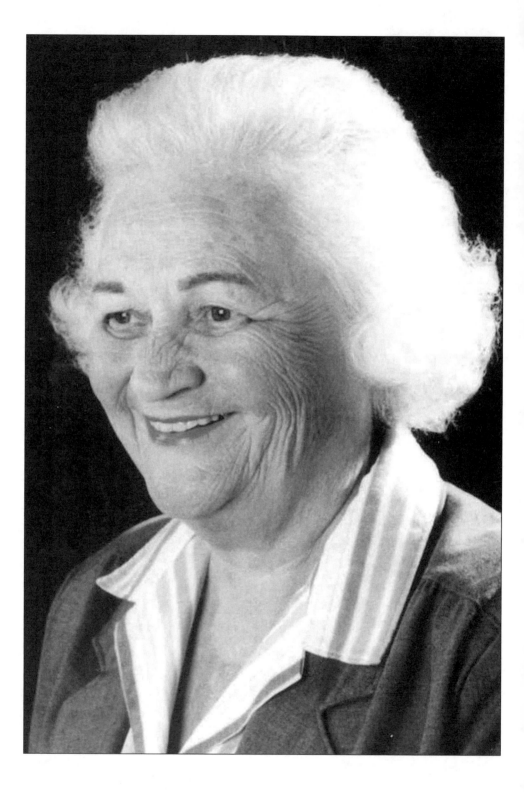

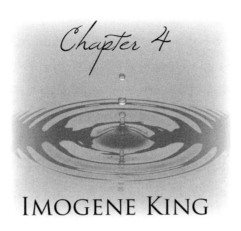

Chapter 4

IMOGENE KING

*"If the students can't do the fundamentals, how
can they use advanced knowledge?"*
—Imogene M. King

Imogene M. King, EdD, MSN, RN, FAAN, was born and raised in a small
Midwestern farming town called West Point, Iowa. The youngest of three
children, she remembers a loving family that dealt bravely with life's challenges. Her father was very influential in her early communication style.
He established a key household rule that centered on open communication
and respect for one another. No matter how difficult the times became, "we
always were respectful of one another," Imogene says. She learned perseverance from challenges she experienced early in life, and these influences
guided her later actions as a nursing leader.

As wonderful an environment as she experienced, her youth spanned
the 1920s to 1930s, when the Great Depression caused hardships for most
families. During this time, even education for young children was viewed
as a luxury only the wealthy could afford. However, Imogene's father

provided her with some of the best education right in her home environment. When she came to him with an issue or a problem, he made her use logic in decision making. Her father would ask her to consider the matter carefully before arriving at a conclusion. "As young children, we learned reasoning and decision making in problem identification and resolution," Imogene says. She credits these early life lessons as her foundation for deriving the goal attainment theory and transaction process model, theories still used today in nursing programs and hospitals striving for the Magnet Recognition Award.

THE CHALLENGE OF THE EARLY YEARS

Imogene King was born in 1923, weighing a healthy 9 pounds. Her family was relieved, as her two older siblings were premature and weighed only 3 pounds. For two premature infants born to one family to survive during the early 1900s was no small miracle.

Like most Midwest families in the early 20th century, Imogene's family farmed for a living. During the late 1920s, they suffered a terrible financial setback. The local banker embezzled money from the bank that held both her father's and uncle's savings. Both families lost all their farming property and had to redesign the life they once knew. As Imogene's parents did not discuss topics of this nature during dinner, she was oblivious as to how challenging the times really were. She remembers hearing only bits and pieces of conversation. It was not until much later that she understood the full effect of the financial problems on her family. All she knew at the time was that her family had to move 9 miles away to Fort Madison, Iowa, so her father and uncle could find employment.

In addition to her father's early teachings in reasoning, her orthography class influenced her conceptual thinking, which later influenced her nursing theory.

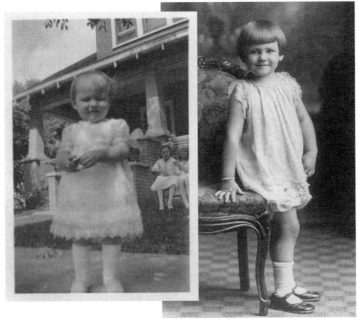

Even though education was viewed as a luxury by some families, it was a priority to her family. Imogene went through Catholic grade school and high school with the Sisters of Notre Dame from St. Louis. They provided her with the wonderful foundational learning she craved. Imogene did not know what her future career path would be, but she loved learning. She participated in theater, debate, and foreign language classes, in addition to the general studies of high school.

One class that had the biggest impact on her life—and still does today—was a course called orthography, which focused on the study of words. This course taught the origin, pronunciation, definition, and spelling of words—basically, the science of language. In addition to her father's early teachings in reasoning, her orthography class influenced her conceptual thinking, which later influenced her nursing theory.

One thing was certain during her early high school years: Imogene had no intention of being a nurse. She felt certain her future would be in the teaching profession, so she set out on that educational track. The two primary professions for women during those years were teaching and nursing. "It was more of an apprentice-style education," Imogene remembers. Education was set up for learning and practicing knowledge all at the same time, in contrast to today's formal college programs.

During the late 1930s, the United States was still experiencing the economic hardships of the Great Depression. The majority of women who graduated from high school did not consider college education as an option. Financial survival was the priority for most families. This was also true for Imogene. Upon graduation from high school, she accepted a position as a secretary and entertained ideas of marrying her high school sweetheart.

But life turned upside down as World War II was declared. Local dancing events were one of the few outlets for fun during those stressful years. Imogene, like many others, took to dancing the jitterbug, which she remembers as a type of competitive sport. Hours were devoted to perfecting new steps, the ideal diversion for those left behind when others went off to war.

Imogene did not marry her young sweetheart, as her boyfriend was drafted into the service and became a pilot overseas. During this time, Imogene's uncle, who was the town surgeon, asked her to consider going to St. Louis to become a nurse. He offered to pay the tuition. Initially, she declined his offer. All Imogene knew about the nursing profession was that her aunt was a nurse, and her sister really wanted to become a nurse. She would have nothing to do with her uncle's offer. Nearly a month later, she reconsidered.

NURSING SCHOOL

"Times were tough and I wanted to get out of town. There were no men left anyway, so this started to sound like a better idea," Imogene says. In a way, going to nursing school was her ticket out of a small town.

With a grade point average that would make any parent proud, Imogene knew she stood a good chance of getting into a nursing program. She went off to nursing school somewhat blind to what lay ahead. She was not quite sure what she was getting herself into, but she planned to have fun and packed her uncle's car with her golf clubs and tennis racket. "Oh, they got a good laugh out of me when I arrived with all my toys," she says. The first thing Imogene told the nursing director was that the tennis courts were badly in need of repair. As reality would have it, she brought her athletic equipment home on Thanksgiving break because nursing school did not allow much time for fun.

She went off to nursing school somewhat blind to what lay ahead. ... "Oh, they got a good laugh out of me when I arrived with all my toys," she says.

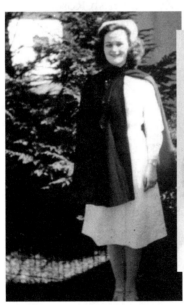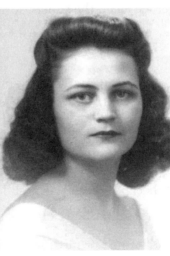

IMOGENE KING IN HER FORMAL NURSING UNIFORM AND IN HER NURSING SCHOOL GRADUATION PHOTO. BOTH PHOTOGRAPHS WERE TAKEN IN HONOR OF HER 1945 GRADUATION FROM ST. JOHN'S HOSPITAL SCHOOL OF NURSING IN ST. LOUIS, MISSOURI.

Imogene compares the nursing programs of the 1940s to today's standards and explains that in each class, students only had one book to study.

"There were really no specialty areas like we have today with oncology and neurology," she says, "because during these years we did not have this breadth of knowledge. All that progress came after the war." Consequently, each nursing student knew those few books very well.

Even today, Imogene can recall her first patient assignment, a very vocal woman who had been on the ward for a while. Imogene walked into the patient's room and said, "I'm Miss King and have been assigned to give you your morning care." The patient did not respond right away, but then asked, "Are you one of those 'probies'?" Imogene said, "Yes, in fact you are my first patient." The patient gave a big sigh. Imogene asked her if she was from Ireland. She snapped back, "What do you know about the Irish?" Imogene let the patient know that her grandparents had come to the United States many years ago and had taught her about the "old country." Before long, the patient asked Imogene to sing "My Wild Irish Rose." The two were singing together when the supervisor walked into the room to ask what was going on. The patient spoke up and said, "Please assign her to give me care every morning."

In the 1940s, all nursing students were required to work in the dietary department. Imogene had to spend 4 weeks in the special diet kitchen. In her first week, she was assigned to cook and mash potatoes. She cooked the potatoes and placed them in the potato masher. "I turned it on and potatoes started to fly out, because there was no lid on the machine." The rest of the day she spent cleaning mashed potatoes off the walls and floors.

Because most of the trained professional nurses had gone to war, the nuns who were RNs were left to work in the hospitals as nurses. In addition, the students were responsible for long shifts and weeks that included working all 7 days. These long hours were essential in providing the additional support and nursing care that patients needed. The pace was grueling, but it allowed Imogene to rise to a leadership position early in her career.

Tuition for nursing school was minimal in those days. Imogene remembers each year costing about $100, but students were also working 7 days a week. "I loved what I was doing, so I did not view it as abusive, but they were very long weeks." During the war, nursing programs accelerated the pace at which students took classes, so they were able to complete their education in 2 years.

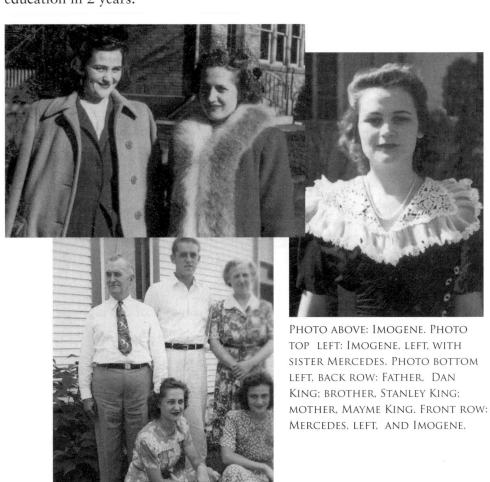

PHOTO ABOVE: IMOGENE. PHOTO TOP LEFT: IMOGENE, LEFT, WITH SISTER MERCEDES. PHOTO BOTTOM LEFT, BACK ROW: FATHER, DAN KING; BROTHER, STANLEY KING; MOTHER, MAYME KING. FRONT ROW: MERCEDES, LEFT, AND IMOGENE.

Today, nurses discuss the differences between the associate degree program and the baccalaureate degree program. During the 1940s, nurses had the same discussion about diploma programs. Although she was not aware of it at the time, her first "real" leadership position was during her senior year of the diploma program, when she provided relief for RNs who were off to war. Imogene was promoted to head nurse on a medical-surgical floor during her last semester at St. Louis.

HIGHER EDUCATION

Hearing the debate about what nursing education and standards the profession should adopt, Imogene knew she must complete her baccalaureate degree in nursing. After finishing her diploma program, Imogene worked in a medical-surgical unit to support her way through St. Louis University's BSN program. She heard that the Jesuits of St. Louis Province selected their best teachers to instruct these serious college students who were veterans of World War II. Imogene received a liberal arts education combined with professional studies. When she had only three credits left before graduation, the director of her diploma program at St. John's approached her about returning to teach students in the program.

> *Hearing the debate about what nursing education and standards the profession should adopt, Imogene knew she must complete her baccalaureate degree in nursing.*

There was no doubt she would accept the position. Because Imogene had firsthand knowledge of St. John's faculty and curriculum, she eagerly jumped at the opportunity. She fondly remembers the director, Sister Rene, who coached her on the side with skills in interpersonal relations and diplomacy. There were physicians and nuns who had taught nurses for years at St.

John's, so making the change to lay nursing professors was a difficult situation, to say the least.

ASSOCIATION LEADERSHIP

While Imogene was working at St. John's, Sister Rene provided her with another leadership opportunity. She asked her to attend the district meeting of the state nurses association. Even though the nuns had a hospital car and driver, Sister Rene asked Imogene to drive her to the association meeting and casually added, "Maybe you would like to stay and hear the

> *Sister Rene said, "Imogene, I have an application for you to fill out, because it sounds to me like you should be a voice for the profession. This is the way you become a voice."*

discussion." Since it was Imogene's first meeting and she was not a member, she did not feel it was appropriate to question those who were making the decisions. But on the car trip home, she asked Sister Rene, "Why did the president of the district hardly give anyone a chance to speak? The environment seemed so controlling." Imogene could not understand why no one had challenged the process and decisions being made that evening. Sister Rene said, "Imogene, I have an application for you to fill out, because it sounds to me like you should be a voice for the profession. This is the way you become a voice."

"That was 1948, and I have been a member of the American Nurses Association ever since," Imogene says.

Sister Rene gave Imogene other opportunities to refine the skills she later become so well-known for in nursing. One of the first times Imogene remembers implementing her skills in conceptualization (even before it became a theory) was when she suggested that the nutrition and pharmacology teachers meet to discuss an approach for medical-surgical nursing

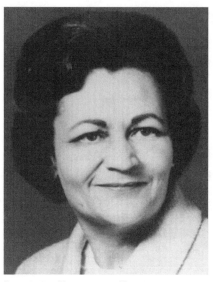

instructors to relate and integrate the content in the three courses. This way, "students could see the interrelationships of how the sciences and nursing education worked together," Imogene says. She observed that when these subjects were taught separately, students had great difficulty with the principles of pharmacology, because they did not have the foundational knowledge to anchor their new learning. When the change was implemented, students began to pick up the content more quickly and the complaints diminished. Students preformed so well on their state board exams they asked Imogene if she had advanced knowledge of the questions. "I knew that I was onto something, and this was the start of it," she says. At the time, her approach was considered innovative teaching.

FURTHERING EDUCATION

A baccalaureate degree was not enough for Imogene. In the mid 1950s, while working toward her master's degree at St. Louis University, she was introduced to new research demonstrating that community colleges prepared students specifically to take and pass their state board exams to become RNs. Information on this topic was being published in nursing journals. While it was controversial, the topic fascinated her. She knew that during the war, nurses had completed their training in 2 years, so this research study inspired her to pursue her doctorate.

The study proposed a 2-year nursing program within an educational institution, instead of a hospital setting. As it was proposed, the curriculum looked very organized. "I went to Sister Rene and told her that I must travel to Teachers College in New York to study with Dr. Mildred Montag, as she had published this research," Imogene says.

"I am lucky because I love to learn, so I am not one to just sit back and do what is necessary to get by."

From the time Imogene arrived on campus at Teachers College, she sought Dr. Montag as her advisor. She was very organized and had already planned her entire first and second semester. Imogene informed Mildred that she intended to work hard so she could complete her doctoral studies in 2 years, since she was responsible for caring for her mother. Not only did Imogene pressure herself to take a heavy load of courses, but she also had to make A's in the first semester to qualify for a fellowship. She succeeded in getting enough money to cover her first and second semester at school. "I am lucky because I love to learn, so I am not one to just sit back and do what is necessary to get by," she says.

While attending one of her first graduate education courses, Imogene met a gentleman who appeared to be a bit of a lost soul. He was a frustrated artist striving to become a professional artist. As they developed a friendship, Imogene learned that he had started teaching high school students instead of pursuing his dream of becoming a professional artist. At that point, he decided to attend graduate school at Teachers College and major in art history. Imogene recognized his potential, even if he did not. As he struggled to "find himself," she would find him on the steps of the dorm—usually hung over.

One day, she approached him with an idea she thought would give him a sense of purpose in life. "I said, 'John, instead of going out with the boys and coming up with what looks like a hangover, a group of us would love it if you would take us around New York and really give us lessons in art appreciation.'" Since New York City is filled with fabulous architecture and artwork, it was a natural request. At first he thought she was kidding, but she told him their payment would be to treat him to lunch those days. He was delighted, and for the next 3 months, he spent every Saturday giving Imogene and her three friends "the tour." They learned about the hidden art treasures in New York City. "We did not have any money as graduate students, so our lunches amounted to $5 meals," she says. The artist called Imogene a few years after graduation to thank her for pulling him out of his miserable slump. While he was not a mentor to Imogene, his passion for art influenced her to join an art class and learn the process for painting beautiful pictures, a hobby she continues in her retirement.

The focus of her independent study was to research the history of baccalaureate education. As Teachers College was in the forefront of baccalaureate education, Imogene had access to all the old books and materials containing the history of nursing and nursing education. Even the documents pertaining to education from the American Nurses Association were housed at Teachers College. Imogene thoroughly enjoyed all she was learning in her doctoral program, and she focused her efforts on preparing to become an expert in curriculum and instruction.

"Mildred facilitated my movement as a graduate student in a way I don't see our professors doing today," Imogene says. Mildred kept her on track to finish in 2 years and made sure she met the approved timelines for her dissertation.

Imogene was thoughtful about selecting her dissertation committee. She had heard the warnings and caution about choosing one's committee wisely. Mildred Montag was the chair of her committee, along with another nurse faculty member and an educator. "I could never have wanted for a better committee," she says. It took only 2 weeks to gather agreements from all committee members and set up her proposal defense. Imogene had already started working on her topic before pulling the committee together and was fortunate it went so smoothly.

With very few doctorally prepared nurses, Imogene found that her education almost scared her peers away.

As part of her dissertation, Imogene worked with faculty at the University of Illinois to develop a master's program in nursing. As it turned out, the faculty members were not of one accord and did not use Imogene's model for their program. "Even though the program did not use my dissertation material, I learned from the experience," she says.

Imogene was successful in completing and defending her dissertation, but graduated with only $250 to her name. Upon graduation, she went home to Iowa to spend time with her family. After completing her doctoral studies in such a short time, she was exhausted and took a month off before being interviewed for a faculty position in Chicago.

POSTDOCTORAL CAREER PATH

As it happened, Imogene did not have to look far to find employment. Very few nurses held a doctorate degree during the 1960s, and Imogene was appointed assistant professor at Loyola University Chicago. "Let me tell you, the faculty was very intimidated by people like me in those days," she says. With very few doctorally prepared nurses, Imogene found that her education almost scared her peers away. But Imogene was persistent in making changes and trying to share her knowledge in a way that would make others comfortable.

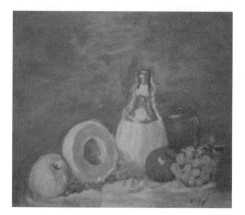 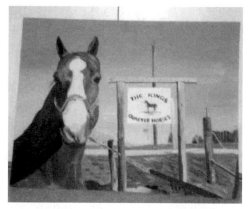

IN THE 1970S, IMOGENE BEGAN A LIFELONG LOVE AFFAIR WITH PAINTING THAT HAS BROUGHT HER MUCH PLEASURE. ON THE LEFT IS HER FIRST OIL PAINTING STILL LIFE. ON THE RIGHT IS HER REPRODUCTION OF A PHOTOGRAPH OF HER NEICE SUSAN'S HORSE BACK IN FORT MADISON, IOWA.

Imogene remembers her first teaching assignment at Loyola University. In addition to teaching in the classroom, she planned the clinical experiences in hospitals. On one particular day, a colleague observed her working with students and questioned why Imogene made them practice bed making until they could do it safely and comfortably. Imogene replied, "If the students can't do the fundamentals, how can they use advanced knowledge?" She thought that important communication and assessment occurred while the nurse made a bed. "Never underestimate how much a nurse can learn about the patient in those few minutes," she said. She stressed nursing knowledge and skills to her students, and the hospital nursing staff noticed she was different from the other university instructors.

Imogene never described herself as a "teacher practitioner." Instead, she called herself a "practitioner teacher," because of her philosophy that a nurse who teaches students needs to be actively practicing. This philosophy allows a nurse to stay current in both knowledge and skills. "To me, if a student was doing something incorrectly, it was important to step in with up-to-date knowledge and teach the appropriate way." Because healthcare and nursing have so many changes, it is critical that the person in the role of educator be up-to-date, or the skill level and knowledge base of the students who graduate will be deficient.

Imogene has a love for lifelong learning. Even after completing her doctoral program, she found herself desiring more knowledge in the area of statistics and research methods. The more Imogene published and researched the literature on a particular subject area, the more knowledge she craved. In 1985, she completed a 2-year continuing education program in measurement in nursing sponsored by the University of Maryland.

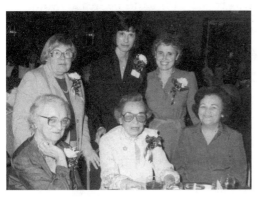

FAMOUS NURSE THEORISTS GATHERED AT A DINNER IN MAY, 1985 AT THE NURSE THEORY CONFERENCE IN PITTSBURGH, PENNSYLVANIA. BACK ROW, FROM LEFT TO RIGHT: DORTHEA OREM, ROSEMARIE PARSE, AND SISTER CALLISTA ROY. SEATED, FROM LEFT TO RIGHT: HILDEGARD PEPLAU, MARTHA ROGERS, AND IMOGENE.

CITY GOVERNMENT

Early on, Imogene realized the power of getting involved and having a voice—not only in the nursing arena, but in politics as well. While teaching graduate students at Loyola (1972-1980), she bought a condominium in the city of Wood Dale. When she purchased it, she was told two more buildings were going up in the near future. A deep foundation was dug for the second building, but the investor had a family tragedy and the project was put on hold. This incomplete building became a public hazard. Two children rode their bikes into the hole and required emergency medical care. At the time, Imogene was president of the condo board and went to city hall to present the situation of the public hazard and ask for help from the city. She spoke with the mayor about her concerns, but to no avail. The

Early on, Imogene realized the power of getting involved and having a voice—not only in the nursing arena, but in politics as well.

mayor suggested that if she didn't like the responses she was getting, perhaps she should run for office herself. After serious consideration, she filed the paperwork and was placed on the ballot to run for the empty alderman seat in her ward. She won by an overwhelming number of votes, even though no woman had ever been elected to the city council.

Imogene knew how important it was to stand up and be heard. Some of the older men had difficulty accepting a woman in this position, but she was able to turn them around. Imogene was proud she could demonstrate honesty in government, a keen ability to identify problems and ways to solve them, and goal setting for the community of 10,000 citizens.

EXPERTISE IN CURRICULUM AND INSTRUCTION

Imogene's philosophy is that a nurse should not have to choose between nursing practice and nursing education. She believes that nursing education is a prerequisite for being a professional practicing nurse. The two are interrelated and should be thought of and practiced as such. Throughout her career, Imogene would never allow herself to entirely abandon her clinical nursing in lieu of a faculty role. She continued to work in the medical-surgical area while teaching nursing students.

For someone with a strong background in curriculum and instruction, the opportunities were plentiful. Imogene was appointed assistant professor at Loyola University in Chicago and appointed chair of the RN to BSN program in 1961. She was appointed as chair of the basic baccalaureate program in 1962. In 1963, in addition to her duties as chair, she worked with faculty to plan and implement curriculum leading to a master of science degree in nursing.

Imogene believed that the faculty committee should identify a conceptual framework for the graduate program at Loyola. "At that time, there were no programs in the country using this information in nursing schools," she says. It was difficult to find research in nursing. Only one journal, *Nursing Research*, published information about nursing research, and few libraries had resources on the topic. Imogene knew she had to expand the effort to collect research sources. She used the educational network to solicit deans across the country to send their lists of dissertations, as well as research resources. Dr. Peg Kaufman's dissertation was titled "Identification of a Theoretical Basis for Nursing Practice." This intrigued Imogene, and she was able to work with the faculty committee to use Kaufman's three concepts of time, stress, and perception as the conceptual framework for the new MSN program.

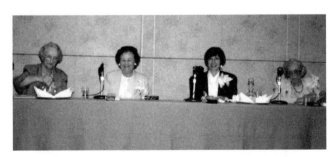

FROM LEFT: HILDEGARD PEPLAU, IMOGENE KING, ROSEMARIE PARSE, AND MARTHA ROGERS AT THE 1991 NURSE THEORY CONFERENCE IN TOKYO, JAPAN.

During this time period, Imogene became active with the Illinois Nurses Association. At the time, proposals to create 2-year associate degree in nursing (ADN) programs at community colleges were being acted on at the state level. Since she had studied under Mildred Montag, who is credited with creation of the ADN programs, Imogene served as the nurse educator on the Illinois Nurses Association committee that developed the first community college nursing program in Chicago.

At the same time the ADN programs were taking off, the advanced practice movement was gaining strength, and the clinical nurse specialist (CNS) and nurse practitioner (NP) roles ultimately were created. "Today, we have so many nursing degrees right through the doctorate level, and we continue to create more nursing education programs," she says. "It only confuses other health professionals about nursing education for the professional nurse. Nursing education has become a hodgepodge in terms of degrees and initial education for beginning professional practice."

Imogene's interest in theory began as an undergraduate student, when she studied theories of learning in an educational psychology course.

Imogene believes the profession needs to make some decisions about the multiple ways and programs that prepare for nursing practice. The proliferation of nursing programs does not allow the nursing discipline to be represented in higher education in a manner similar to other disciplines.

Imogene published *Curriculum and Instruction in Nursing* in 1986, focusing on curriculum principles related to teaching and learning. In the book, she presented an approach for articulating an associate program and a baccalaureate program. Throughout her career, she has consistently looked for ways to organize knowledge and programs to facilitate learning and application to practice.

CONCEPTUAL SYSTEM AND THEORY

Imogene's interest in theory began as an undergraduate student, when she studied theories of learning in an educational psychology course. She reviewed the literature to understand how nursing was being described at that time. From this review, she identified 15 concepts and developed a conceptual system (initially called a conceptual framework) showing the interaction of individuals as personal systems, small groups as interpersonal systems, and large groups as social systems. She selected 10 of the 15 concepts and developed her theory of goal attainment. Using four of the concepts (perception, communication, interaction, and transaction), she derived a transaction process.

When this process is used in nurse-patient interactions, the critical variable is mutual goal setting, which, in most instances, leads to goal attainment or outcomes. Outcomes represent evidence-based practice. In addition, nurses' notes represent data that can be used to design studies relating practice to research in nursing. These four concepts in the transaction process provide basic theoretical knowledge used to implement the nursing process method of assess, nursing diagnosis, plan, implementation, and evaluation.

According to Imogene, nurses should be conscious of both the patient's and their own perceptions as they plan nursing care. For quality nursing care and outcomes, she encourages the use of her transaction process, which leads to goal attainment. The critical variable in this process is *mutual* goal setting with patients.

INTERNATIONAL REACH

Imogene's conceptual system and theory of goal attainment have been employed nationally and internationally by nurse practitioners, researchers, educators, and administrators. Several hospital officials seeking Magnet recognition status have implemented her conceptual system as the basis for organizing nursing as an integral part of multidisciplinary healthcare.

Internationally, Imogene has presented her theory at conferences and consulted in various practice and educational settings all over the world, including Canada, Japan, Germany, and Sweden. Imogene served on the editorial board of *Theoria: Journal of Nursing Theory* in Sweden. However, this journal was discontinued in 2006. She continues to write, speak, and consult about nursing theory. She would like to serve on a committee to develop the discipline of nursing, such as the nursing doctorate (ND) for professional practice, PhD for research, and EdD for education.

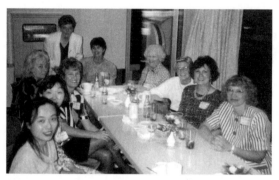

IMOGENE KING (SEATED ON THE RIGHT SIDE OF THE TABLE CLOSEST TO THE WALL) AT THE 1993 HONOR SOCIETY OF NURSING, SIGMA THETA TAU INTERNATIONAL RESEARCH CONGRESS IN MADRID, SPAIN.

The demand for her consulting services increases after every speaking engagement. After Imogene presented her ideas at a theory conference in Alberta, Canada, during the 1980s, a director of nursing and two supervisors from a Toronto medical center invited her to serve as consultant as they implemented theory-based practice using her ideas. She accepted their proposition

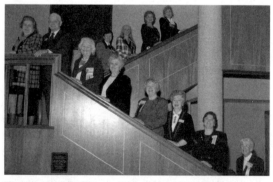

THE FIRST GROUP OF VIRGINIA HENDERSON FELLOWS TAKEN IN 1993 AT THE HEADQUARTERS OF THE HONOR SOCIETY OF NURSING, SIGMA THETA TAU INTERNATIONAL. IMOGENE IS THIRD FROM THE LEFT.

and worked with them for 2 years. She consulted with several nurses in other Canadian hospitals who have published their work in nursing
journals. The year she retired from her faculty
position at the University of South Florida, a
major teaching hospital in Tampa decided to
implement her theory and asked her to serve as a consultant.

*The ideas she formu-
lated and published in
the 1970s and 1980s
are still applicable and
sought out in the 21st
century.*

THE RETIRED NURSE

Imogene remains active in what she calls "retirement." She travels around
the country consulting at hospitals and for nursing schools, mentoring
nurses who seek her advice, presenting and speaking, and attending book
signings. She laughs as she asserts she should never have retired from a
faculty position. "During my retirement, I am writing a book to update my
theory of goal attainment to illustrate how nurses who use the transaction
process can demonstrate effective nursing care and evidence-based practice," she says. The ideas she formulated and published in the 1970s and
1980s are still applicable and sought out in the 21st century.

Working with nursing students is the part of her career Imogene loves
the most. Educating those coming up through the ranks allows her to give
back to the profession. "I
can't recall that I was ever
discouraged in my work," she
says, "but I was sometimes
disappointed in the behavior
of individuals I worked with
in practice and education."

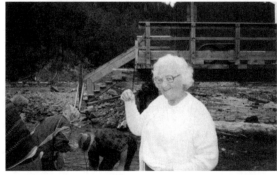

IMOGENE PANNED FOR GOLD IN ALASKA IN 1994
AND CAME AWAY WITH SOME REAL GOLD.

Imogene hopes that associate degree nurses recognize the value of education and return to school for their bachelor's degree in nursing, so they can be oriented to any nursing position or situation in which they are expected

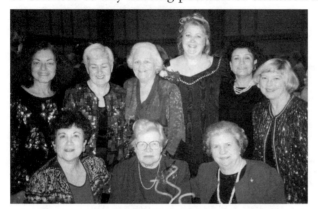

to function. "If nurses don't understand the rules and regulations," she says, "they need to step up and ask questions before acting." She fervently believes that all nurses should continue to learn at every opportunity.

IMOGENE KING AT THE AMERICAN ACADEMY OF NURSING 1996 FELLOWS INDUCTION CEREMONIES. IMOGENE IS IN THE BACK ROW, THIRD FROM LEFT.

As Imogene looks back over her career, she acknowledges that speaking her mind and having a voice in change involved the biggest risks. Speaking out often meant going against popular opinion, but today, she has no regrets. She laughs at her recollection that when she raised a question or concern, even a crowded room would fall silent.

At the 100th-anniversary convention of the American Nurses Association in 1996, Imogene was awarded the Jessie Scott Award, which is given for the demonstration of the interdependent relationships among nursing education, nursing practice, and nursing research. She was scheduled to give a speech. However, the U.S. president at the time, Bill Clinton, was to make an appearance later that same day. There was tremendous security around the convention, and as a result, Imogene's presentation was moved to a different location. Her friends had a taxi waiting for her to return to hear President Clinton's remarks.

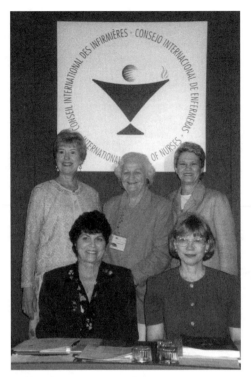

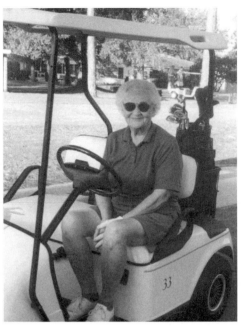

IMOGENE AT ONE OF HER LONG-TIME FAVORITE PASTIMES—GOLFING. HERE, SHE'S COMPETING IN THE BAY POINTE GOLF COURSE LADIES LEAGUE IN 1999.

1999 INTERNATIONAL COUNCIL OF NURSES MEETING WHERE KING'S THEORY WAS PRESENTED. BACK ROW FROM LEFT: MARY KILLEEN, IMOGENE, MAUREEN FREY. SEATED FROM LEFT, PATRICIA MESSMER AND CHRISTINA SIELOFF.

The young girl who never intended to go to nursing school grew up to be a renowned nurse who has contributed much to the profession. She was inducted into the Florida Nurses Association Hall of Fame in 2003 and the American Nurses Association's Hall of Fame in 2004, and she was named a "Living Legend" by the American Academy of Nursing in 2005. Imogene's constant search for excitement in learning and building relationships in nursing organizations drove her desire and passion. Despite her many awards and honors, she considers her most important accomplishment to be teaching thousands of nursing students and watching them become expert practitioners, teachers, and researchers over the years.

"That is the biggest honor of all," Imogene says.

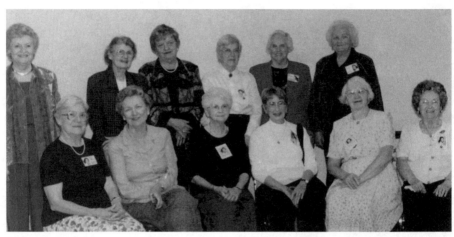

THE 55TH REUNION OF THE 1945 ST. JOHN'S HOSPITAL SCHOOL OF NURSING CLASS WAS HELD IN 2000. IMOGENE IS STANDING ON THE FAR RIGHT IN THE BACK ROW.

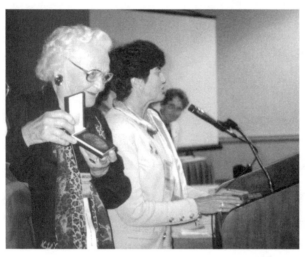

PATRICIA MESSMER PRESENTS IMOGENE WITH THE STATE OF FLORIDA GOVERNOR'S MEDAL FOR HER CONTRIBUTIONS TO NURSING.

REFERENCES

King, I.M. (1986). *Curriculum and instruction in nursing.* Norwalk, CT: Appleton-Century-Crofts.

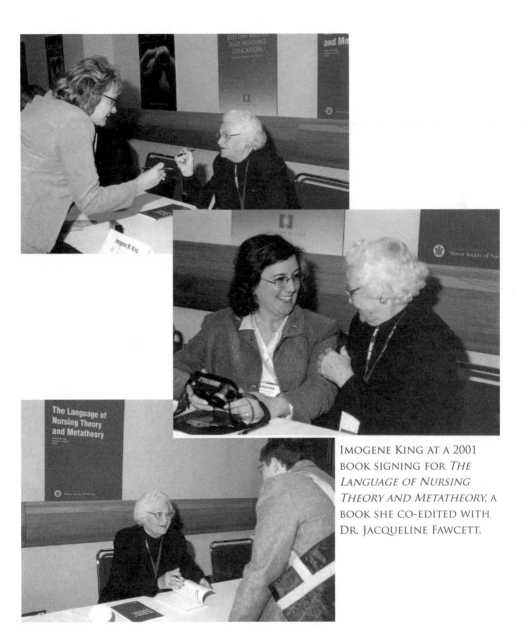

IMOGENE KING AT A 2001 BOOK SIGNING FOR *THE LANGUAGE OF NURSING THEORY AND METATHEORY,* A BOOK SHE CO-EDITED WITH DR. JACQUELINE FAWCETT.

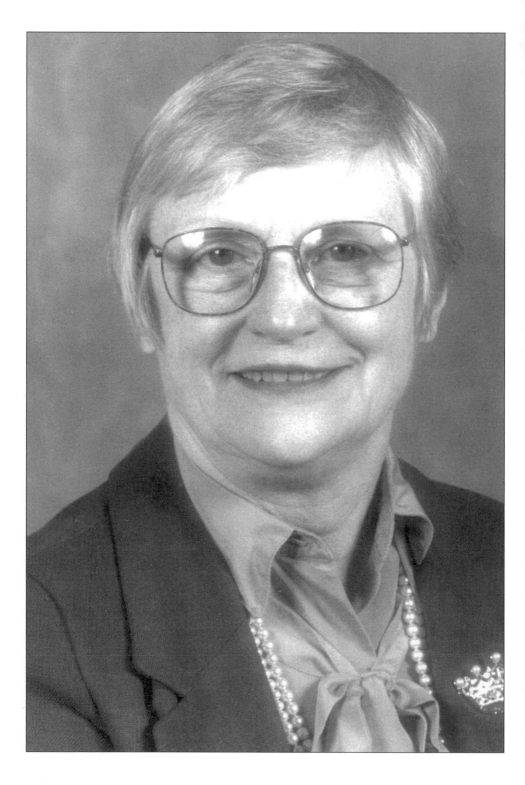

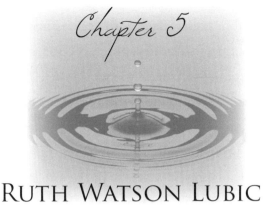

Chapter 5

RUTH WATSON LUBIC

"[The childbearing experience] strengthens families because every time a baby comes into this world, hope comes back again, doesn't it? And, when the power is shared with the people, it grows exponentially."

—Ruth Watson Lubic

Ruth Watson Lubic, CNM, EdD, FAAN, FACNM, grew up 21 miles north of Philadelphia in Bristol (Bucks County), Pennsylvania, where the Delaware Canal empties into the Delaware River. Growing up during the Great Depression and World War II, Ruth developed a strong work ethic and drive that would serve her well throughout life. Along the way, she experienced some difficult times and learned some early life lessons that proved pivotal in building her character. She is an innovative leader who developed our country's first accredited free-standing birthing center, allowing women to take the childbirth process from the rigors of a hospital into a comfortable, homelike atmosphere.

Ruth has received honorary doctorate degrees from five universities, as well as two adjunct professorships, and has conducted invitational lectureships in several countries around the world. In 1971, she was in the first class of members elected to the Institute of Medicine of the National Academy of Science, and in 1993, she was the first nurse to be awarded the prestigious MacArthur Fellowship (known as the "genius" award). When the Institute of Medicine presented her with the esteemed Gustav O. Lienhard Award, Gordon DeFriese, PhD, quoted a colleague, who said of Ruth: "She is a leader who also scrubs the floor. She leads by example. She never forgets that her work is about real women having real children in real communities" (Institute of Medicine, 2001, p. 10).

THE EARLY YEARS

Born in 1927, Ruth was strongly influenced by her surroundings and the era in which she grew up. Her mother's family was Episcopalian, while her father's family was devout Baptist. Her parents brought together unusual and interesting backgrounds. Her maternal family members, with the sur-

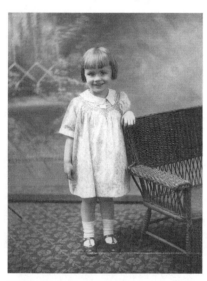

name Kraft, were listed in the Philadelphia Social Register, while her father's side was of more humble, albeit professional, origins, having immigrated to Pennsylvania in Colonial times. Education was highly regarded by both parents. At the time of her parents' marriage, Ruth's father had graduated from the Philadelphia College of Pharmacy and had started medical school. He was, however, compelled to withdraw and return home to

RUTH AS A YOUNG CHILD

operate the family pharmacy when his father developed kidney disease. In regards to Ruth's mother, she completed her secondary education and then assisted her father, the Bristol tax collector, until marrying Ruth's father, at which point she began working in the pharmacy. During the 1920s, it was not a common—or even acceptable—practice for women to go to college.

Ruth's life was busy and difficult. "In those days, when you had your own pharmacy, you just lived around the store," recalls Ruth. It was open 80 hours a week—from 9 a.m. until 10 p.m. weekdays and until 11 p.m. on Saturday. Virtually the only family time was on Sunday afternoons. In addition, unemployment was high in those years, and bills were paid late or not at all. However, Doc Watson never denied anyone on that account, as service to the community was considered to be a personal and philosophical obligation of the family.

The workload at the drugstore was shared. When there was a break in the traffic of customers, Ruth could do her homework in the back room. But more often than not, there was an excess of chores—such as stocking shelves, packaging containers of citronella, and dividing Ichthyol ointment (black salve) for retail sale. Homework had to be completed on time, and she squeezed it in somehow.

Faced with much responsibility, Ruth grew up quickly. It was not uncommon for children to work while attending school full time so the family could make ends meet. Her daily responsibilities became more difficult when her father died suddenly at the age of 48, just after World War II broke out. "My mother tried to hire a pharmacist, but all the pharmacists were being called off to war," Ruth says. It was impossible to find qualified personnel, but the enterprise continued as an over-the-counter drugstore, with Mrs. Watson in charge.

There was nothing that Ruth, only 14 years old at the time, could have done to prepare herself for losing her father, with whom she had a particularly close relationship. Any remaining childhood came abruptly to an end, and out of necessity, she was called upon to assume adult responsibilities. She had become accustomed to long days and hard work, but now she was needed even more. Her only sister was away at college, and it was up to Ruth to fill the gap. Somehow, she and her mother managed to accomplish what had to be done.

At age 15, Ruth became engaged to a high-school classmate who was leaving to join the Marine Corps. While he was serving in the South Pacific, she continued her frenetic pace of working in the pharmacy, while occasionally helping the war effort at the local Selective Service Board and the Fleetwing Airplane plant and, of course, finishing school. She graduated second in her class.

Her fiancé returned from the war in 1945, and they were married in Bristol. She was 18. Together, she and her new husband ran the family drugstore. After several years of marriage, however, differences arose that resulted in separation and then divorce.

Ruth was in her early 20s. Being divorced carried quite a stigma in those times, especially in small towns. She did have, however, a great deal of life experience, a small-business background, and a genuine thirst for knowledge. Having been a good student, she wanted to further her education. Hard work had permitted her to accumulate sufficient savings to help pay her own way through school.

A local physician, Dr. Charles Sampsel, befriended Ruth. He understood her personal difficulties and attempted to guide her into a professional career path. When she could break free from her responsibilities, Dr. Sampsel would invite her to join him on patient house calls. This nurturing relationship and his guidance proved to be significant in Ruth's decision to enter nursing. In yet another misfortune in her young life, Dr. Sampsel was killed in the line of duty while serving in the South Pacific. A second significant mentor in choosing a career path was Ruth's Aunt Alice, a graduate nurse who had a vibrant professional career in the healing arts in Philadelphia. With her mind made up, she decided to apply for admission to the Pennsylvania Hospital School of Nursing.

While Ruth experienced adversity, hardship, and tragedy early in her life, her tenacity and perseverance were evident as she prepared herself for the extraordinary career obstacles she would face in the future.

The Trials of Nursing School

Ruth was not a typical nursing student of this era. She was 25 years old and divorced and had helped run a business. Ignoring her excellent academic record and powerful motivation, the administrators of the Pennsylvania Hospital School of Nursing refused to accept her into the nursing program because, astonishingly, they felt her "worldliness" might be a negative influence on younger classmates. Taken aback but persistent, Ruth explored other options and decided to apply to the diploma nursing program at the Hospital of the University of Pennsylvania. The more progressive admission officials at the hospital better understood the value of her life experiences, and she was permitted to enroll. To this day, Ruth is very proud of the education and experience she gained on the diploma track, and she believes such programs had value in the wide spectrum of nursing education.

At school, Ruth was a natural. Quickly elected as a leader in student government, she soon experienced the perils that can go along with leadership. Prior to her enrollment, a group of nursing students had organized a protest to the mandated 44-hour clinical work week. Subsequently, when the issue came to a head, the director accused her of instigating the students and exacerbating the conflict—accusations that were incorrect. She believes to this day that she was used as a scapegoat by the director. The irony was that the 44-hour work week was a breeze compared to the 80-plus hours she had been working in her family's drugstore. But in her role as a student government officer, she had to "take the heat."

"I sat there in the hospital director's office in disbelief that this woman would accuse me this way," Ruth says. "Worst of all, I was disappointed in not even being given the opportunity or having the courage to defend myself. I was compelled to just sit there and listen."

Leadership Lesson Learned

Ruth learned a difficult lesson in leadership—timing can be critical when one assumes a new leadership role. The school psychologist told her that some day she would be grateful for these experiences, and she would have to learn to deal with people who were willing to sacrifice others to suit their personal ambitions. She took those words very much to heart.

Upon leaving the meeting, Ruth was distraught and burst into tears. Sensibly, she visited the school's staff psychologist for advice. "The whole situation was so dishonest," she says.

Ruth continued to stand out among her peers. She excelled in both academic and clinical areas and was happy with her decision to attend nursing school. She dreamed of someday making a contribution to the profession—but what that contribution would be was still a mystery to her.

Ruth managed the academic challenges and physical routines with alacrity, but she struggled with the ominous "life and death" aspects of nursing practice. Because of her difficulty in adjusting to patients who were terminally or chronically ill, she continued to work with the school psychologist. "It might have been related to my father's death, but I had to try to overcome the sense that perhaps in some way, I could have done more to help him," Ruth says. On one hand, she felt fear and disappointment when taking care of critically and terminally ill patients. On the other hand, she was exhilarated when a grateful, well-attended patient made progress.

Ruth chuckles as she reflects on how much nursing has changed from those early days. Aside from patient care, there were strict, militaristic rules to be followed. All the wheels of parked stretchers had to be turned a certain way, pillowcases had to be draped a certain way, and window shades in patient rooms had to be pulled to a certain height. This uniformity appeared to give a sense of absolute order and control. Even flowers could not remain in private patient rooms, because they might in some way disturb the environment of the sick room. The duty nurse was responsible for an entire floor, without the assistance of electronic or mechanical devices available today. She was expected to be able to accurately survey the whole floor in a glance and to attend to every situation, including emergencies.

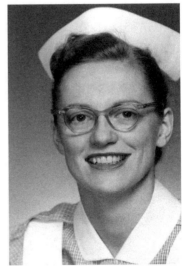

RUTH LUBIC AS A YOUNG NURSE

Introduction to Maternity Care

When Ruth first worked in maternity as a student, it was not "love at first sight." She remembers the maternity rotation as her worst nursing experience, probably because there was little preparation. "I knew little about childbirth, and the first morning on duty I was placed in a room with four women, all being induced with Pitocin," she says. "In those days, Demerol, scopolamine, and caudal anesthesia were mostly used for labor management." One result was that women would remember little, if anything, about their delivery experience.

One experience did leave a favorable impression. A medical student's wife delivered her child using so-called "natural childbirth" techniques. Having a husband present in the delivery room was very unusual in those days, but it was permitted in this one case. Ruth watched this patient go through labor without being induced by drugs or sedated with analgesia and anesthesia. The joy of this birthing experience was a powerful moment for Ruth, and little did she realize the extent to which it would impact her future.

In 1952, a high school friend arranged a New Year's Eve blind date for Ruth with a young New York attorney, Bill Lubic. Bill and Ruth lost their way in the Philadelphia suburbs, got stuck in 20 inches of snow, and arrived 2 hours late, but nothing could smother the sparks of delight that flew between them. Perhaps arriving at their destination at the stroke of midnight made the moment magical. However, she was still in nursing school in Philadelphia, and he was just starting the practice of law in New York. Bill had completed his service in the Navy as a hospital corpsman and had graduated from Columbia University and the University of Pennsylvania Law School.

It was a commuter courtship. Ruth laughingly admits that "for 2 1/2 years, he chased me until I caught him." With special dispensation, they married a month before graduation in her hometown, and she became the first openly married student nurse at the school.

Ruth maintained her high grades, notwithstanding the distraction of the commuter courtship and her leading role in the student cancan chorus line. At graduation in 1955, her stellar academic record and professional talents were recognized by the faculty. She was awarded both the Florence Nightingale medal for her nursing qualities and the prize for the highest academic performance. The prize included a check for $600, which represented a substantial part of the net worth of the young couple.

LIFE AS A NEW NURSE

After graduation, Ruth and Bill moved to a small apartment in New York. As a staff nurse at Memorial Hospital for Cancer and Allied Diseases, Ruth earned about $80 per week. Bill, who had decided to join a small, general practice law firm, earned half that amount. During those lean years, they set up their household.

Memorial Hospital at that time was divided into systems, such as thoracic, GI, breast, and head and neck. Ruth worked mostly in the oncology area on the medical floor, taking care of patients with lymphomas and other nonsurgical cancers. She quickly rose to the head nurse position. Her difficulties caring for the critically ill continued, but she slowly acclimated. At this time in history, nurses had their place, and it was much below the doctor's "station." Ruth tells a tale about an evening on the surgical floor when she was caring for a female patient with a new colostomy. Seeing stool on her abdomen, the patient panicked and was terrified. She pleaded to know what was happening to her. Ruth informed her about the colostomy and told her that she could easily learn to self-manage the discomfort. "The patient had not been told by anyone the nature and consequence of the surgery that she had," Ruth recalls. Later, when the surgeon met up with her, he "really let me have it," she says.

At that time, a nurse was not even permitted to tell a patient his or her temperature, blood pressure, or any other basic information. It was within the strict province of the doctor to relay that information. Not being permitted to intervene and teach patients about their own care, if not their condition, seemed unnatural and inhumane. It was not her way to have a patient be overcome, perhaps even exploited, by fear of the unknown. This was another lesson that was ingrained in Ruth's mind.

While on staff at Memorial Hospital, she took some evening courses at Hunter College for 3 years and then decided to continue her education full time. A well-conceived federal scholarship program allowed her to enter Teachers College at Columbia University, where she earned her bachelor's degree. She graduated in 1959, just before her first child was born. When son Douglas was 6 months old, she returned to Teachers College to continue work on a master's degree in medical/surgical nursing, which was the area of her experience.

MATERNITY CARE AND MIDWIFERY

Ruth would never have imagined it back in nursing school, but maternity care would soon become her destiny. By now, she had experienced two very positive births. One was the natural childbirth experience she observed as a student, and the second was the birth of her son, Douglas. Ruth's obstetrician was considered very progressive for his time. He had been a psychiatrist, but he became interested in postpartum depression and went on to do a residency in obstetrics.

As progressive as Cornell Medical Center was in 1959, fathers were not allowed in delivery rooms. In this case, however, Ruth's doctor let her know that if the right nurses were on shift and there were no administrators around, he would allow Bill to "gown up" and come into the delivery room. All these "stars" lined up, and Bill was at her side throughout a long, 30-hour labor and delivery. As a result of her birth experience, Ruth looked at the potential for maternity nursing through a different lens. She remembers that she and Bill were left with their newborn son for more than an hour in the delivery room. During this time, she began breast-feeding her son, and the family was allowed to bond together—although it was not called bonding in those days.

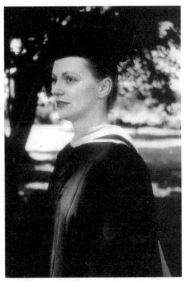

RUTH LUBIC RECIEVED HER MASTER'S DEGREE IN 1961

As an aside, in some painful moments for Ruth, she preferred not to elaborate or to relive the awful moments of an episode that could have been tragic in the lives of this young couple. Their beautiful child developed serious health issues with a long, treacherous aftermath. Suffice it to say Doug did well, and he is now married to his Princeton classmate. They have two children, and he practices law in New Jersey.

During her Preparation for Childbirth Classes at Cornell Medical Center, Ruth became aware of nurse-midwives who were graduates of the Maternity Center Association (MCA) program in midwifery. They served only as maternity nurses and were not permitted to manage intrapartum care. No hospital would allow midwives to practice in those years, except for the Frontier Nursing Service in rural Kentucky. This service, founded by Mary

Breckinridge, was initially staffed by British nurse-midwives. These nurses lived and worked in Appalachia, riding on horseback or in jeeps to deliver babies in isolated areas, almost always in the home.

Case in Point

NEVER STOP LEARNING

After receiving her master's degree and while working on completing her program in midwifery, Ruth provided prenatal care to a particular patient who taught her a valuable lesson. The patient shared her history and her unique labor pattern. She said she would dilate to 2 fingers (4 cm), then she would give one push and the baby would arrive. Being well-schooled in midwifery by this time, Ruth patiently explained that labor just did not work this way—there were several stages to the process.

By coincidence, Ruth was in the delivery ward when the patient was admitted with regular contractions. The patient was 4 cm dilated when examined, so Ruth pointed out to her that the baby had not yet arrived, and thus her theory was not correct. With that, the patient groaned and out came the newborn infant.

The valuable lesson learned was the importance of listening to and respecting the words of the patient. "It dispelled any professional arrogance I might have had at the time," Ruth says.

Douglas was only 2 when Ruth decided to earn her certificate in midwifery. She went back to school and joined an MCA class of five midwifery students. Their practical, hands-on midwifery experience was at Kings

County Hospital in Brooklyn. The clinical arm of that institution, known for a time as the Lobenstine Clinic, conducted a highly regarded, well-reported home delivery service in New York City from 1931 to 1959. Among its graduates and staff were a number of pioneer nurse-midwives who forged the early path for others to follow, including Vera Keane, Betty Hosford, Eunice K.M. (Kitty) Ernst, and Ernestine Weidenbach. At that time, there were eight schools in the country offering midwifery programs; today, approximately 50 schools offer such programs. In 1961, the training took 1 year and there was no formal certifying exam—all graduates were called certified nurse-midwives. Today, graduates of these programs earn certification by taking a national certification exam sponsored by the American College of Nurse-Midwives.

JOURNEY AS THE EXECUTIVE ADMINISTRATOR

Ironically, for all her contributions over the years to the midwifery profession, Ruth's postgraduate clinical practice was rather limited. She was, however, extensively involved in teaching parent education classes. When she completed her midwifery program in 1962, positions were difficult to find and midwives in most hospitals were not permitted to practice beyond the scope of maternity care nurses. Thus, Ruth ventured into administration, accepting a part-time position as the first executive director of the American College of Nurse-Midwives, while still employed by MCA as a parent educator and counselor.

Ruth enjoyed and learned much from these positions, and they influenced her decision to earn a doctorate degree. She chose to study applied anthropology because of her experiences with low-income women, especially Latino women in Brooklyn and on the lower East Side. She believed that health professionals should be more in tune with cultural differences between clients and providers. With these insights, she decided to develop a curriculum that would help health professionals better understand cultural differences. She was on a quest for more knowledge.

Ruth began doctoral studies at Columbia University in 1967 and managed to complete her coursework in 1970, while she and Bill were raising a son, renovating and moving into a brownstone on the west side of Manhattan, and dealing with student upheaval and disruptive events on the Columbia campus during the Vietnam War. Maintaining her focus and intensity, she continued to impress those around her and was finally offered the position of general director at MCA. At that time, she was president-elect of the American College of Nurse-Midwives. She resigned that position, knowing she could not simultaneously do both jobs well.

MCA, a venerable not-for-profit organization (now known as Childbirth Connections, with a somewhat altered focus), was initially organized and always operated by women since 1917. The first general director was Frances Perkins, who became the first woman cabinet member when President Franklin Roosevelt named her secretary of labor. The clear focus of MCA was on mothers, babies, nursing, and midwifery. Ruth was convinced that if she did not take the position of general director, for which several physicians had already been interviewed, MCA might lose or change its direction. By then she had already become aware of the growing political tensions between physicians and midwives, which made her realize the importance of her choice.

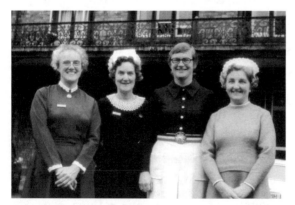

MIDWIVES FROM THE UNITED KINGDOM AT AN INTERNATIONAL CONFEDERATION OF MIDWIVES MEETING IN CHILE, CIRCA 1969. RUTH IS SECOND FROM RIGHT.

ESTABLISHING BIRTH CENTERS IN THE UNITED STATES

Until 1975, the only facility in the United States that resembled the concept of a "birth center service" was the Catholic Maternity Institute (CMI), a home birth service in Santa Fe, New Mexico. One of the buildings at CMI, La Casita, had two dedicated obstetric beds to serve Native American and Latino women who lived too far away or in conditions inadequate for home births. This service allowed the women a safe harbor in which to deliver their newborns.

Ruth's definition of a birthing center, however, went beyond that. "A birth center is a facility in which women are seen in a homelike setting as early and as often as possible in their pregnancy, in order to provide them with continuing, nurturing midwifery care and enough education so they can take control of aspects of their own health," Ruth says. In her opinion, a birth center is a whole program, not simply a different place to have one's baby. A homelike birth room furnished with curtains, pretty bedspread, and easy chair, as advertised by many hospital administrators, hardly fulfills the necessary criteria. Ruth was founder and executive director of three very separate and distinct birth centers, each with unique populations, which will be described later.

Sometimes physicians would refer patients to a center for delivery simply because they thought the patient would prefer it to a hospital birth. Those requests would be routinely denied, because "the care given within a birthing center is an entirely different type of care than the conventional hospital experience, and women need to have preparatory prenatal care and education for a safe and satisfying birth. It can be a difficult concept for some to grasp," Ruth explains.

In the early 1970s and later, there was a scarcity of facilities available to midwives for their practice and hands-on experience. Kitty Ernst, a pioneering nurse-midwifery graduate of the Frontier Nursing Service, learned of the Booth Maternity Hospital in Philadelphia. Originally a Salvation Army facility, it had been set up to privately serve unwed mothers. Because the number of unwed mothers seeking the isolation of a maternity hospital was decreasing, it was being closed down. Together, Ruth and Kitty established a partnership with a progressive obstetrician named John Franklin, and the team set up shop. The obstetrician moved his entire practice to the Booth Maternity Center—formerly the Booth Maternity Hosptial. With a staff of nurse midwives, it operated successfully for a number of years.

Because midwives had been very limited in finding facilities in which to practice clinically, MCA, with Ruth and Kitty in charge, created a refresher-course program in nurse-midwifery at Booth Memorial. The Commonwealth Fund awarded a grant to fund MCA and refresher programs at the University of Mississippi and the Downstate Program in Brooklyn. These refresher courses, along with the one at Booth, allowed many British and American nurses who had never had a chance to apply their knowledge and skills in the United States to be brought back into the profession.

Ruth's reputation was growing. In 1973, she received the high recognition of being the only woman and the only nurse to be part of the first official American medical delegation to the People's Republic of China (PRC) during President Nixon's administration. Team members, who were among the most prominent healthcare providers in the United States, were official guests of the PRC as they visited a number of medical and health facilities in various parts of the country. With a few exceptions, healthcare in China was found to be rudimentary, with little Western sophistication, but it was nevertheless universally available. Ruth questioned why basic healthcare could not be made available to all U.S. citizens as well. As an outgrowth of the China venture, Ruth developed many lasting personal and professional relationships.

After returning home from China, her MCA team and a dedicated, courageous board of directors composed of visionary women began work on her concept of establishing a free-standing birth center on East 92nd Street, on the first two floors of MCA's beautiful brownstone home in Manhattan. Called the Childbearing Center (CbC), this was to be the first state-licensed and accredited free-standing birth center staffed by nurse midwives in the United States. Problems were indeed many. Kitty played an important role in CbC's concept and design. There were frustrations with the impediments to its legal establishment by the "nay-sayers" in the district office of the American College of Obstetricians and Gynecologists and the New York City Department of Health. Not to be denied, Ruth had the knowledge, energy, relationships, and reputation to successfully approach the state authorities in Albany on this issue.

The families that chose to come to the birth center were mostly middle class and highly educated, including women in various professions. They resented the increasing cesarean section rates, did not approve of the depersonalized and highly medicated maternity care given in hospitals, and had genuine concern about the periodic outbreaks of staphylococcus infections that occurred in hospitals.

In spite of the benefits that families received from MCA's CbC, the political battles were raging. Some members of Ruth's medical advisory board, consisting of the chairs of most of the obstetrics and gynecology departments in the city, resigned as a group. Among other things, women were told that they and their babies would die if they let midwives deliver care, and that "bad" babies were being buried in the backyard of the center. "There was nothing gentlemanly about it," Ruth says. She describes the untruths about the CbC and the efforts to have the center's license taken away as tactics of segments of the organized medical community. Rumors were spread about increases in malpractice insurance and the danger of lawsuits to instill fear in the midwives who were planning to work at the CbC.

She believes that when families are invited to become part of the birthing process, there is a very special and precious bonding that occurs not only between parents and newborn, but also with grandparents, in-laws, and other family members.

These repression tactics had such a profound impact that they became the basis of her doctoral dissertation at Columbia, titled "Barriers and Conflict in Maternity Care Innovation." (Tongue-in-cheek, Ruth says the subtitle should have been, "What the Boys Did to Us.") It is interesting to note that this dissertation is now required reading in the Community-Based Nurse-Midwifery Education Program (CNEP).

Despite the political battles, the Manhattan CbC was successful. Ruth immediately began to consider how that model could be transported to other communities, particularly those less well-to-do than Manhattan's Upper East Side Carnegie Hill area. She believes that when families are invited to become part of the birthing process, there is a very special and precious bonding that occurs not only between parents and newborn, but also with grandparents, in-laws, and other family members. Later on, this concept was verified for Ruth and put into practice in the South Bronx Birth Center. There, she had the exhilarating experience of hearing from her staff the details of a newborn being passed from hand to hand in a large Muslim family circle, with murmurs of joy and love as the words of Allah were whispered in the ear of the newborn.

Moving on to the South Bronx

By the mid-1980s, during Ruth's tenure as general director, MCA had a staff of more than 50. She and other nurse-midwife leaders had spearheaded significant advancements in the field, including development of innovative classes designed to prepare children for the birth of a sibling and to attend the birth when parents so desired (1979); establishment of the National Association of Childbearing Centers, a professional association for out-of-hospital birth centers (1983); and establishment of the Commission for the Accreditation of Freestanding Birth Centers (1985), to ensure high standards of operation for out-of-hospital birth centers across the United States (Childbirth Connection, 2006). Also, with the help of her husband, Bill, the American College of Nurse-Midwives Foundation was incorporated and legally established. The foundation continues to flourish to this day.

> *"We are not here for the greater glory of midwifery ... we are here to serve people who have been underserved, and that is why we are such strong advocates."*

Ruth's vision of extending the principles and benefits of the CbC beyond Manhattan gained ground. Over a period of 8 years, she obtained a substantial financial commitment from MCA's courageous board, confirmed a relationship with the Morris Heights Health Center, and secured additional foundation funding. She then assembled a develop-

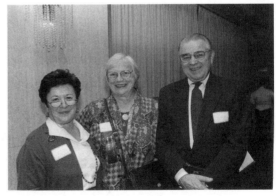

Ruth Lubic (center) and her husband, Bill, at the 1996 Archon Award ceremony, sponsored by the Honor Society of Nursing, Sigma Theta Tau International. At left is Joyce E. Roberts, then-president of the American College of Nurse-Midwives.

ment team, selected and renovated the site (including repairing bullet holes in the ceilings), and obtained licensing. In 1988, staffing was put in place, and the Childbearing Center of Morris Heights opened its doors. This neighborhood-based birth center was set up to serve low-income families in the South Bronx, a community then characterized by fear, crime, and extreme poverty. Ruth believed that if you gave women and families the chance to take charge of their own birthing experience, they would take that feeling of empowerment back to the community. In a remarkable videotape about the South Bronx CbC, titled *Hope Reborn, Empowering Families in the South Bronx,* Ruth tells the Morris Heights Community Advisory Committee: "It (the childbearing experience) strengthens families because every time a baby comes into this world, hope comes back again, doesn't it? And, when the power is shared with the people, it grows exponentially" (Maternity Center Association, 1994).

THE DC DEVELOPING FAMILIES CENTER

Despite all the publicly funded and free programs offered to mothers in the District of Columbia (DC), the area nevertheless had the highest infant and maternal mortality rates in the United States. Upon arriving in DC in 1994, Ruth was well aware of statistics that showed that in Ward 5, 25 infants died for every 1,000 live births, compared with the national rate of 7 deaths per 1,000 births. After receiving the MacArthur Fellowship in 1993—with a no-questions-asked, annual stipend of $75,000 for 5 years—and her severance pay from MCA, she set out to use the funds in an attempt to replicate the two successful birth centers in one of the most underserved areas in the nation. Twenty years earlier, Ruth had seen the sickly babies in tenant farmers' homes in rural Mississippi and could never get the vision out of her mind.

Resigning her position at MCA, Ruth decided to devote all her time to this overwhelming project. Ruth and Bill have since commuted to DC almost weekly using the New York City to Washington shuttle.

Work on the Developing Families Center began in 1994. Initial efforts centered on finding community-based partners that were established in Wards 5 and 6, which had been designated by the DC Department of Health as being underserved and having families in need. One such organization is the Healthy Babies Project (HBP), which serves as an outreach case management and educational nonprofit partner. At the time, HBP had been serving the community for 6 years, but it did not offer clinical healthcare. Dolores Farr, a nurse who then was head of the project, eagerly pointed out an empty supermarket as a potential home for both the birth center and HBP. When she looked at the site, Ruth realized the building could house not only healthcare (the Family Health and Birth Center) and social supports (the HBP), but also an early childhood development program. Nation's Capital Child & Family Development became the third partner for the center.

The owner of the property in question was Hechinger Enterprises, operated by John W. Hechinger Sr., a businessman with a reputation for community involvement and charitable acts. Ruth tried to speak to him directly, but his real estate manager would not permit her to do so. It was during this period that Ruth served as *pro bono* expert consultant to Philip R. Lee, MD, assistant secretary for health in the Department of Health and Human Services (DHHS). A chance meeting with Donna Shalala, secretary for health in the Clinton cabinet,

The Hechingers donated 1.2 acres of land and the 15,600-square-foot building, which had been vacant for almost 20 years, to house Ruth's collaborative project.

resulted in Secretary Shalala writing a personal note to Hechinger suggesting that Ruth had something important to say. He then agreed to meet with her. After numerous attempts over a span of 3 years, Ruth's persistence and drive had finally resulted in a meeting with Hechinger, who was quickly won over.

"He told me that I was like a pit bull who wore him down with the rightness of my cause" (Loose, 1998, p. 1), Ruth recalls. The Hechingers donated 1.2 acres of land and the 15,600-square-foot building, which had been vacant for almost 20 years, to house Ruth's collaborative project. When it was discovered that the roof could not be repaired, Hechinger volunteered to pay for a new one. Ruth had her property, and it had cost nothing but time and determination.

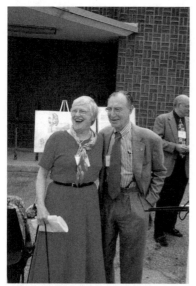

RUTH LUBIC AND JOHN W. HECHINGER, SR. AT THE GROUNDBREAKING CEREMONY FOR THE DEVELOPING FAMILIES CENTER IN WASHINGTON, DC. HECHINGER ENTERPRISES DONATED THE BUILDING AND LAND FOR THE CENTER.

One battle had been won, but there were a few more ahead. It was necessary to transform the abandoned building into a sunlit, communal space for women's reproductive healthcare, birthing, child care, check-ups for women and children, mentoring for teen fathers, welfare-to-work services, parenting classes for teen mothers, and an early childhood development program for children from 3 weeks to 3 years. The budget for the renovation project was $1.2 million, but unfortunately, all building estimates came in well over that. Ultimately, funds were raised from foundations, corporations, and individuals to match a $785,000 grant promised by the DC

Department of Community Development, and work began. A not-for-profit "umbrella" corporation was organized to take title. Shortly after Ruth's and Bill's 73rd birthdays in the year 2000, the Developing Families Center (DFC) opened its doors.

To pretend that health is somehow separate from people's social conditions is madness

It took more than 6 years of preparation, negotiation, and construction nightmares before the grand opening took place. Ruth's dream of "setting healthcare in its social context" had become reality through a $2.15 million facility located in northeast Washington, DC. The collaboration among three nonprofit entities—DC Birth Center, Healthy Babies Project, and Nation's Capital Child and Family Development—was unique, and it was the first center of its kind in the nation.

Ruth estimates that at full occupancy, the Family Health and Birth Center staff will attend about 250 births annually. No patient is turned away, regardless of health status or insurance. "To pretend that health is somehow separate from people's social conditions is madness," Ruth says. She reached out to neighborhood women to consult about everything from the use of lavender-colored paint for the building façade to services to be rendered and the nature of day-care needs.

The center is a replicable model that has attracted much interest in the United States and elsewhere, including the Middle East and Africa. Ruth reports that over the years, many hundreds of visitors—including foundation board members, public health figures, and federal and state officials—have viewed the gleaming interior of the center, its bustling programs, and the delightful children (from babes in arms to toddlers).

INTERNATIONAL MATERNITY CARE

Ruth retired as executive director of MCA in 1995, after 25 years at the helm. The DFC did not open until 2000, but all the while Ruth had the opportunity to travel around the globe, observing and consulting on maternity care practice standards. When asked where the best system of maternity care can be found, she replies, "France is recognized to be the best system in the world—not because of midwifery, in my estimation, but because of their approach to care." The French call their system *Protection Maternelle et Infantile,* meaning protection of mothers and babies—not aid *to* or assistance *for.* Mother and baby are protected by the system and allowed access to all levels of care. The United States does not have that approach to maternity care, nor does Ruth see it changing anytime soon. The French hold the entire maternity, childbearing, and childrearing experiences as critically important. Once a child is born, the French provide early childhood development education and several types of day care that are convenient for mothers (Richardson, 1994).

The French model influenced the vision of the project in Washington, DC. "If I had not gone to France on a French-American Foundation study tour early in 1994, I never would have thought to include the whole child-care concept with the reproductive health and maternity care services," Ruth says. Midwives are typically involved through the 6-week checkup and with the woman's inter-conceptional care, but usually do not deal with child-care issues beyond assuring successful breast-feeding. Ruth changed her conceptual thinking as to what should be included in the "one-stop shop," which now includes outreach and day-care sectors. She hopes the structure of this demonstration will have a significant impact on all such services in the United States.

Although France has a mixed private and public healthcare system, it allows for choices. Every pregnant woman can get maternity care free of charge and knows where she can get child care. Home care for children and infants is available through a *puericultrice*, which is similar to a pediatric nurse practitioner. The government also provides for prenatal care in the home of the mother, when necessary. The French seem to understand that providing preventive care will ultimately reduce healthcare costs. Most professionals in the United States acknowledge this fact, but the concept does not drive current practices, particularly in Congress.

> *The number and type of practitioners are based on the needs of women, rather than on the needs of professions.*

Ruth also has memories of numerous trips to Germany, Japan, Sweden, and Russia. In Stockholm, Sweden, a birth center based on the CbC concept was established. Nurse-midwives provide 85% of maternity care, which demonstrates that only 15% of Swedish women require obstetrical management by a physician. This is the case throughout most of Europe. The number and type of practitioners are based on the needs of women, rather than on the needs of professions.

In the 1990s, a typical Russian maternity hospital, or *rodom,* was grim by comparison. "It is like going into a prison," Ruth says. A room might have two labor beds and a delivery table. One woman might be in labor while another is delivering an infant. If the woman who is delivering gets into medical difficulty, the laboring patient witnesses the entire crisis. "It is unbelievably inhumane," Ruth says. Also, a woman in either the labor or postpartum ward cannot see her children during this time, as labor and delivery are off-limits to her family.

Ruth had the good fortune to meet a Russian midwife who wanted to make the maternal experience more positive and caring for the mother. The midwife set up a birth room in *rodom* and made the necessary changes to enhance the experience. This midwife understood at least that it was possible to make a difference for some delivering mothers.

Ruth believes that U.S. aid to undeveloped and developing countries is not always focused on these basic, primary needs. Instead, the United States frequently sends trained teams into low-tech settings to introduce expensive, high-technology equipment and techniques. "We go at it from the point of view that the technology for complicated cases is of greater importance than developing a balanced program," Ruth says. She believes that carrying technology everywhere, rather than determining what people need from a cultural and practical perspective, is a great disservice to the healthcare needs of those people. Highly developed technology simply is unaffordable or unsustainable in many countries.

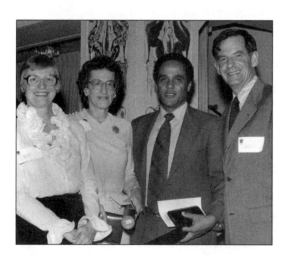

In 1981, Ruth Watson Lubic, left, and Phyllis Farley received the Rockefeller Public Service Award for Innovation in the Health Care Delivery System for their roles in establishing the Manhattan Childbearing Center. Ruth was general director and Phyllis was chairman of the board of Maternity Center Association (MCA). Also pictured are award-recipient Richard Smith, third from left, and presenter William G. Bowen, president of Princeton University.

AWARDS AND HONORS

Ruth is a member of the Institute of Medicine. Named in 2001 as a Living Legend by the American Academy of Nursing, she holds fellowships in the American Academy of Nursing, the American College of Nurse-Midwives, the New York Academy of Medicine, the Association for the Advancement of Science, and the Society of Applied Anthropology. Ruth has been awarded honorary doctorates by five universities and commendations from two others, and has received many awards from national, local, professional, and community groups. She was particularly gratified to receive the Rockefeller Public Service Award, presented by Princeton University. She was surprised to be named an honorary member of Alpha Omega Alpha, often referred to as the Phi Beta Kappa of the medical profession.

The MacArthur grant allowed the white-haired grandmother from New York City to pack her travel bags and move her professional work to DC.

The prestigious (and useful) MacArthur Fellowship, recognized internationally, is given to individuals from a large variety of professions and backgrounds. Ruth, the first nurse to receive a MacArthur award, still does not know who submitted her name, as nominations are made anonymously by a team of "finders." She remembers coming home after dinner to a voicemail message asking her to call the MacArthur Foundation. "My immediate reaction was that they must be seeking my opinion about somebody who was being considered," she says. No certificate or medal accompanies this honor, just a 5-year, unrestricted stipend. This award has opened many doors and impressed many influential people. Her family decided that she should use it all to make her dream of the Developing Families Center in Washington come true and to attack the worst maternal and infant mortality outcomes in the United States. The MacArthur grant allowed the white-haired grandmother from New York City to pack her travel bags and move her professional work to DC.

The Lubics continue to reside in New York, and Bill still practices law at his Manhattan law firm. Years ago, he was the first person designated as an "Honorary Nurse-Midwife," and he also received the Public Advocate

Award from the National Association of Childbearing Centers (now the American Association of Birth Centers) in honor of his pro bono legal work over the years to the cause of midwifery. Throughout Ruth's career, Bill has always been her supporter, booster, and helper. He joins with her in her objective to make the world a little bit better than it was before. During their more than 50 years of married life, Ruth and Bill have been significantly involved in various forms of public service.

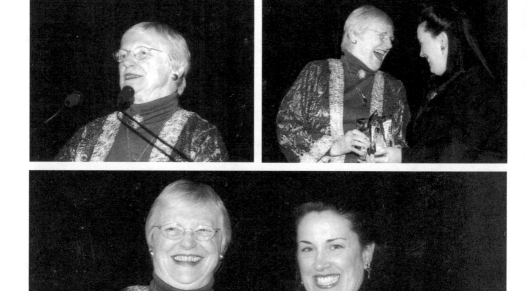

RUTH LUBIC, LEFT, RECEIVED THE 2003 LILLIAN WALD AWARD, PRESENTED BY NINA HENDERSON, DIRECTOR AND CHAIRMAN OF THE DEVELOPMENT COMMITTEE OF THE VISITING NURSE SERVICE OF NEW YORK'S BOARD OF DIRECTORS.

LEADERSHIP LESSONS

In addition to perseverance, one key to Ruth's success in leadership has been her bountiful sense of humor. Especially when tensions are greatest, Ruth says, "I am not above pouring on the charm and getting a laugh to get attention, so that our agenda is heard." When she received the Lienhard award from the Institute of Medicine, she spoke about midwifery's focus on the social, emotional, spiritual, and political aspects of health. She colorfully noted that according to the Old Testament, it was midwives who saved the baby Moses from Pharaoh's persecution.

On another occasion, while on a panel discussion at the Institute of Medicine, she listened to a physician use the football team concept to describe social work, nursing, and medicine. He used the analogy of the physician as quarterback and also captain of the team and said social work and nursing were often blocking each other out. When he finished his descriptive story, Ruth responded from the audience, "You may be the captain and the quarterback, but I am the tight end—you are not going to get the ball over the line unless I am there." The audience broke down in laughter, but she had clearly made her point about the essential role of the team approach.

Leadership Lesson Learned

"It is important to realize that you will require a lot of help from a lot of people when advancing a forward-looking agenda," she says. "You can't afford to make enemies, and confrontation doesn't help much."

Other key leadership attributes are Ruth's ability to visualize the larger picture and maintain her composure under the most trying of circumstances. In addition, she is creative and irrepressibly optimistic. "It is important to realize that you will require a lot of help from a lot of people when advancing a forward-looking agenda," she says. "You can't afford to make enemies, and confrontation doesn't help much."

For example, when the first birth center in New York was established, Ruth could not get Medicaid reimbursement for the center's patients. Only about 5 to 10% of the people who came to the birth center in New York were eligible for Medicaid. Mostly they were students who were temporarily poor as well as people from impoverished backgrounds. Ruth pushed this issue on the principle that Medicaid-eligible women should be able to access the same prenatal services as affluent women, if they so desired. That barrier was finally broken down when she caught the ear of Ed Koch, who was then a congressman but later was elected mayor of New York City. His staff argued that poor people were being denied something to which rich women had access. So, in a sense, not allowing Medicaid reimbursement for the birth center was discriminatory.

Ruth appreciates that professional practices and practical economics can cause conflict and stress among professions. Physicians in particular have spent an enormous amount of time, energy, and money to acquire their knowledge and skills and achieve their important status in society. They may feel threatened when others suggest that women want something different from what was done in the past. Understanding and tact must be used when dealing with these issues, Ruth says.

Keeping her goal clearly focused on the community, not on the profession, has made her message more powerful and more credible.

Over the years, midwives have become accustomed to resistance toward their profession from some physicians and hospital administrators. Unfortunately, a share of this resistance can be attributed to strife within the profession. Currently, "turf" battles remain among maternity care registered nurses and midwives working in the hospital setting. Ruth's long-term view is that the practice of a maternity nurse, while certainly adequate to the task, would be immensely enriched and more satisfying with midwifery training. "We midwives don't need to be fighting with maternity nurses; we need to be supporting them, because we are all there for one thing—to help families," she says.

Throughout her career, Ruth's message has always been: "We are not here for the greater glory of midwifery; we are here to serve all the people, including the underserved, and that is why we are such strong advocates and why they are our advocates." Keeping her goal clearly focused on the community, not on the profession, has made her message more powerful and more credible.

LATER YEARS

The Developing Families Center in Washington, DC, is the pinnacle of this nurse-midwife's career. The center sums up who Ruth Lubic is and what she stands for as an individual. From her early Great Depression days, when she worked in her father's pharmacy and gave free supplies to needy families in her Pennsylvania community, to her later work ensuring that women's healthcare services are provided for the underserved, Ruth has dedicated her career to providing quality care for all families, including the underprivileged, wherever they may be.

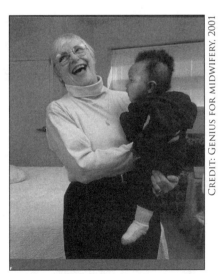

CREDIT: GENIUS FOR MIDWIFERY, 2001

RUTH LUBIC USED THE FUNDS SHE RECEIVED FROM THE MACARTHUR FELLOWSHIP TO OPEN THE DEVELOPING FAMILIES CENTER IN WASHINGTON, DC.

When asked about retirement, she shakes her head as if she would love to. However, the reality is that much work remains to be done. Retirement, as defined by most, is nowhere in Ruth's immediate future. She still holds a vision for what women's healthcare should be, and it does not appear that she will stop working anytime soon.

Ruth is more than just words—she is a woman of remarkable courage and action. Perhaps her most powerful leadership lesson is to set a vision first and then act on it as life's passion. She has set down a number of self-guiding principles that ensure a successful professional career. Her favorite is, "Nursing prepares you for excellence … be proud you are a nurse."

REFERENCES

Childbirth Connection. (2006, March 10). *History.* Retrieved October 27, 2006, from http://www.childbirthconnection.org/ article.asp?ck=10076&ClickedLink=0&area=3

Genius for midwifery. (2001). *Science & Health, The magazine of SUNY Downstate Medical Center, 1.*

Institute of Medicine. (2001, October 15). *Presentation of the Gustav O. Lienhard award.* Retrieved October 24, 2006, from http://www.iom.edu/ Object.File/Master/5/054/2001leinhardpresentation.pdf

Loose, C. (1998, September 30). A battle won, a center born: Nurse-midwife to open birthing facility for D.C's poor, *The Washington Post*, p. 1.

Lubic, Ruth W. (n.d.). *Brainy quote*. Retrieved October 25, 2006, from
http://www.brainyquote.com/quotes/authors/r/ruth_w_lubic.html

Maternity Center Association. (Producer). (1994). *Hope reborn, empowering families in the South Bronx*. [Videotape]. (Available from Maternity Center Association, Publication Department, 281 Park Ave., 5th Floor, New York, NY 10010.)

Richardson, G. (1994). *A welcome for every child: How France protects maternal and child health*. Arlington, VA: National Center for Education & Child Health.

American Association of Birth Centers

America's Birth Center Resource

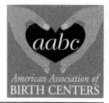

3123 Gottschall Road ~ Perkiomenville, PA 18074 ~ Tel: 215-234-8068 ~ Fax: 215-234-8829 ~ aabc@birthcenters.org ~ www.birthcenters.org

Selected Bibliography on Birth Centers

Albers, L.l. & Katz, V. L. (1991). Birth setting for low-risk pregnancies: An analysis of the current literature. Journal of Nurse-Midwifery, 36(4), 215-220.

American Public Health Association (1983). 8209 (PP): Guidelines for licensing and regulating birth centers. American Journal of Public Health, 73(3), 331-334.

Ballard, R.A. (1979). Changing the environment for birth, an alternative birth center in the hospital. In Lindheim, R. (Ed.), Environments for humanized health care (pp. 83-89). Berkeley, CA: University of California.

Ballard, RA, Ferris, C, & Clyman, RI (1985). The hospital alternative birth center: is it safe? Experience in 1000 cases from 1976 to 1980. Journal of Perinatology, 5(61-64).

Bennetts, A. (1982). The first national collaborative study of birth centers. Cooperative Birth Center Network News, (February/May), 12-13.

Bennetts, A.B. & Lubic, R.W. (1982). The free-standing birth centre. The Lancet, February 13, 378-380.

Campbell, R. & MacFarlane, A. (1986). Place of delivery: a review. British Journal of Obstetrics and Gynecology, 93, 675-683.

Campbell, R. & MacFarlane, A. (1987). Where to be born. Oxford: National Perinatal Epidemiology Unit Publication.

Chamberlain, M., Nair, R., Nimrod, C., Moyer, A., & England, J. (1998). Evaluation of a midwifery birthing center in the Canadian north. Circumpolar Health, 57(1), 116-120.

Cunningham, J.D. (1993). Experiences of Australian mothers who gave birth either at home, at a birth centre, or in hospital labour wards. Social Science & Medicine, 36(4), 475-483.

Declercq, E. R. (1984). Out-of-Hospital Births, U.S., 1978: Birth Weight and Apgar Scores as Measures of Outcome. Public Health Reports, 99(1), 63-73.

DeJong, R. N., Shy, K., & Carr, K.C. (1981). An Out-of-Hospital Birth Center Using University Referral. Obstetrics & Gynecology, 58(6), 703-707.

DeVries, R.G. (1983). Image and reality: an evaluation of hospital alternative birth centers. Journal of Nurse-Midwifery, 28(3), 3-9.

Dickinson, C.P., Jackson, D.J. & Swartz, W.H. (1994). Mainstreaming the alternative: maintaining a family centered focus at a freestanding birth center for low-income women. Journal of Nurse-Midwifery, 39, 112-118.

Eakins, P.S. (1989). Free-standing birth centers in California; program and medical outcome. Journal of Reproductive Medicine, 34(12), 960-970.

Faison, J.B., Pisani, B.J., Douglas, R.G., Cranch, G.S., & Lubic, R.W. (1979). The child bearing center: an alternative birth setting. Obstetrics and Gynecology, 54(4), 527-532.

Feldman, E. & Hurst, M. (1987). Outcomes and procedures in low risk birth: a comparison of hospital and birth center settings. Birth, 14(1), 18-24.

Ferris, C. (1976). The alternative birth center at Mount Zion hospital. Birth and Family Journal, 3(1), 127-128.

Fleming, A.S., Ruble, D.N. & Anderson, V. (1988). Place of childbirth influences feelings of satisfatction and control in first-time mothers. Journal of Psychosomatic Obstetrics and Gynecology, 8, 1-17.

Fullerton, J. D. T. (1982). The choice of in-hospital or alternative birth environment as related to the concept of control Journal of Nurse-Midwifery, 27(2), 17-22.

Fullerton, J.T., Jackson, D., Snell, B.J., Besser, M., Dickinson, C., Garite, T. (1997). Transfer rates from freestanding birth centers; a comparison with the national birth center study. Journal of Nurse-Midwifery, 42(1), 9-16.

Fullerton, J.T. & Severino, R. (1992). In-hospital care for low-risk childbirth; a comparison with results from the national childbirth center study. Journal of Nurse-Midwifery, 37(5), 331-340.

Garite, T.J., Snell, B.J., Walker, D.L., & Darrow, V.C. (1995). Development and experience of a university-based, freestanding birthing center. Obstetrics and Gynecology, 86(3), 411-416.

Gilson, G.J., O'Brien, M.E., Vera R. W., Mays, M.E., Smith, D. R., & Ross, C.Y. (1988). Prolonged pregnancy and the biophysical profile; a birthing center perspective. Journal of Nurse-Midwifery, 33(4), 171-177.

Gilson, G.J., O'Brien, M.E., Vera, R.W., Block, A., & Grubb, P.N. (1988). Expectant management of premature rupture of membranes at term in a birthing center setting. Journal of Nurse-Midwifery, 33(3), 134-139.

Gottvall K, Winbladh B, Cnattingius S, Waldenstrom U.. Birth centre care over a 10-year period: infant morbidity during the first month after birth. Acta Paediatr. 2005 Sep;94(9):1253-60

Hodnett ED, Downe S, Edwards N, Walsh D. Cochrane Database Syst Rev. 2005 Jan 25:(1):CD000012.

Hodnett, E.D. (28 September 1998). Home-like versus conventional institutional settings for birth (Research Rep. No. 1, 2000). : The Cochrane Library.

 formerly the National Association of Childbearing Centers (NACC)

Holz, K., Cooney, C., & Marchese, T. (1989). Outcomes of mature primiparas in an out-of-hospital birth center. Journal of Nurse-Midwifery, 34(4), 185-189.

Institute of Medicine and National Research Council (1982). Research issues in the assessment of birth settings. Washington, D.C.: National Academy Press.

Jackson, D. et al, Outcomes, safety and resource utilization in a collaborative care birth center program compared with traditional physician-based perinatal care. American Journal of Public Health, Vol 93 No 6, 999-1006, June 2003

Jackson, D.J., Lang, J.M., Dickinson, C.P., & Fullerton, J.T. (1994). Use of the nurse-midwifery clinical data set for classification of subjects in birth center research. Journal of Nurse-Midwifery, 39(4), 197-213.

Laube, D.W. (1983). Experience with an alternative birth center in a university hospital. Journal of Reproductive Medicine, 28, 391-396.

Lieberman, E. and Ryan, K. J. (1989). Birth-Day Choices. The New England Journal of Medicine, 321, 1824-1825.

Lindheim, R. (1981). Birthing centers and hospices: reclaiming birth and death. Annual Review of Public Health, 2(1), 1-29.

Lubic, R (1982). Evaluation of an out-of-hospital maternity center for low-risk patients. In Akien, L (Ed.), Health policy and nursing practice (1st. ed.) New York, New York: McGraw- Hill.

Lubic, R.W. (1999). Giving birth is powerful. Bulletin of Zero to Three: National Center for Infants. Toddlers and Families, 19(4), 20-24.

Lubic, R.W. & Ernst, E.K.M. (1978). The childbearing center: an alternative to conventional care. Nursing Outlook, December, 754-760.

Maternity Center Association (1989). The economic rationale for the freestanding birth center: a case study. New York, New York: Maternity Center Association.

McClain, C. S. (1983). Perceived Risk and Choice of Childbirth Service. Soc. Sci. Medicine, 17(23), 1857-1865.

Murdaugh, S.A. (1976). Experiences of a new migrant health care clinic. Women and Health, 1, 25-29.

Olsen, O. (1997). Meta-Analysis of the Safety of Home Birth. Birth, 24(1), 4-13.

Olsen, O. & Jewell, M.D. (20 April 1998). Home versus hospital birth (Research Rep. No. 1,2000): The Cochrane Library.

Paneth, M., Kiely, J.L., Wallenstein, S., & Susser, M. (1987). The choice of place of delivery. American Journal of Diseases of Children, 141, 60-64.

Proctor, S. (1998). What determines quality in maternity care? Comparing the perceptions of childbearing women and midwives. Birth, 25(2), 85-93.

Public Health Service (1999). In (Ed.), Progress Review: Maternal and Infant Health (Healthy People): Department of Health & Human Services.

Rice, A. & Carty, E. (1977). Alternative Birth Centers. The Canadian Nurse, November, 31-34.

Richards, M.P.M. (1978). A place of safety? An examination of the risks of hospital delivery. In Kitzinger, S. & Davis, J.A. (Eds.), The Place of Birth (1st. ed.) (pp. 66-84). Oxford, England: Oxford University Press.

Rooks, J. (1999). Journal Review: The Stockholm Birth Centre Trial. Journal of Nurse-Midwifery, 44(2), 159-161.

Rooks, J.P., Weatherby, N.L., & Ernst, E.K.M. (1992). The national birth center study: part I-methodology and prenatal care and referrals. Journal of Nurse-Midwifery, 37(4), 222-253.

Rooks, J.P., Weatherby, N.L., & Ernst, E.K.M. (1992). The national birth center study: part II-intrapartum and immediate postpartum and neonatal care. Journal of Nurse-Midwifery, 37(5), 301-330.

Rooks,J.P., Weatherby, N.L., & Ernst, E.K.M. (1992). The national birth center study: part III-intrapartum and immediate postpartum and neonatal complications and transfers, postpartum and neonatal care, outcomes, and client satisfaction. Journal of Nurse-Midwifery, 37(6), 361-397.

Rooks, J.P., Weatherby, N.L., Ernst, E.K.M., Stapleton, S., Rosen, D., & Rosenfeld, A. (1989). Outcomes of care in birth centers; the national birth center study. The New England Journal of Medicine, 321(26), 1804-1811.

Scupholme, A., McLeod, A.G.W., & Robertson, E.G. (1986). A birth center affiliated with the tertiary care center: comparison of outcome. Obstetrics and Gynecology, 67(4), 598-603.

Smith, S. (1980). Adapting the birthing center concept to a traditional hospital setting. Journal of Obstetrics, Gynecological, and Neonatal Nursing. (March/April), 103-106.

Soderstrom, B., Stewart, P.J., Kaitell, C., & Chamberlain, M. (1990). Interest in alternative birthplaces among women in Ottawa-Carleton. Canadian Medical Association Journal, 142(9), 963-969.

Spitzer, M.C. (1995). Birth centers: economy, safety, and employment. Journal of Nurse-Midwifery, 40(4), 371-375.

Stern, C., Permezel, M., Petterson, C., Lawson, J., Eggers, T., & Kloss, M. (1992). The royal women's hospital family birth centre: the first 10 years reviewed. Australian and New Zealand. Journal of Obstetrics and Gynecology, 32(4), 291-296.

Stone, P.W. & Walker, P.H. (1995). Cost-effectiveness analysis: birth center vs. hospital care. Nursing Economics, 13(5), 229-308.

Tew, M. (1978). The case against hospital deliveries: the statistical evidence. In Kitzinger, S. & Davis, J.A. (Eds.), The Place of Birth (1st. ed.) (pp. 55-65). Oxford, England: Oxford University Press

Waldenstrom, U. & Nilsson, C.-A. (1994). Experience of childbirth in birth center care; a randomized controlled study. Acta Ostetricia et Gynecologia Scandinavica, 73, 547-554.

Waldenstrom, U. & Nilsson, C.-A. (1993). Characteristics of women choosing birth center care. Acta Ostetricia et Gynecologia Scandinavica, 72, 181-188.

Waldenstrom, U. & Nilsson, C.-A. (1993). Women's satisfaction with birth center care: a randomized, controlled study Birth, 20(1), 3-13.

Waldenstrom, U., Nilsson, C.-A., & Winbladh, B. (1997). The Stockholm birth centre trial: maternal and infant outcome British Journal of Obstetrics and Gynecology, 104, 410-418.

Zabreck, E., Simon, P., & Benrubi, G. (1983). The alternative birth center in Jacksonville, Florida: the first two years. Journal of Nurse-Midwifery, 28(4), 31-36.

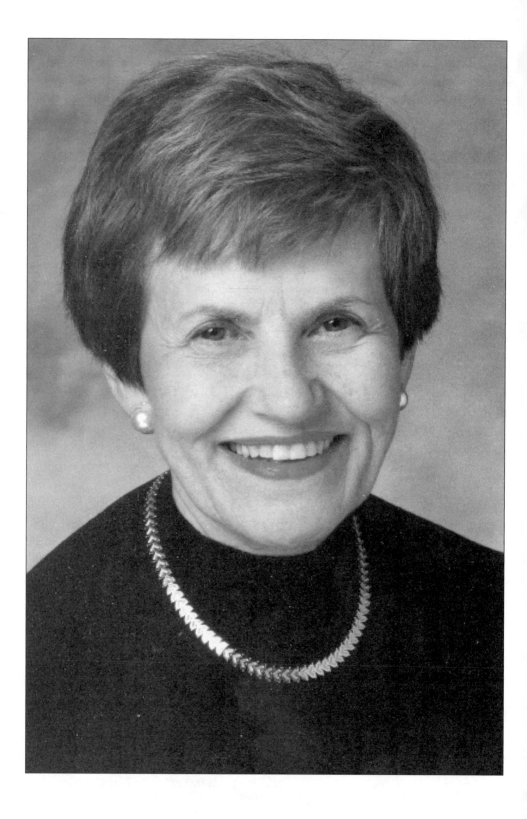

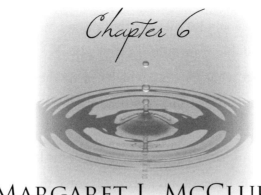

Chapter 6

MARGARET L. MCCLURE

I love being a nurse, every piece of it.

—Margaret L. McClure

Margaret McClure, RN, EdD, FAAN, fondly known as Maggie to her friends, is an internationally recognized nurse leader with exceptional success as a nurse executive. However, she may be best known for a seminal research study she and several colleagues conducted that evaluated hospital work environments. This study laid the groundwork for what are now known as "Magnet hospitals" throughout nursing and healthcare.

When asked to recount her leadership journey, she muses, "You know, I am not very interested in the past because that is gone, but I am very interested in tomorrow. Ask me about tomorrow." In many ways, however, it is her past leadership that has helped to create future leadership opportunities for professional nursing, as Magnet status and recognition become increasingly important throughout the United States and the world. The Magnet framework empowers, develops, and validates the contribution of direct-care nurses as partners with other disciplines and departments in healthcare.

Maggie's message includes the idea that nurses must learn to accept credit for their invaluable contributions to healthcare. In her words: "Nurses don't respect what they do, which is why they say, 'I am only a nurse'! Can you imagine? The most important job in the hospital, and we discount our value?"

Maggie believes nursing is the cornerstone to healthcare. To emerge as healthcare leaders, she believes nurses must resolve the debate concerning educational requirements for entry into practice. "The truth is, there really should be no debate," she says. "The nursing profession needs to break away from the educational model of the 1950s and join our interdisciplinary colleagues by raising the required educational preparation for entry into practice, even in the face of a workforce shortage.

"I love being a nurse, every piece of it," she adds. She loves the profession enough to push for excellence and has created a legacy committed to elevating the status of nursing.

EARLY INFLUENCES

Samuel McClure was 53 when he married Lois (Jean) Doane. Two years later, on 24 January 1937, Jean gave birth to Maggie. In 1942, Maggie's sister, Carol Jean, was born. Samuel told anyone who would listen that his girls were "perfect." Maggie believes that her father's adoring manner fueled an early self-confidence that she credits as her ego strength, enabling her to tackle difficult circumstances, even when the odds were against her.

Samuel was born in Northern Ireland and grew up a Scotch-Irish Presbyterian. As a young boy, he contracted polio and was left with lifelong physical limitations. Despite his restrictions, Maggie describes him as a "corker" with loads of spirit and few complaints. Although he did not earn a college degree, he became a public accountant and founded the McClure and Company accounting firm in Philadelphia. While the McClure family lived on a modest income, their home was rich with love.

Maggie's mother was born and raised in Canada. She immigrated to Hudson City, New York, at 16 to enter nurse training at Hudson City Hospital. Upon completing school, Jean moved to Philadelphia to work in a physician's office. It was in Philadelphia that she met Samuel. After their marriage, Jean decided to forgo employment to stay with her children. However, when Maggie was about 4 years old and World War II was raging, Jean took a position as a medical/surgical nurse and worked nearly every night of the week. The strong work ethic and cheerful disposition embodied by both parents heavily influenced the McClure girls. "Carol and I can't understand people who don't see a responsibility to work hard," Maggie says. "We are workaholics and are happiest that way."

Both daughters were also influenced by their mother's passion for nursing. Jean loved taking care of others and knew she was making a difference every day. A conversation with her mother had a lasting impression on Maggie. Jean pointed out that physicians could perform autopsies to know the impact of their work on patients. Jean was both fascinated and frustrated with this, because it was not possible to perform any test or procedure to understand how nursing practices affected patient outcomes.

Jean delighted in describing Maggie's early leadership qualities—even as a toddler. Jean often recounted that other mothers complained that Maggie remained immaculate by making the other kids do the dirty work. Maggie confesses that she was born bossy. "If people would just pay attention to me, the world would be a better place," she says with a smile. While she acknowledges there are many different ways to get things done, her leadership gift has been to inspire others to see her vision. Maggie is clear that leaders don't have to be perfect, but they do have to be effective while maintaining integrity.

THE POWER OF LEADERSHIP

Maggie was voted "Most Ambitious" and "Most Likely to Succeed" by her classmates at Germantown High School in Philadelphia. It was obvious to others that she would be a leader in any area she chose to pursue. Initially, music was her passion, but she quickly switched to nursing when she realized that caring for people better suited her abilities.

Maggie started nursing school at the Lankenau Hospital School of Nursing in Philadelphia. It was a well-established diploma program experiencing great change and conflict when she arrived. The year before she entered school, the hospital had moved into a new building high on a hill in suburban Philadelphia and left behind a 100-year-old inner-city building. The move was difficult for all involved. Additionally, the school underwent a leadership change. Historically, the nursing school had been led by a group of Lutheran sisters. Now, a non-Lutheran sister was in charge for the first time. According to Maggie, it didn't go over well. One day, the entire faculty, with the exception of one instructor, Lida White, quit without notice. Lida was left teaching every course, from nursing arts and microbiology to anatomy and physiology, until J. Margaret "Ada" Mutch was recruited from Presbyterian Hospital in New York City.

When Ada arrived, both the hospital and school saw immediate change. According to Maggie, "Everything just started to improve. She [Ada] touched every corner of the lives of the students and patient care too." No longer were poor performances tolerated, and those in leadership roles were empowered by Ada to create positive change. Students were given more liberty to have a life outside of school and were treated with greater respect. Maggie was amazed that one person could so dramatically transform a work environment in what seemed such a short time. Maggie's original plan had been to teach, but Ada's leadership ability convinced her that one day she wanted Ada's job. Even then Maggie understood that this leadership responsibility required a baccalaureate degree, at a minimum, and preferably a master's degree.

In 1956, at the end of Maggie's second year of nursing school, a nurse recruiter addressed her class about a new Army Reserve program. The students were told they would receive $80 each month and be classified as privates on active duty while attending school. At the time, this was very appealing because Maggie's allowance, which she felt was a financial burden on her family, was only $20 per month. Upon graduation, the participants would owe the Army Nurse Corps 2 years of service and be commissioned as officers. Additionally, Maggie believed the Army would support her desire to get a baccalaureate degree. For her, it made perfect sense and was an easy career decision.

It was all quite foreign and, in her words, "really hilarious to see healthcare providers trying to figure out the military part."

After graduation from Lankenau, Maggie was stationed at Fort Sam Houston in San Antonio, Texas, for 6 weeks, where she learned to march and salute. She laughs as she remembers the chaos created by nurses and doctors attempting to fall into formation and shout out commands. It was all quite foreign and, in her words, "really hilarious to see healthcare providers trying to figure out the military part." Following this orientation course, she was stationed for 2 years at Madigan Army Hospital in Tacoma, Washington. The Army was lightly staffed for nurses, and it was not unusual for

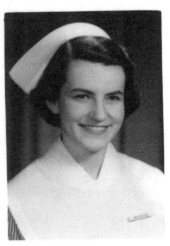

MARGARET (MAGGIE) MCCLURE UPON GRADUATING FROM LANKENAU HOSPITAL SCHOOL OF NURSING IN PHILADELPHIA, PENNSYLVANIA.

Maggie to be the only nurse on a shift to care for a 66-bed surgical unit. It was common for nurses to rotate shifts, work double-back shifts (work the evening shift one day and the day shift the next day), and sometimes work 7 days in a row. Because of Maggie's strong work ethic and the Army's willingness to accommodate her baccalaureate studies, she didn't mind the grueling hours. Overall, she found it to be a great opportunity to develop her skills. She was surrounded by high-quality professionals who were very committed to continuing education. The Army provided the foundation for her future professional goal—excellence in practice.

The opportunity to work with a great leader who would willingly mentor her career seemed more important than the perfect position.

In 1960, Maggie finished her active duty commitment and moved on to become the school nurse for Moravian College in Bethlehem, Pennsylvania. This position provided her the opportunity to finish her BSN at Moravian while getting free room and board and tuition. In 1961, when she finished her degree, Maggie reconnected with Ada Mutch to seek employment as a head nurse at Lankenau Hospital. While Ada suggested she consider a faculty position, Maggie was able to convince Ada to give her 1 year as a head nurse.

Maggie was a skilled head nurse, and Ada not only kept her in the role, she supported her plan to pursue a master's degree, even if it meant leaving Lankenau. In 1963, Maggie enrolled in the Nursing Service Administration master's program at Columbia University's Teachers College in New York. Upon completion of the program in 1965, Maggie returned to Lankenau Hospital. She made this decision for one reason—Ada Mutch. The opportunity to work with a great leader who would willingly mentor her career seemed more important than the perfect position. Initially, Maggie returned as the medical-surgical supervisor but within 1 year was promoted to assistant director of nursing. Ada was grooming her as a nurse executive.

Leadership Lesson Learned

Visionary leaders identify strong talent and mentor them to the next level—the good deed often comes home again.

In seeking a career move, consider more than just the position. Consider the leader who promises to grow the position.

Maggie recalls a particularly difficult day when nothing had gone as planned. She knocked on Ada's door and asked, "Is there anyone in this hospital who is not allowed to yell at me? If so, I would like to meet that person." Together, they roared with laughter, and Ada took the opportunity to validate and inspire Maggie's leadership. She brought out the best in her people, even in the worst of times, and Maggie believes that is a "powerful quality in a leader."

She had begun to wonder if doctoral studies should be the next step in her professional journey. She questioned if nurse leaders needed the highest education to make a difference in the future. Then, a grateful patient answered the question for her. The patient was an executive with General Electric and was so pleased with his care that he wanted to give something back to the hospital. He offered to conduct efficiency studies

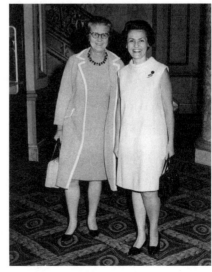

MAGGIE, RIGHT, WITH J. MARGARET "ADA" MUTCH IN 1968.

on nursing care and identify methods to streamline operations. The offer was accepted, and study results showed that each unit needed a head nurse and only one other nurse. Everything else, it had been determined, could be done by nurses aides. Maggie looked at the findings and pointed out key missing variables, such as patient monitoring and clinical judgment. The hospital chief executive officer (CEO), however, had the General Electric experts telling him their findings, and there was no way she could refute the findings in a quantitative manner. Maggie knew that the report was wrong for patients, and she did not intend to be placed in this position of intellectual disadvantage again. She enrolled once again at Teachers College, Columbia University, to earn a doctorate in research in nursing service administration.

Maggie never returned to Lankenau Hospital, but Ada Mutch remains a force in her life even today. Ada was a remarkable mentor and prepared Maggie for the rest of her career. Maggie learned the art of leadership from a master and knew it was time to establish her own leadership.

Launching a Nurse Executive

Maggie arrived at Teachers College with an interest in understanding why nurses stayed at their jobs. However, she quickly concluded that this was not a practical dissertation topic. First, she was concerned that nurses might not be prepared to articulate why they stayed in their respective positions, because they probably hadn't thought about it very much. Second, and most important, was the fear that she might create turnover by introducing the query "why do you stay at your job?" to nurses who might not have given it any thought. She feared the "That is a good question" response, which could create a catalyst for employment change. "What doctoral student wants to leave a wake of resignations in her path?" she asked.

Instead, she titled her dissertation "The Reasons for Hospital Staff Nurse Resignations," and hoped one day she could get to the core of her original question.

In 1972, with her doctorate in hand, Maggie began to review her career options. She applied to the University of Vermont and George Washington University for executive nurse positions in their hospitals. The University of Illinois, University of Iowa, and Case Western University all recruited her for nursing service administration positions. In all cases, she was either turned down or she turned them down because the fit was not right.

Even though she had a doctorate in nursing, a rarity at the time and almost always a direct entrée into deanships or other faculty positions, administration and operations were still her dream. Thus, with little hope of a good fit, Maggie applied for an advertised chief nurse officer (CNO) position at Maimonides Medical Center (MMC).

Maggie's interview was scheduled with the MMC personnel director at 2 p.m. on a Friday. Her instincts told her this would be a short interview, because CNO candidates are not typically vetted by personnel directors and because Orthodox Jewish organizations typically closed Fridays at sundown in observation of the Sabbath. At the interview, she met briefly with the personnel director, who excused himself to call the CEO from the next room. She overheard him say, "Lee, you'd better meet this one; she seems pretty good."

Lee Schwenn, the CEO, was new in his position and had no previous hospital experience. He had been at MMC for a very brief period when the previous CEO was fired and Lee was unexpectedly promoted. The organization needed a strong CNO, and Lee knew it.

So you are telling me that if the charge nurse calls in sick on a Saturday night, you want to be called at home to figure out who to put there?

Maggie toured the building with the associate director of nursing while Lee pulled together the medical chiefs of service. She remembers thinking it was the oddest building she had ever seen. Three construction phases—1902, 1920, and 1950—had been completed, and the old construction did not blend with the new. By the time she returned to the conference room with all the assembled medical chiefs of service, she was convinced this was not the position for her. As soon as the discussion began, she identified that Lee was a good leader with a great heart. She recalls thinking he was "100% Boy Scout" and it was impossible not to like him. During the course of the interview, the director of pediatrics stated that he wanted the pediatric nursing staff to report to him instead of the CNO, trying to make the case that pediatrics was different from the other services. Looking him squarely in the eye, Maggie said, "So you are telling me that if the charge nurse calls in sick on a Saturday night, you want to be called at home to figure out who to put there?" He stammered, "Well, no." With complete candor and respect, she responded, "If you can't stand the heat, stay out of the kitchen." With that, they were in her thrall. Monday morning, Lee called Maggie with an offer. She let him know that one of her reservations about the position was that Maimonides didn't have a nursing school connection. He asked, "Is that all that is bothering you?" Lee called back that afternoon to say he had gotten a faculty appointment for her at the SUNY (State University of New York) Downstate School of Nursing. Maggie was impressed that he had been able to move so quickly for something he wanted and needed. She decided that if Lee could do that, then working with him would be an adventure. She accepted the position and has never regretted the decision.

Among the many lessons learned at Maimonides was the value of mutual mentoring. She taught Lee about hospital operations and how they relate to attaining quality patient care. Maggie's determination did not intimidate Lee, and he was commonly found on the units interacting with staff and patients—learning what he needed to know to be successful. Lee also taught many lessons to Maggie, including political savviness. For example, he told her on any board or decision-making body, you only need one vote, and it is important to make sure you are satisfying that person. "Get to know who that one vote is and make sure you are aligned with that person," he said.

Lee was often her one vote, but he counseled her on how to handle high-profile situations when he was not the one vote. She noticed that each year, Lee would put on his best suit and tie and meet with a member of the board of trustees. While this man did not outwardly appear to be a person of power, his influence extended to many voting members of the board. Lee would speak to this retired leader about his evaluation, because he knew this person was the one vote. For the second time in her career, Maggie had the good fortune to be mentored by a great leader who incorporated the art of leadership into professional practice. Lee invested in Maggie's career by teaching her to always look beyond the obvious.

Maggie remained the CNO at Maimonides Medical Center for 7 years. In 1979 she was simultaneously recruited by the University of Pennsylvania Hospital and New York University (NYU) Medical Center as their CNO. Maggie considered returning to Philadelphia, but her mother was battling esophageal cancer and receiving treatment in New York City. Thus, she chose to go with NYU.

During her 7-year tenure at Maimonides, Maggie established herself as a nurse executive capable of managing the conflict of a union environment and elevating nursing practice to excellence. Moreover, she launched her national professional presence during the mid-1970s as she and Claire Fagin led the campaign for the passage of the 1985 proposal.

THE 1985 PROPOSAL—GATEWAY TO NATIONAL LEADERSHIP

The 1985 proposal was a New York State legislative initiative that aimed to change the educational requirements for the nursing licensure exam. The proposal mandated that by the year 1985, 10 years from the proposed legislation date, nurses preparing to take the registered nurse (RN) exam must have completed a baccalaureate in nursing. Additionally, licensed practical nurses (LPNs) seeking licensure must have completed an associate's degree in nursing by this same time.

Whether nurses like it or not, the truth of the matter is the powerful players in healthcare are physicians, so if you go to a legislator or any other policy leader and ask for support related to a healthcare issue, they turn around and ask the physicians, "What do you think?" even if it is solely related to nursing.

The 1985 proposal gained national attention and was one of the first efforts to raise the educational requirements for nursing licensure. Maggie, an advocate for the legislation, was suddenly speaking nationally on the subject. The concept was controversial, but it was supported by many in the nursing community. Ultimately, the measure died in committee. Maggie regrets not being clever enough to form the proper coalitions to get the legislation passed. She recognizes that there was no chance of getting this important measure enacted into law without medicine on the side of reform, and they never went to physicians to ask for their support.

"Whether nursing likes it or not, the truth of the matter is the powerful players in healthcare are physicians, so if you go to a legislator or any other policy leader and ask for support related to a healthcare issue, they turn around and ask the physicians, 'What do you think?' even if it is solely related to nursing." She believes that if physicians had stepped forward with the message that this reform was necessary for healthcare and patients, the legislation might have passed. Maggie is clear that nurses might hate this change, "but it is reality, and we must live with it and use it to our advantage as we move into the future." She learned to form the proper coalitions early and not resist the reality of the process—use it instead. Maggie recommends that when leaders commit to a concept, they should be flexible about methods they use to make it a reality.

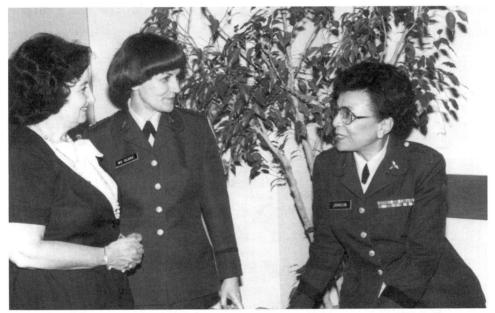

ARMY NURSE CORPS CONFERENCE IN SAN ANTONIO, TEXAS, 2-5 MAY, 1983. FROM LEFT, THELMA SCHORR, THEN PRESIDENT AND PUBLISHER OF THE *AMERICAN JOURNAL OF NURSING*; U.S. ARMY RESERVE LIEUTENANT COLONEL MARGARET L. MCCLURE, EXECUTIVE DIRECTOR OF NURSING, NEW YORK UNIVERSITY MEDICAL CENTER; AND BRIGADIER GENERAL HAZEL JOHNSON, CHIEF OF THE ARMY NURSE CORPS.

Maggie's leadership during the 1985 proposal earned her selection as a fellow of the American Academy of Nursing (FAAN) in 1976. The national reputation she developed for her commitment to improving practice through higher educational standards placed her among nursing's elite leadership group. Maggie went on to hold key leadership positions within the American Academy of Nursing (AAN), including the chair of the Task Force on Nursing Practice in Hospitals (1981-1983), a member of the Governing Council (1993-1996), secretary (1996-1998), president-elect (1999-2001), president (2001-2003), member of the Commission on Workforce (2000-present), and co-chair of the Committee on the Educational Preparation of the Workforce (2005-present).

While time-consuming and sometimes contentious, holding national and international leadership positions was an honor. "Whenever I spent time working with and among professional organizations, I always got more than I gave." She valued the ability to work with some of nursing's finest leaders, such as Muriel Poulin, Joyce Clifford, Yvonne Munn, Angela McBride, Claire Fagin, and many others, who helped further develop her leadership skills.

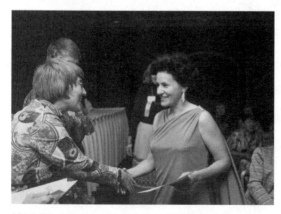

MAGGIE, RIGHT, BEING INDUCTED AS A FELLOW INTO THE AMERICAN ACADEMY OF NURSING IN 1976. ELLEN EGAN PRESENTS THE HONOR.

According to Maggie, the role of a nurse executive is often a lonely position. There is little opportunity to talk to colleagues, because there are few peers at that level. The vice president for nursing is often the only woman and the only nurse at that level. The executive culture is complex and sometimes less than transparent, and you have to learn a new way to interact with other leaders. "This is commonly a man's world with a man's perspective on communication," Maggie says. She points out that the other vice presidents often do not understand nursing issues, such as dealing with 12-hour shifts. "They don't get it, nor do they really care," she says. "Additionally, there is no executive-level hands-on training, so you have to make your own way—it is a sink or swim situation." Maggie found as a nurse executive that her peer group support often came from colleagues in professional organizations, which was valuable to her career. Maggie's association with the AAN supported and facilitated her participation in the study defining hospital work environments that attracted and retained quality nurses.

IN SEARCH OF EXCELLENCE

In 1980, the United States was experiencing a nursing shortage that had captured the attention of many stakeholders, including the AAN. The AAN had been established 7 years earlier and was seeking to become an influence on healthcare policy, similar to the Institute of Medicine. Studying the elements of a hospital work environment that might contribute to the nursing shortage seemed like a perfect opportunity to make an important and relevant contribution to easing the nursing shortage, and thereby improving care to patients.

The AAN Governing Council created a task force on nursing practice in 1981 and invited several fellows to examine characteristics that impeded or facilitated nursing practice in the acute care setting. Maggie, then-executive director of nursing at NYU Medical Center, was appointed chair of the task force. The three other fellows were Muriel Poulin, EdD, RN, professor at Boston University's School of Nursing; Margaret (Marg) Sovie, PhD, RN,

These ideas focused the team on evaluating the elements of a work environment that created the ability to attract and retain professional nurses with "magnet" strength.

chief nursing officer at Strong Memorial Hospital at the University of Rochester; and Mabel Wandelt, PhD, RN, professor at the University of Texas at Austin's School of Nursing.

The task force was asked to determine how the AAN might assist in solving the nursing shortage. The first meeting was held at the NYU Medical Center. The idea for the Magnet hospital study was developed the first day as the task force team members reviewed the possibilities. They concluded that everyone knew what was wrong with nursing, and the last thing needed was another paper pointing out what was wrong.

The dialogue was guided by Maggie's 1972 doctoral dissertation, "The Reasons for Hospital Staff Nurse Resignations" and Mabel's study on nursing turnover. Mabel had discovered a disparity in nursing turnover in Texas hospitals. She had observed that hospitals in close geographic proximity often had very different nurse staffing outcomes. One hospital might have an employment waiting list, while a nearby hospital could not adequately staff its nursing units. Mabel was very interested in those hospitals that were not having trouble with high turnover and vacancies. These ideas focused the team on evaluating the elements of a work environment that created the ability to attract and retain professional nurses with "magnet" strength.

The task force team did not use the term "Magnet hospitals" until late in the planning stage. During one of their many planning discussions, Marg identified that in Rochester the school system had a program called Magnet schools, which identified unique and innovative public schools based on their extraordinary outcomes. The out-of-industry comparison made sense to all the members, and so the term "Magnet hospitals" was adopted and became synonymous with the study.

The team formulated a study methodology and returned to the AAN board at the annual meeting in 1981 for final approval. Maggie presented the study plan at the business meeting. She proudly stood at the microphone and carefully outlined the plan for conducting a qualitative study of superior hospitals by interviewing the chief nursing officers and representative staff nurses from the selected institutions.

What hospitals shall we select as the comparators? Who would volunteer to be the bad work environment hospitals? There has to be some feasibility!

Maggie and her team believed they were bringing forward a solid method to better understand the magnetic pull of selected hospitals. Other academy members were invited to express their opinions during an open discussion period after Maggie's presentation. Maggie began to "sweat bullets" as some of nursing's most revered researchers stepped to the microphone and aggressively challenged the study methodology. The challenge was centered on the validity of the study, as there was no comparison group—the debate of hard science (randomized controlled trials) versus soft science (qualitative discovery). Maggie attempted to explain that the proposed study was a qualitative design. After a time, she finally blurted out in frustration, "What hospitals shall we select as the comparators? Who would volunteer to be the bad work environment hospitals? There has to be some feasibility!"

Maggie was completely blind-sided by the negative reaction from the nurse researchers. Prior to the task force proposal, the AAN had only produced white papers on salient topics. The team believed its suggestion of conducting a study would be viewed as a bold statement that the AAN was investing in the science and solutions to the nursing shortage. She admits they were so pleased with the proposal that they were unprepared to effectively defend the dismantling of the study. They had neglected to prepare for the worst.

Leadership Lesson Learned

"Leaders must not become so enamored by a project that they forget to examine closely those aspects that may derail the project," Maggie says. "You are continually attacked by things you didn't even think had teeth." She advises that the wise leader should think through who might be opposed to their ideas (and why), and carefully prepare the response.

After the open academy business meeting, the board requested the task force members report to a private and confidential meeting. It was the four M's—Maggie, Muriel, Marg, and Mabel—against some of the finest nurse leaders in the United States. They entered the small hotel room and "stood like soldiers" as they awaited the board's decision. With relief, they heard that the board had approved the plan. The study was to go forward as presented.

The next major challenge was that the AAN had sparse funds for the study. The AAN had a membership of approximately 130 who paid minimal dues ($75-$100/year at the time), resulting in a "minimal budget" that didn't even allow for full-time office staff, much less funding for studies. Maggie and the team wrote more than 15 grant proposals to such organizations as the Kellogg Foundation, Robert Wood Johnson Foundation, and

Commonwealth Fund, all without luck. Not one funding source would invest in the study.

In hindsight, the problem clearly was a case of known versus unknown. "We weren't well-known in the research world, and professional reputation was paramount to funding success at that time," Maggie laments. "I was young and foolish and believed that the quality of the study would pique the interest of foundations and funders. It turns out they have to know you, and this was a major lesson learned."

AAN was too new to carry any funding influence, and task force members quickly understood that they must be innovative to finance the study. They personally funded some of the expenses and called in favors from colleagues around the country to act as site coordinators, supplying space, food, and graduate student assistants for the regional data collection sessions. The task force members stayed in the least expensive hotels with double and triple occupancy, took the cheapest flights, and avoided additional expenses whenever possible. Maggie laughs today about how crazy it was trying to conduct a national study with no money, but they were too stubborn to give up on a good idea.

OPERATIONALIZING THE STUDY

The first step was to identify which hospitals were considered by staff nurses to be good places to work. The study design called for geographic grouping as designated by the Bureau of Labor Statistics (BLS), except that regions I and II were combined as were regions VII and VIII, creating eight study regions. Letters were sent to six AAN fellows from each region who were not formally connected with a hospital. These fellows were asked to use their formal and informal contacts to identify and nominate nurse-friendly work environments. They were then asked to write a paragraph explaining the selection. The fellows took the request seriously, and 165 hospitals were nominated. Much to their surprise, there was almost no overlap of nominations.

The task force members had expected to select hospitals with the most nominations, but with little overlap, the logical methodology failed and forced them to consider an alternative plan for sampling. Under Plan B, a pilot study would be conducted with a handful of the nominees, based on what the fellows had written. All four task force members were going to be at a meeting in Washington, DC, so this was to be the pilot study site.

They invited the six Washington, DC-area nominees with the most compelling nomination write-ups to participate in the pilot study. Each of the six hospitals received a letter requesting the CNO and a staff nurse who was involved full time in direct patient care (not in a leadership role) to attend an off-site session with the task force. The CNO was invited to the morning session and the staff nurse to the afternoon session. Thus, the staff nurses in the sample did not need to worry that their comments would be shared with the CNOs. Both the CNOs and staff nurses were asked to adhere to the same rules. Specifically, everyone in the session would eventually answer all nine questions (see Figure 6.1). The questions did not have to be answered in order, and the participants were allowed to ask questions and interrupt one another.

As it turned out, the CNO responses and the staff-nurse responses were starkly different, with very few exceptions. For example, some staff nurses indicated there were serious problems in the work environment, whereas the directors of nursing stated quite the opposite. The team realized immediately that the sampling method lacked validity. For them, it was back to the drawing board.

INTERVIEW QUESTIONS

1. What makes your hospital a good place to work?

2. Can you describe particular programs in your situation that you see leading to professional/personal satisfaction?

3. How is nursing viewed in your hospital and why?

4. Can you describe nurse involvement in various ongoing programs or projects whose goals are quality of patient care?

5. Can you identify activities and programs calculated to enhance, both directly and indirectly, recruitment and retention of professional nurses in your hospital?

6. Can you tell us about nurse/physician relationships in your hospital?

7. Please describe staff nurse/supervisor (various levels) relationships in your hospitals.

8. Are some areas in your hospital more successful than others in recruitment/retention? Why?

9. What single piece of advice would you give to a director of nursing who wishes to do something about high registered nurse vacancy and turnover rates in her or his hospital?

Source: McClure, Poulin, Sovie, & Wandelt, 1983, p. 8.

FIGURE 6.1—THE NINE QUESTIONS THE PILOT GROUP MEMBERS WERE REQUIRED TO ANSWER.

In response to the pilot study failure, the task force reverted to the organization questionnaire completed by each CNO following the hospital's nomination. The questionnaire included information regarding staff nurse

> *People can write anything they want about how great things are, but we found the bottom line was the turnover rate. The turnover rate tells you whether the nurses are happy working there or not.*

demographics, educational preparation, staffing patterns, skill mix, ancillary support, turnover and vacancy rates, and professional practice models to establish which organizations were high performers. The team was convinced that the nomination process did not accurately measure magnetism and believed that the truth was in the data. They pored over the data and selected study participants strictly by turnover and vacancy rates. According to Maggie, this method of decision-making was defining. It was easy to see that there were distinct data differences among the nominated hospitals.

"People can write anything they want about how great things are, but we found the bottom line was the turnover rate," Maggie says. "The turnover rate tells you whether the nurses are happy working there or not." As a result of the more rigid method of sample selection, 46 hospitals were formally invited to participate in the Magnet hospital study. Five of the invitees declined involvement for a variety of reasons, so the final sample size was 41 hospitals (see Table 6.1). Because the study was qualitative in design, the researchers were not looking for anything; they had a blank page with no preconceived notions. They wanted to create an atmosphere where the CNOs and staff nurses could describe the hospital without being influenced by the questions—in other words, in a totally open-ended manner, much like you would ask a child to "tell me about your picture."

Now that the selection process was over, daylong interviews were scheduled in 1982 in each region. The interviewing process took nearly two-thirds of the year and included eight U.S. cities: Seattle, Washington; San Francisco, California; Sioux City, Iowa; Oklahoma City, Oklahoma;

Table 6.1

MAGNET HOSPITAL STUDY PARTICIPANTS

Alta Bates Hospital—Berkeley, California

Arlington Hospital—Arlington, Virginia

Bess Kaiser Medical Center—Portland, Oregon

Beth Israel Hospital—Boston, Massachusetts

Charlton Methodist Hospital—Dallas, Texas

El Camino Hospital—Mountain View, California

Evanston Hospital—Evanston, Illinois

Fairfax Hospital—Falls Church, Virginia

Family Hospital—Milwaukee, Wisconsin

Fort Sanders Regional Medical Center—Knoxville, Tennessee

Franklin Square Hospital—Baltimore, Maryland

Henrico Doctors' Hospital—Richmond, Virginia

Hillcrest Medical Center—Tulsa, Oklahoma

Iowa Methodist Medical Center—Des Moines, Iowa

Lutheran Medical Center—Wheat Ridge, Colorado

Memorial General Hospital—Union, New Jersey

Meridian Park Hospital—Tualatin, Oregon

Morristown Memorial Hospital—Morristown, New Jersey

Park Plaza Hospital—Houston, Texas

Presbyterian Hospital—Oklahoma City, Oklahoma

Prince George's General Hospital and Medical Center—Cheverly, Maryland

Rochester Methodist Hospital—Rochester, Minnesota

Sacred Heart Medical Center—Spokane, Washington

Saint Francis Hospital—Roslyn, New York

Saint Joseph Hospital—Saint Charles, Missouri

Saint Joseph Hospital—Kansas City, Missouri

Saint Mary's Hospital and Health Center—Tucson, Arizona

Saint Michael Hospital—Milwaukee, Wisconsin

Seton Medical Center—Austin, Texas

Shady Grove Adventist Hospital—Rockville, Maryland

Stanford University Hospital—Palo Alto, California

Strong Memorial Hospital—Rochester, New York

University Hospital—Augusta, Georgia

University Hospital—Seattle, Washington

University Hospitals of Cleveland—Cleveland, Ohio

University of California, San Francisco—San Francisco, California

Valley General Hospital—Renton, Washington

Veterans Administration Medical Center and Regional Office Center—Cheyenne, Wyoming

Virginia Mason Hospital—Seattle, Washington

Women's Hospital—Baton Rouge, Louisiana

Worcester Hahnemann Hospital—Worcester, Massachusetts

They all realized they were experiencing something special, no matter how many hours it absorbed.

Milwaukee, Wisconsin; Atlanta, Georgia; Baltimore, Maryland; and Boston, Massachusetts. The pilot structure of interviewing CNOs in the morning and staff nurses in the afternoon had worked well and was repeated. Two task force members facilitated every session, which meant each member participated in approximately four sessions. The sessions were held at a centrally located university in each of the regions. The deans of those nursing schools arranged for graduate students to assist with note taking and provided lunch as well. The interviews were taped but seldom transcribed due to lack of funds. During the process, Maggie developed tendonitis in her shoulder from excessive note taking that persists even today—a constant reminder of the "no pain, no gain" maxim.

As had been hoped, these interviews revealed strong common threads between the CNOs in the morning meetings and the staff nurse discussions in the afternoons. "The overall story was the same, and the overlap between the CNO and staff nurse groups was amazing," Maggie says. With only one suspicious hospital in the mix, team members knew they had hit the mark. Maggie believes that she became a better nurse executive as a result of being exposed to the leadership and concepts that bubbled up during the data collection. She was witnessing nursing practice excellence in a variety of presentations from across the nation, and she was a sponge.

The four team members held down their respective full-time nurse executive or faculty position while conducting the study. They all realized they were experiencing something special, no matter how many hours it absorbed. Still, none of them realized the magnitude of importance of this work.

Producing the Book

With the timeline set and chapters assigned, Maggie made plans to attend a conference hosted by the American Society of Nursing Service Administrators (ASNSA), known today as American Organization of Nurse Executives. She was so sure that the project was on course that she agreed to be the master of ceremonies to roast Joyce Clifford, the outgoing president of ASNSA. Maggie knew she would have to review the final draft of the manuscript and get it to the publisher prior to flying to San Diego for the ASNSA conference. To her astonishment, the book was not ready for publication, and Maggie was concerned that the deadline would be impossible to meet without intense, concentrated work. The content itself was fine, but the writing styles were not compatible. There was no time to send it back to the original authors. So, she unpacked her bags and set to work rewriting the manuscript. There would be no trip to San Diego this time.

Maggie had already recruited Edith P. Lewis, known as Pat to her friends, to do the final editing of the manuscript. Pat had spent many years as editor of *Nursing Outlook,* and the two of them had worked together in the past. Maggie describes Pat as a gifted writer and editor. She recalls waiting for *Nursing Outlook* each month, primarily to read Pat's "magnificent editorials." Pat was also a member of the academy and knew of the study. After reworking the manuscript for one week—all day, every day, working late into the night—Maggie sent it to Pat. They met at Pat's house and Maggie was overwhelmed when she discovered nearly every page of the freshly reworked manuscript was littered with Pat's yellow stickers, indicating additional work was needed. Maggie would have cried if she had more time. She had been attempting to preserve the original work of the authors, but Pat was blending the writing styles—at all costs. The enormous lesson Maggie learned was to "assume nothing," and never minimize the amount of editing that an undertaking of this magnitude requires.

The manuscript was finally mailed to the ANA for publication on 3 January 1983. Making it to this point in the project was no small feat. Even when the study was complete, there were no funds available to have the manuscript printed. Several publishers were eager to publish it, but it would take them a year or more after receipt of the manuscript to publish the book. The ANA was the only publisher that could promise a quick turnaround, but the organization lacked the funds to produce the book. There was real concern that lack of finances would delay the study findings. Finally, funding came through (see Figure 6.2) and made publication possible.

Selecting ANA as the publisher required more than financial considerations. The choice created a true dilemma, as ANA had alienated many hospital administrators and trustees when the association became involved in union activities. This was unfortunate, as hospital leadership was a target audience for this work environment study. The task force members questioned whether the study findings would be diluted or judged fairly due to the connection with ANA. However, waiting 12 or more months for another publisher to produce the book almost guaranteed the findings would be diluted by the three studies that promised to precede them. The team members decided to let the study stand on its merits.

An unexpected ANA controversy occurred in the final hours. Maggie was given an advance copy of the book and noted that the task force members were not listed as the authors. The credit was being given solely to the academy. Maggie made several attempts to correct the situation through the highest levels of ANA, without success. The compromise was to paste in a new title page with their names above the academy logo. However, the Library of Congress citation credits AAN as the author, instead of the four nurse leaders who gave their time, money, reputation, and knowledge for nearly 2 years to produce the landmark study. Prior AAN publications had listed the principal authors while giving the academy due credit for sponsorship. This was a professional disappointment to the team, but a valuable lesson learned.

As often is the case with significant projects, the people supporting Maggie kept her and her other obligations on track. She believes that she

NEW YORK UNIVERSITY MEDICAL CENTER
A private university in the public service

550 FIRST AVENUE, NEW YORK, N.Y. 10016
CABLE ADDRESS: NYUMEDIC

(212) 340- 5507

January 10, 1983

TO: American Academy of Nursing
             Task Force on Nursing Practice in Hospitals

FROM: Margaret L. McClure

Just a note to let you know that the manuscript was mailed to ANA on January 3, 1983. I did attempt to incorporate everybody's comments in the final draft.

Jeanette Draper called me from ANF with some very good news. EXXON has given us a grant for $22,000 which will pay for our publishing costs. As a result, our contributions to date are as follows:

EXXON	$22,000
American Association of Critical Care Nurses	10,000
Sterling Drug Company	2,500
National League for Nursing	1,000
Association of Operating Room Nurses	1,000
Loretta Ford	1,000
Stanford University Medical Center, Nursing Department	200

I think we can all breathe a little easier as a result of these donations.

Hope you had happy holidays. I will be in touch with you soon.

MLM:gr

cc: M. Poulin, M. Sovie, M. Wandelt

TTY Phone for Deaf (212) 673-6974

FIGURE 6.2—MAGGIE'S LETTER TO TASK FORCE MEMBERS ANNOUNCING THE BOOK HAD BEEN SENT TO ANA AND IDENTIFYING THE FUNDERS.

could never have participated in the study had it not been for Patricia L.
Valoon, her second-in-command at NYU Medical Center. Patricia was

instrumental in keeping operations running smoothly while
Maggie devoted inordinate
hours to the study. Additionally, Maggie's administrative assistant, Grace Rauer, fondly referred to as the "best administrative assistant in the world,"
typed every single word of the
manuscript and kept Maggie's
professional life in control.

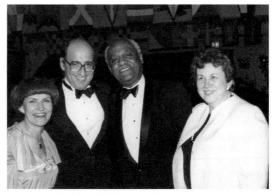

FROM LEFT TO RIGHT: MAGGIE; RICHARD
BERMAN, EXECUTIVE VICE PRESIDENT, NYU
MEDICAL CENTER; EVERETT FOX, VICE PRESI-
DENT FOR HOSPITALS, NYU, AND PATRICIA
VALOON, MAGGIE'S SECOND-IN-COMMAND,
IN 1985.

THE NURSING SHORTAGE ABATES

It would be decades later that the full effect of the Magnet Study would
be realized in the healthcare industry. The research team had uncovered a
framework of excellence that defined superior patient, nurse, and organizational outcomes. This work would lead to the future transformation of
hospital strategic planning, interdisciplinary relationships, nursing empowerment, and work environment cultures. Nurses would be expected to
lead through crisis and the four M's had created the tool box of possible
solutions.

In 1984, the task force members presented the study at the ANA annual
convention. The study findings created professional interest, but the urgency of the topic was waning because the nursing shortage was beginning to
abate. The year the study was published, Peters and Waterman released the
bestselling book *In Search of Excellence*. Maggie remembers thinking how

exciting it was that the business elements of the Peters and Waterman work were so aligned with the identified qualities of Magnet work environments in the AAN study. In fact, Marlene Kramer and Claudia Schmalenberg conducted subsequent research that was published in a two-part article in 1988 in the *Journal of Nursing Administration*, comparing Magnet principles to Peters and Waterman's principles of excellence, with complete alignment in all but one category.

KNOWING YOUR TALENT

Knowing your talent can be difficult, and Maggie didn't always want to be a nurse. Her early dream was to be a "solo singer." Along with her academic preparation, she majored in music in high school until it became clear that singing was not her talent. "I wasn't solo material, even though I wanted to be," she says. Moreover, what she learned from the music experience was that "even when you possess the talent, you can't just go out and sing. You have to practice every day and find a good coach so that you may develop the expert skill set that differentiates you from other talent." It didn't matter how much she practiced, Maggie realized she was not center stage material, and she wouldn't be happy teaching music to small children. What she learned was that at some point, talent and personal happiness must intersect.

Maggie believes that the best way to merge talent and personal happiness is by identifying strengths. She identifies personal strengths as "your toolbox"—those things that make you unique and successful. "People who tell you to focus on your weaknesses have it all wrong," she says. "You can only make marginal progress focusing on weaknesses. Your strengths are your natural talents that form the basis of your leadership style." She has witnessed many leaders who focus on improving their weaknesses to the extent that they forget to exploit the strengths that made them successful. The failure to identify and develop strengths becomes a barrier for many people. Maggie advises leaders to "seize on the identified strengths and make them stronger; no one will even notice the weaknesses. We all have weaknesses. The key is to minimize them by allowing your strengths to stand out and become your identifying characteristics." Great leaders have people around them whose strengths compensate for their own weaknesses.

Maggie identifies one of her strengths as "being blessed with a lot of energy" and natural curiosity. She uses these strengths to connect with others, including her staff. Experience as a nurse executive taught her that "staff members do not believe you know what is going on in the units unless they have told you, even though you may have heard it 100 times." The importance of being connected with staff was validated in the Magnet study when she observed that "each one of those nurse executives, whether the hospital was 900 beds or 99 beds, figured out how to make the staff feel heard." Prior to the study, when Maggie was CNO at Maimonides Medical Center, she conducted "around-the-clock meetings," where staff members could come to the administrative conference room and tell her what was on their minds. After the study, Maggie realized that her method of connecting with the staff was flawed. The same people always came, and those who did not come were never heard. Maggie knew they all had something to say, so the communication format needed to be addressed. She was not afraid to critique her leadership style and change quickly when needed.

> When you practice a profession, it means you are studying all the time and reviewing what you have done with an understanding that as you do that, you will continually get better.

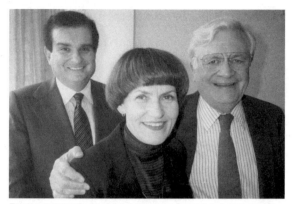

FROM LEFT TO RIGHT: MARTIN BEGUN, ASSOCIATE DEAN AND VICE PRESIDENT FOR EXTERNAL AFFAIRS; MAGGIE; AND SAUL J. FARBER, DEAN AND PROVOST, NYU MEDICAL CENTER

Maggie did change her modus operandi and started making appointments on the units, with intentional extra coverage so everyone could participate. She began these meetings by saying, "OK, this is your meeting. What do you think I need to know?" She thanked them and told the staff how much she respected what they did every day. Maggie often used her gift of humor to ease the tension and break down the barriers of communicating about tough subjects. She was honest with her communication—never making promises she could not keep and acknowledging those things they could be assured would be acted on. This was her leadership style, and it integrated well with her talents.

One of her observations is that some executive leaders do not treat their career like a practice. She points out that "when you practice a profession, it means you are studying all the time and reviewing what you have done with an understanding that as you do that, you will continually get better." Her concern is that some professionals don't practice the way musicians do; instead, they just work. These leaders predictably do the same thing all the time, and they never review or learn from the experience. Some leaders, she believes, are "tone deaf" when it comes to communication and don't understand why the staff does not respond or improve. "So, if we think about the notion of talent, then the truth of the matter is everybody doesn't have the talent to do every job, and you are doing them a favor to find a job that fits their talent." Just because someone is in a certain role does not mean the individual is able to lead as a practicing professional. It may require your leadership courage to properly align the talent with the role, rather than perpetuating "tone deaf" outcomes.

ODD JOBS

Maggie advises nurses to be open to developing new and unexpected skills. When Maggie was in doctoral studies with Eileen Zungolo, they had a conversation that led her in unexpected directions. Eileen mentioned she was working for *The Guiding Light*. Maggie, believing Eileen was working with blind patients, responded with profuse praise. Eileen, curious about what was so wonderful about her working for *The Guiding Light*, kindly informed Maggie that *The Guiding Light* was a New York-based soap opera, and not a service for the blind. One thing led to another, and Maggie found herself in the role of medical adviser for a soap opera. The money was a nice supplement to her doctoral stipend, and the role has provided numerous laughs over the years.

TAIL WAGGING THE DOG

One of the accomplishments Maggie is most proud of was the elimination of 12-hour shifts at NYU Medical Center. Patients were unhappy that they did not see the same nurse twice, and this was a result of 12-hour shifts. When Maggie would bring up this patient complaint during staff meetings, the response was always, "I am competent and give great care during my 12 hours, and that is all that should matter." Maggie would respond with, "Yes, that is important, but we all want continuity in our lives, even for the small things—*especially* for the small things because they are what build comfort and confidence."

Maggie provided the staff with the example of something as simple as a visit to her hairdresser. She counted on her hairdresser to know how to shampoo and cut her hair. If there was a turnover problem at the salon, and Maggie was required to explain the preferred shampoo and conditioner each time, she became dissatisfied with the service. Then she would say to the staff, "Now imagine you are a patient who depends on the nursing staff to keep you safe and improve your health condition." She would point out that patient care is commonly complex. "Let's say you as the patient have a difficult dressing that everyone changes differently, and you don't want it done differently, nor do you want to have to explain every shift how you want it done." Maggie would point out other simple things, such as when the patient wanted to receive medications and what the routine was for ambulation. These simple matters can create anxiety to the point where patients and family ask with angst, "Are you going to be back tomorrow?" What they are really saying, Maggie points out, is, "Please come back tomorrow so I can feel confident in my care."

The personal needs of the staff were driving how patient care was being delivered, and there was something wrong with that picture.

Maggie would show staff nurses data supporting the premise that patients and families do not like the discontinuity of care created by 12-hour shifts. In turn, staff nurses would share with her their desire to continue 12-hour shifts. The management team noted that 12-hour shifts also had a negative impact on shared governance. Nurses generally lived a great distance from NYU Medical Center and would not return on their days off to attend committee meetings and other events. Management concluded that the "tail was wagging the dog," and patient-care concerns were not driving the nursing care at NYU Medical Center. The personal needs of staff were driving the delivery of patient care, and this was not acceptable. The conversation between staff and management had been going on for years, and now it was time to do the right thing and return to 8-hour shifts.

As 1995 rolled around, other hospitals were redesigning and restructuring to reduce expensive registered-nurse skill mix. In contrast, Maggie hired all the nurses she could manage within her budget, and she hired only nurses with a BSN. In September 1995, she and the management team announced that 8-hour shifts would return in February 1996. The nurse management team expected a mass exodus of staff in reaction to this change, but only a few staff left.

The courageous leadership necessary to create the shift change also exposed some unexpected benefits of 8-hour shifts. Attendance at educational offerings improved, and nurses were more willing to participate in committee work when they were not working such long hours and were on campus more days each week. Workplace socialization began to change as well. When nurses were working 2 to 3 days per week, their social structure was focused at home. Maggie noticed that staff began to go out together for social activities after their 8-hour shifts, and relationships grew stronger.

Leadership Lesson Learned

If the "tail is wagging the dog," it is time to look for alternatives, even if those alternatives appear to be monumental and have the potential to create chaos. Unexpected benefits may surface and surprise even the resisters.

The management team also noted a marked decline in patient complaints. Now the real question focused on how the staff was tolerating the change. When Maggie attended her first unit meeting after the change, staff members handed her the agenda. The first item was, as expected, the conversion to 8-hour shifts. Maggie steeled herself to defend the change for the good of the patients. Instead, she was surprised to receive an acknowledgment from the staff and appreciation for the change. As it turns out, the nurses were now well-rested and realized for the first time just how tired they were when working 12-hour shifts.

The change was filled with angst, but the outcome had been worth the risk. Ultimately, 12-hour shifts returned to NYU Medical Center in the late 1990s as a result of the nursing shortage, which once again overrode what was best for patients.

HINDSIGHT IS 20/20

Looking back on her career, Maggie holds individual academic preparation as an important element to overall professional status. She had a unique perspective on the evolution of academic preparation in nursing from Teachers College at Columbia University, where one of her professors was Mildred Montag, RN, EdD—the "mother" of the Associate Degree in Nursing (ADN). According to Maggie, the development of the ADN was Mildred's doctoral dissertation, and her intent was to move nursing education into the higher educational system and away from apprentice-type training. However, Maggie believes that in some ways, the ADN concept backfired and in fact has stymied the advancement of basic nursing education.

The only time the nurse executive heard from patients or family was in extreme cases of things going very well or very poorly, and it was primarily the latter.

Maggie indicates that Mildred intended the ADN to be a "terminal" degree, modeled after engineering, where there are two levels of practice—technical and professional—with different job expectations. Maggie believes that this two-level concept works in engineering because the work involves strictly inanimate materials that allow for defined bundles of duties between the technician and professional to create the final product. Healthcare work involves a complex human being. Therefore, it is not possible to expect the neat, predictable bundling of care needs that fits nicely into a technical or professional domain. The conceptual blurring was further exacerbated by allowing ADN and BSN nurses to sit for the same licensing exam.

The development of the ADN program occurred in the 1950s, when the healthcare knowledge base was considerably smaller than today. Additionally, the emergence of high technology in healthcare has demanded a higher level of critical thinking than could ever have been predicted 5 decades ago. According to Maggie, it is time for the nursing profession to recognize that this multi-tiered academic preparation has not kept pace with healthcare changes, and the concept is no longer serving patients and healthcare well. She is firm that entry into practice should be elevated to a minimum of baccalaureate preparation, even in the face of a workforce shortage.

Maggie also realized that her leadership as a nurse executive could be measured by the number of patient complaints. She called it her "validity measure," as the only time the nurse executive heard from patients or family members was in extreme cases of good and bad. When Maggie first arrived at Maimonides, there was a new CEO and seven different CNOs had been in place over the prior 6 years. The number of patient complaints was high, and it took 7 years of changes in practice to slow the complaints to a trickle. In her first 18 months at NYU Medical Center, Maggie had not seen any patient complaints. She asked Pat Valoon, her second in command, how letters of complaint were being handled. Pat asked, "What letters of complaint?" Maggie was dumbfounded when only one complaint letter could be found. She concluded that when the standards are high and the job is being done well, the outcomes follow. She cautions that it is a mistake for nurse executives not to closely monitor the quantitative and qualitative nature of patient complaints as the barometer of nursing practice.

Maggie learned from Ada Mutch that leaders should retire at the age of 65. Ada believed that if you stay after 65, you do not know when to go. People wish you would leave, but they do not know how to tell you. Maggie remembers that she was 63 years old when she realized it was time to retire. She had risen to the dual COO and CNO leadership role for NYU Medical Center; however, the center had merged with several other hospitals, and her position was changed to that of nurse executive for the new system. The new position was going well. As she walked the halls one day, doing what she had done thousands of times before, she recalled Ada's words that retirement should occur on a high note in a career. Then and there she made her decision. She laughs, however, as she speaks of retirement, because she has never been busier professionally. The difference is that "now I only do what I want to do, not what I have to do, and there is a tremendous difference in quality of life."

ASK ME ABOUT TOMORROW

Maggie is clear that hospital administrators must understand that nursing is very important to patient outcomes. Pay for performance is very attractive to those who finance healthcare. The principle that good patient outcomes deserve higher reimbursement rates than poor outcomes seems to make sense. Her concern is that those organizations that do not qualify for quality performance payouts will become financially trapped by their poor outcomes and will have too little money to invest in improving quality.

Maggie is emphatic that quality matters; it matters to the person who is purchasing the care, and it matters in a monetary way to hospital CEOs. She uses "failure to rescue," a mortality variable dependent on nursing surveillance and early intervention, as an example of the impact of nursing care on hospital and physician outcomes. According to Maggie:

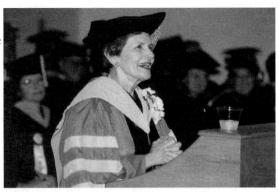

MAGGIE SPEAKING AT THE HOODING AND RECOGNITION CEREMONY AT DUKE UNIVERSITY'S SCHOOL OF NURSING COMMENCEMENT EXERCISES IN 2002.

"The day might not be far away when we find CEOs and physicians blaming nursing for not having improved our education, which will be rightly connected to quality outcomes. CEOs historically have not encouraged nurses to attain higher education for fear the nursing workforce will command a higher salary." She believes physicians have an innate sense about the value of nurses to patient outcomes but lack the motivation to push for higher education. Maggie is sure that pay for performance will define what nursing really contributes to quality outcomes, because "there is nothing like having somebody's pocketbook impacted to get their attention."

Maggie is keenly aware that for any organization, if there is no margin there is no mission. The nursing division is one of the largest cost centers in the hospital, which places great pressure on nurse executives to defend and adjust the budget during times of financial stress. On the other hand, she says,

Everything a nurse executive does requires explicit and refined communication skills, and underlying those skills is the ability to build good relationships.

"If nurses aren't delivering decent care, then the hospital doesn't make money, because high-quality care is the most inexpensive care." Patient care and finances must work together to balance the margin and the mission. This dual responsibility has sent many nurse executives back to school for a Master of Business Administration (MBA), which Maggie thinks is a serious error. "They didn't hire nurse executives because they had a financial head," she says. "They hired them because of their ability to lead nurses and nursing practice and to provide leadership around patient care." Maggie thinks that nurse executives should focus on developing communication skills, because the staff must understand leaders' views of clinical practice and how priorities need to be set as a result. "Everything a nurse executive does requires explicit and refined communication skills, and underlying those skills is the ability to build good relationships," she advises.

Maggie indicates that the most important relationship for a nurse executive is with the hospital CEO. The CNO must be philosophically aligned with the CEO to create and sustain clinical excellence. She points out that the quickest way to convert a Magnet hospital to non-Magnet is to change the CEO. This importance of leadership was supported in the original Magnet study. Maggie's experience has taught her that "when you hear that a CNO has been fired, the next question should be 'Where is the CEO?' Nine out of 10 times, you will hear there is a new CEO." Maggie's advice is to pick your CNO position in accordance with your belief that the CEO will be there for the long term and that your visions are aligned.

SUMMARY

Maggie is recognized for her extraordinary accomplishments in the leadership domains of research, executive nurse management, and professional organizations—most leaders devote an entire career to one domain without achieving the formidable outcomes Maggie has in several different domains. She has led with courage and candor. Maggie is a master communicator, and at the center of her conversations is the patient.

> *She wants the world to know that there is nothing more rewarding than being a nurse.*

Maggie's leadership journey caused the professional bar to be raised to improve work environments so that nurses can thrive and patients can expect consistent excellence. Her professional publications are extensive and compelling. She has presented on topics of practice excellence and leadership around the world. Maggie has received some of nursing's highest recognitions—president of the AAN (1990-1991), president of the AONE (1984-1985), Lifetime Achievement Award from AONE (2004), and several honorary doctorates. She would humbly tell you that is history and tomorrow is all that counts.

She may have been a peripheral player in *The Guiding Light* but there is no question that Maggie is one of nursing's brightest beacons. The Magnet Study has been a tremendous influence on professional nursing emerging onto the global center stage to take a lead in today's healthcare challenges. Her pride and passion for the nursing profession are palpable. She wants the world to know that there is nothing more rewarding than being a nurse. Many thanks, Maggie, for helping to create the platform where nurses can substitute "I am just a nurse" with "Look at me, I AM A NURSE!"

AFTERWORD

THE ANA MAGNET STUDY

In 1994, the American Nurses Credentialing Center (ANCC) designated its first nursing organization as a program of excellence. This designation as a "Magnet hospital" was the first time in ANCC history that a nursing organization—as opposed to individual nurses—had been eligible for recognition for excellence in practice. The landmark event would elevate the importance of nursing in the hospital setting as never before.

Today, "Magnet fever" sweeps the nation in response to a daunting nursing shortage. In 2001, the American Hospital Association reported 126,000 hospital nurse vacancies across the United States (Reilly, 2003). The U.S. nurse vacancy rate is expected to grow from 800,000 to 1.5 million by the year 2020 (Bleich, Hewlett, Santos, Rice, Cox, & Richmeier, 2003; Health Resources & Services Administration, 2002; Peter Buerhaus, personal communication, April 2, 2003). The Health Resources & Services Administration (HRSA) reports that demand for nurses will grow 40% by 2020, while the number of nurses is projected to grow only 6% (HRSA, 2002).

The question "Who will care for America's sick?" has become a legitimate concern that has prompted many to identify the current nursing shortage as a public health crisis (Kimball & O'Neil, 2002). The impact of the nursing shortage on quality of care and patient safety has all stakeholders concerned (Needleman, Buerhaus, Mattke, Stewart, & Zelevinsky, 2002).

Crisis invites opportunity. The Magnet framework, and its tested ability to attract and retain quality nurses, offers a sense of hope to nurse executives and hos-pital administrators as they deal with this seemingly hopeless workforce shortage.

THE MAKING OF THE MAGNET DESIGNATION PROGRAM

The ANA Magnet study completed by McClure, Poulin, Sovie, and Wandelt (1983) provided a distinct understanding of common themes in a hospital work environment that consistently attracted and retained quality nurses. These Magnet hospitals often had a waiting list of nurse applicants during the nursing shortage, while other organizations of like size and location could not get nurses in the door, much less hold onto them.

The following decade, Linda Aiken, RN, PhD, and the team of Marlene Kramer, RN, PhD, and Claudia Schmalenberg, RN, MSN, provided quantitative evidence that Magnet organizations produced superior patient, nurse, and organizational outcomes. Both groups of researchers published solid research supporting improved outcomes and developed tools to measure the magnetic components that were believed to contribute to this unique work environment. In addition, each group of researchers made important individual contributions that strengthened Magnet understanding and credibility.

Aiken's research discovered the "all or nothing" aspect of Magnet. She attempted to conduct an individual item review of the Magnet variables that contributed to improved outcomes; however, she discovered it was the synergistic effect of all the variables that created the outcome. Her work contributed to the "all or nothing" evaluation of the ANCC Forces of Magnetism.

In 1988, Kramer and Schmalenberg wrote a two-part article in the *Journal of Nursing Administration* titled "Magnet Hospitals: Institutes of Excellence." The article reported the results of their study that compared 16 Magnet organizations (from the original Magnet hospital study sample) to the eight characteristics of America's best-run corporations studied in the Peters and Waterman bestselling book, *In Search of Excellence*. Magnet hospitals aligned closely to seven of the eight corporate success characteristics. The only exception was the "stick to the knitting" principle—the idea that you should stay with what you know works. However, survival in healthcare at that time depended on agile leadership and swift change when necessary. Thus, that principle did not apply to healthcare. The outcome of this study was Magnet validation and brand-name correlation at a high-profile level.

The evidence was formidable and growing that Magnet organizations from the original study had the structure, processes, and outcomes that were worthy of recognition and modeling. The Magnet characteristics could be measured and reproduced. Why not follow this trail of success?

A nursing shortage prompted the ANA Magnet hospital study. The ANCC Magnet designation program was initiated to inspire nursing practice excellence. The purpose of the program was to provide a framework that any hospital could reproduce in its quest for nursing excellence.

SEEKING SOLUTIONS

In the early 1990s, the American Nurses Association (ANA) asked its Council on Nurse Executives (a special ANA interest group at that time) to evaluate ways to motivate excellence. Mary S. Tilbury, EdD, RN, CNAA, BC, was chair of the council. She recalls that there was considerable discussion around moving the Magnet hospital study evidence to a "program that

Once the eight interview sessions were completed, graduate students from the University of Texas (UT) at Austin began to perform content analysis of the interview materials. When the preliminary analysis was completed, the task force members convened at UT Austin for close to a week to finalize the analysis. Themes were clearly identifiable from the interviews. These themes would later be identified as the "14 Forces of Magnetism" that evolved into the American Nurses Credentialing Center (ANCC) Magnet Recognition Program.

At the end of the analysis, task force members divided the writing responsibilities into teams. Maggie and Muriel agreed to collaborate on two chapters, and Marg and Mabel worked on the other two chapters. They agreed that written materials would be exchanged among partners, and each of the partners would incorporate her own changes to keep the process dynamic. This was designed to blend the writing styles and add a fresh perspective to each chapter. Once again, they had come up with a logical method for supporting an efficient process and quality manuscript outcome. Or so they thought.

There was a sense of urgency around finishing the manuscript, because there were three other national studies on nursing resources all racing to publication. These included the report by the committee of the Institute of Medicine titled *Study of Nursing and Nursing Education*, the Congressionally-mandated *Study on Nursing Recruitment and Retention in the Veterans Administration*, and the report of the National Commission on Nursing. It is important to note that these publications focused on why nurses did not stay in their employment positions, as opposed to what attracted and retained them. The task force and Vernice Ferguson, then president of AAN, were anxious to be the first study to press.

would allow every organization to aspire to those characteristics and attributes." The council sent this recommendation to the ANA board. Mary's term ended shortly thereafter, and she thought it would end there.

In 1992, not long after her term had expired, Mary received a phone call from Marie Reid, who served as the first executive director of the ANCC. Marie asked Mary to join a committee to "make the Magnet recognition program happen." Mary was charged with the design and implementation of the program. Committee members determined early on that the program would be based on the ANA Standards for Organized Nursing Services, known today as the ANA Scope and Standards for Nurse Administrators. The committee reviewed every single criterion within the ANA Standards for Organized Nursing Services to determine what was fundamental to nursing excellence. These fundamental criteria became the core criteria in the original Magnet program and had to be present for any organization to achieve nursing excellence. The core Magnet criteria were scored "yes" or "no" for achievement. The application ceased to move forward if one criterion was scored "no."

The committee also utilized two additional sources to design the program:

1) The National League for Nursing, the source of the language of "verify, clarify, and amplify," and

2) ANCC for the accreditation process for continuing education units.

These models had been successfully implemented and contributed greatly to the infrastructure development of the Magnet program.

The committee completed the design in about 4 months, just in time for Fran Harpine, the newly hired Magnet director, to take the helm. Fran was the first permanent Magnet employee, even though she was only part-time, and was directed to implement the committee design.

In February 1993, the phone rang again. This time it was Marie Reid explaining that Fran had left her position. The ANCC still hoped to launch the Magnet program that summer, if at all possible, and needed Mary's help to do it. Mary had only been a faculty member at the University of Maryland School of Nursing for about a month but felt that Marie was the kind of person you did not turn down. Mary also had a real interest in seeing this program go forward, because she considered it "vital to the future of nursing." She was given the good and bad news about her situation. *The good news:* "You can use the ANCC office and work with an administrative assistant, but only on Saturdays because you will need to borrow someone else's desk." *The bad news:* "There is no budget and the ANCC finances are already stretched thin."

It was to be a team of two: Mary and Stephen Snell, who served as the administrative assistant. Their first priorities were developing manuals, one set for appraisers and another for applicants; creating bylaws for the commission; selecting and training appraisers; and planning a pilot study. Mary and Steve worked together each Saturday in 1993 from February until August to accomplish these goals.

To identify qualified appraiser candidates, the ANCC sent out a call through the state nurses associations. In October 1993, the first 10 appraisers were appointed and trained so they could evaluate pilot study applications. In early 2004, another 10 appraisers were appointed, and together these 20 individuals evaluated applications submitted after the program was opened to all facilities. Accurate records of these 20 individuals are not available, but the following nurses have been verified as members of this pioneer group: Joan M. Caley, RN, MS, CS, CNAA; Sheila P. Engelbardt,

PhD, RN, CNA; Phyllis E. Ethridge, RN, MS, CNAA, FAAN; Frances T. Feldsine, RN, MSN, CNAA; Larry F. Hepner, RN, MSN; Helen Hoesing, PhD, RN, FACHE, CNAA; Anne G. Jones, RN, MS; Jeanette S. Matrone, PhD, RN; Dorothea Milbrandt, RN, MSN; Catherine E. Neuman, RN, MSN, CNAA; E. Carol Polifroni, PhD, RN; and V. Anne Scott, RN, MSN, CS, CNA. The appraisers were trained during a 1-day session held in Washington, DC, at ANCC headquarters. Mary was the instructor, and the day was packed with information. There were no funds for additional training time, although this would have been Mary's preference. She recalls the angst of developing a completely new program with no history to guide the process. She has always espoused that the appraisers were "very committed and brave—true pioneers." They were flying by the seat of their pants, but they had enough professional expertise to know nursing excellence when they saw it.

In the latter part of 1993, a letter went out to the original 41 Magnet hospitals, now called "reputational Magnets," thanking them for their contribution and commitment to the Magnet spirit and offering them the opportunity to reaffirm their status in the new program before other organizations were given the chance to participate. Not one hospital responded with any interest in participating in a formal Magnet designation process. Thus, in January 1994, the ANCC asked reputational Magnets to stop using the term "Magnet designation." The organizations were told they could indicate they were one of the original 41, but they could not advertise they were "Magnet" unless formally designated under the new program criteria.

THE PILOT STUDY

Mary designed a pilot study that used a random stratified sampling technique based on the five bed-size categories used by the American Hospital

Association. One state from each of the four time zones—Washington (Pacific Standard Time), New Mexico (Mountain Standard Time), Alabama (Central Standard Time), and Massachusetts (Eastern Standard Time)—was randomly selected as a pilot study site. Three waves of invitations were sent to hospitals falling into each bed-size sampling cell by sampled state. Once an invitation was accepted, the cell was closed in that state. Some cells were never filled with a participating hospital. This gave the Magnet program an idea of what size facilities would be interested in the recognition award. The pilot revealed that hospitals with 300 or more beds were the primary market. This has remained the case even after a decade of Magnet experience, and Mary hypothesizes that a contributing factor may be that larger organizations have more resources to support the necessary infrastructure. One of the carrots held out for hospital participation in the pilot study was a waiver of application fees. The hospitals were not even required to pay for the appraiser expenses if the application advanced to a site visit. This was essentially a nursing excellence consultation at no cost.

Four applications were submitted for the pilot study. Only the University of Washington Medical Center scored high enough on the written application to earn a site visit. The three hospitals that did not pass were offered a site visit for the purpose of appraiser training, and one hospital agreed. The appraisers worked in teams of two, so this meant eight appraisers conducted a document review and four appraisers gained site-visit experience. This was deemed to be adequate evaluation to gauge if the program process allowed the opportunity for appraisers to determine the presence or absence of nursing excellence within the hospital setting.

Ultimately, the University of Washington Medical Center passed the ANCC vote and was the first Magnet-designated organization under the pilot study. In January 1994, the ANCC and the Magnet program staff—

Mary and Steve—believed the program was ready to launch and publicly announced that applications were welcome. The ANCC still had no funds for the program but did commit to hire one full-time person specifically for the Magnet program. By this time, Mary had been appointed the Magnet project consultant, which essentially functioned as a part-time director, spending at least one day during the week in the ANCC office. She knew she had reached a new status when she was provided with voicemail.

The internal debate at the Magnet program office at the time was, "Who is the market?" Some believed the market was the hospital CEO; others thought it was the CNO. After much debate, there was consensus that the CNO had to be the market, and it was through this role influence that Magnet would flourish or not.

THE LAUNCH AND ASCENT OF THE MAGNET PROGRAM

The first applicant under the official Magnet program was Hackensack University Medical Center in New Jersey. The CNO, Antoinette (Toni) Fiore, RN, MA, confirmed for the Magnet program office that the market was indeed the CNO, as she had sold her CEO on the concept. Toni had watched the 41 hospitals in the original study and closely followed the progress of the Magnet pilot program study. According to Mary, Toni wanted to be a part of this club and was waiting in the wings to submit the document.

Toni appointed Stephanie Goldberg, RN, MSN, as the Hackensack Magnet project coordinator. Stephanie and her team had spent most of 1993 compiling the application information in anticipation of the program going live. She had contacted ANCC to obtain the proposed Magnet criteria and conducted a comprehensive gap analysis of the organization.

Stephanie remembers that from the beginning, the purpose of the Magnet journey at Hackensack was to integrate a framework of work environment success, not to collect an award. Magnet became the Hackensack operational framework long before the application was submitted.

In 1994, when the call for Magnet applications went out, Hackensack was ready. The team submitted 14 3-inch notebooks of documentation representing the systems and infrastructure that Hackensack believed met or exceeded Magnet requirements. The appraisal team was Fran Feldsine and Anne Scott. Hackensack scored high enough on the written application that the facility earned a 3-day site visit. In 1995, Hackensack became the first Magnet-designated hospital under the official program, but second behind the University of Washington in the history of designation.

Many would acknowledge that Hackensack was the first to put the Magnet program on the map. The medical center engaged in a huge advertising campaign that told consumers and healthcare providers in New Jersey that Magnet status set the bar for patient-care excellence. According to Mary, Hackensack publicly trumpeted the receipt of Magnet in a manner that caught fire in New Jersey, and every CEO began to pay attention. It was rumored that CEOs began to pressure CNOs to make Magnet part of their strategic goals. The New Jersey market driver was reversed from the original CNO assumption as a result of the highly competitive nature of the state's healthcare leadership. Magnet designation had raised the stakes, and no hospital wanted to be left behind. Today, New Jersey has more Magnet-designated hospitals than any other state—the power of healthy competition and remarkable outcomes.

Stephanie says the Hackensack nursing division became a mentoring factory, with more than 30 healthcare organizations seeking information and requesting site visits during the first year after the facility received the Magnet designation. Hackensack developed a marketing and mentoring committee run by staff nurses to manage the demand and to showcase nursing "the Hackensack way." Nurse leaders from Hackensack were presenting nationally on the Magnet framework, sending the message that the program was not an award but a way of doing business. Magnet principles were the fabric of the organizational decision-making. The Hackensack data were compelling—no agency nurses, nurse turnover in the single-digit range, few nurse vacancies, and high-quality outcomes—all during a nursing shortage. Nurse executives from around the country were watching the outcomes of "building to Magnet," and the news was encouraging.

Toni became a Magnet commissioner and Stephanie became a Magnet appraiser. Living the experience had created believers, and they were giving back to the profession. According to Stephanie, Magnet not only created a strong work environment within hospitals but also effectively created a generation of nurse executives committed to principles of excellence without compromise. She comments that "it wouldn't matter if my organization was applying for Magnet; I incorporate Magnet principles into every aspect of my job. It is the only way I know how to lead. Magnet has endured the test of a decade with consistent results. How can you ignore that?"

The same competitive spirit that ignited New Jersey spread to Florida as Baptist Hospital of Miami (designated in 1998) and James A. Haley Veterans Hospital (designated in 2001) began to promote the significance of Magnet status in their state and across the nation. Shortly after its designation, Saint Joseph's Hospital of Atlanta (designated in 1995) began holding Magnet conferences in Atlanta to educate others on the application process. Mary remembers attending one of the early Atlanta conferences and was amazed that there were hundreds of attendees very interested in learning more about Magnet nursing. She spoke with Carolyn Lewis, executive director of the ANCC, about hosting an annual conference. Saint Joseph's then stepped away graciously, acknowledging that the work of hosting an event of this size needed to be shared with other Magnet colleagues. Mary gives Saint Joseph's a lot of credit for conceptualizing the conference and carrying the early developmental burden.

Growing Pains

In 1996, the Magnet program encountered an unexpected roadblock: the union. An applicant hospital in Virginia had submitted its documentation, received a site visit, and was designated Magnet by the commission. Carolyn Lewis, ANCC executive director at the time, announced that the hospital had been awarded Magnet status. The Virginia Nurses Association, acting as the nurses' collective bargaining agent, challenged the Magnet process. The Virginia applicant hospital had a labor board violation on record. The union leadership challenged that if Magnet represented a superior work environment, why was there an adjudicated labor violation? On 5 April 1996, the Magnet process came to a screeching halt while an in-depth program evaluation was undertaken.

The program remained in hiatus for nearly 14 months. No new applications were accepted, and the two hospitals in progress were put on hold.

This was a defining and healthy period for the Magnet program. It allowed the program to step back and refine processes, as well as establish systems to enhance greater program rigor. In late 1997, the Magnet program reopened. The decision had been made to hire a permanent Magnet director, Jennifer Matthews. She held a dual director role for Magnet and the accreditation program. Mary could no longer hold a full-time faculty position and manage the growing demands of Magnet. She became a

Magnet appraiser in 1998 and has remained active in providing guidance as the program has evolved.

The resource commitment to grow the Magnet program was hampered by the trickle of applications that came in the first 7 years. From 1994-2000, there were a total of 22 Magnet designations, including the hiatus in 1996. However, between 2001 and August 2004, designations more than quadrupled in just half the years, with 93 new designations. Today, early in 2007, there are more than 238 Magnet organizations—the top 4% of nursing organizations in the United States—and more than 260 organizations are in the Magnet application pipeline for review (ANCC, personal communication, August 2006). The Magnet program office staff has grown to 11, and the appraiser pool is now 167 strong.

Not every organization is motivated to or capable of creating a Magnet work environment. Linda Aiken's contemporary research indicates that 20% of hospitals have characteristics similar to Magnet hospitals, suggesting that about 20% could qualify for Magnet recognition (Aiken, personal communication, September 2006). She has spoken about the "tipping point," where what is now judged to be an excellent work environment will be the norm in the future, and Magnet recognition will set a higher bar. Linda further states that "if 20% of hospitals and perhaps as few as 10% attain Magnet recognition, the tipping point will have been reached for the current standards."

The attention given to the Magnet movement has been aided by health-care journals focused on quality, by schools of nursing encouraging students to seek supportive work environments, and by nurse leaders traveling the globe presenting on the power of Magnet in their own organizations. The commitment to the Magnet journey has been noticed and has reached a fever pitch in many U.S. states.

SUMMARY

Dr. David Satcher, former U.S. surgeon general, once said, "It is important to dream BIG dreams … because those dreams may not end with you." Maggie McClure, Muriel Poulin, Marg Sovie, and Mabel Wandelt had big dreams that became reality in a program to sustain and expand their study findings. Mary Tilbury and her pioneering colleagues had big dreams. These dreams have created a paradigm shift that has empowered direct-care nurses, demanded visionary nursing leadership, embedded data-driven decision-making, facilitated interdisciplinary relationships, and placed nursing in the center of quality initiatives. The beneficiary of these big dreams is the rare trifecta in healthcare—superior patient, nurse, and organizational outcomes.

REFERENCES

Aiken, L.H., Havens, D.S., & Sloane, D.M. (2000). The magnet nursing services recognition program—A comparison of two groups of magnet hospitals. *American Journal of Nursing,* 100(26).

Bleich, M., Hewlett, P., Santos, S., Rice, R., Cox, K., & Richmeier, S. (2003). Analysis of the nursing workforce crisis: A call to action. *American Journal of Nursing, 103*(4), 66-74.

Havens, D.S., & Aiken, L.H. (1999). Shaping systems to promote desired outcomes—The magnet hospital model. *Journal of Nursing Administration, 29*(14).

Health Resources and Services Administration, Bureau of Health Professions, National Center for Health Workforce Analysis (2002). *Projected supply, demand and shortages of registered nurses: 2000-2020.* Retrieved May 3, 2004, from http://bhpr.hrsa.gov/healthworkforce/reports/rnproject/default.htm

Kimball, B., & O'Neil, E. (2002). Health care's human crisis: The American nursing shortage. *Health Workforce Solutions for the Robert Wood Johnson Foundation.* Princeton, NJ: Robert Wood Johnson.

Kramer, M., & Schmalenberg, C. (1988). Magnet hospitals: Institutes of excellence. *Journal of Nursing Administration, 18*(1,2).

McClure, M., & Hinshaw, A. (2002). *Magnet hospitals revisited: Attraction and retention of professional nurses.* Washington, DC: American Nurses Publishing.

McClure, M., Poulin, M., Sovie, M., & Wandelt, M (1983). *Magnet hospitals: Attraction and retention of professional nurses.* Washington, DC: American Nurses Association.

Needleman, J., Buerhaus, P., Mattke, P., Stewart, M., & Zelevinsky, K. (2002). Nurse-staffing level and the quality of care in hospitals. *The New England Journal of Medicine, 346*(22), 1715-1722.

Reilly, P. (2003). Help wanted, desperately. *Modern Healthcare.* 24-25, 32-34.

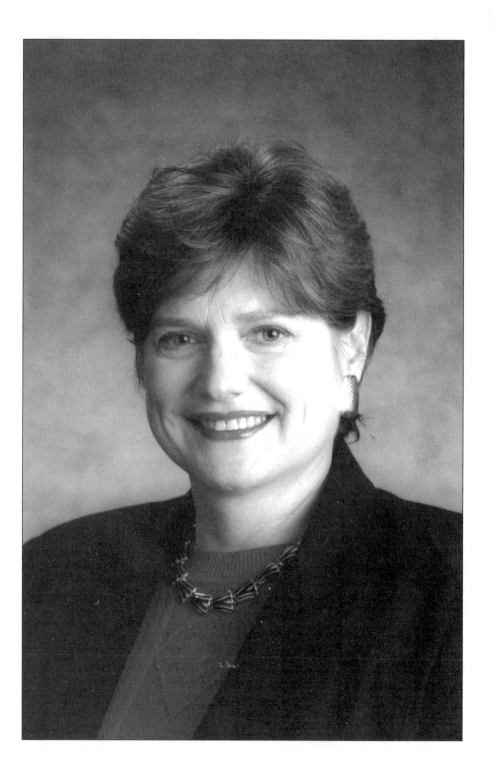

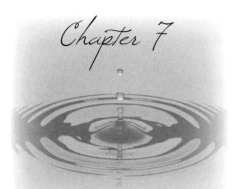

MARLA ELIZABETH SALMON

If there is one thing I could inject in every young nurse, it would be the notion that you should approach possibilities with a "why not" attitude, rather than finding a million reasons for not going forward.

—Marla Salmon

Marla Salmon, ScD, RN, FAAN, is an international ambassador for nursing, public health, and healthcare. In 1995, she was a member of the United States Delegation for the 48th World Health Assembly of the World Health Organization (WHO), and she chaired the Global Advisory Group on Nursing and Midwifery for the WHO from 1997 to 2000. Marla founded the Lillian Carter Center of International Nursing, which she and President Carter dedicated in 2001, and led the development of the biennial Global Health Partners Forums and Government Chief Nursing Officers Institutes, which now bring together senior government leaders from more than 100 countries.

As a 1972-73 Fulbright Scholar at the University of Cologne, Marla studied national health insurance and public health in Germany. She also spent time in Kuwait learning about that country's model of universal healthcare. She is renowned as an expert in international nursing workforce issues.

Marla held the position of chief nurse of the United States in her 1991-97 role as director of the Division of Nursing for the Department of Health and Human Services. As a fellow of the W.K. Kellogg National Fellowship Program from 1984-87, she devoted her project to women's international leadership development. She was elected to the Institute of Medicine for the National Academy of Sciences in 1996 and has been a member of the board of trustees for the Robert Wood Johnson Foundation since 2002. Marla was also a member of the White House Task Force on Health Care Reform in 1993 and chaired the National Advisory Council on Nurse Education and Practice from 1991-97.

This distinguished portfolio of professional accomplishments, as lofty as it may seem, only partially reflects who Marla really is and what has motivated her remarkable leadership journey. She describes her life as unconventional. Working side by side with migrant workers picking fruit in the fields of northern California—"witnessing social injustice" firsthand—inspired her devotion to public health issues. Marla says she wasn't a conventionally good student, yet she earned a double degree in college. Today, she is dean of the School of Nursing at Emory University. She holds a second-degree black belt in tae kwon do, mastering its significant physical and psychological requirements. More impressively, she has repeatedly overcome Capitol Hill roadblocks, earning the President's Meritorious Executive Award and other key federal recognitions that are equivalent to a third-degree black belt in leadership.

As a leader, Marla does not need to get out of the box, because for her the box never existed. She sees the world in multiple dimensions when some see it as flat. Marla has the rare ability to focus on an object yet still capture the foreground and background in a way that explains the entire picture.

Marla has been the translator and bridge builder among disciplines, industries, and nations for solutions to healthcare problems. Her colleagues say that Marla has pushed nursing's boundaries and introduced nursing to a bigger world through her leadership.

Quite simply, Marla is an international pathfinder for the health of people worldwide, particularly those who are most vulnerable. She says that "doing the right thing is an important part of defining who I am." She is a leader who has committed her career to doing the right thing for people, with remarkable results.

EARLY INFLUENCES

Marla was born 2 May 1949 in Vermillion, South Dakota, to Everett Lloyd Salmon and Marceline Louise Adamson Salmon. The second of four children, she has an older brother, Barry, a younger sister, Jana, and a younger brother, Jared. Everett was in medical school when Marla was born, and Marceline was a practicing nurse. (Interestingly, Marceline worked for a physician who was the father of Dr. Judith Ryan, executive director of ANA for many years and a nursing leader herself.) By the time Marla entered kindergarten, the Salmon family had moved to Sebastopol, California, a rural community of approximately 5,000 people about 60 miles north of San Francisco. The community's two claims to fame were that it was the home of Morning Star—the nation's first commune—and Charles Schultz, the cartoonist.

Her parents and the community were both influential in shaping Marla's integrity, vision, work ethic, compassion, and societal conscience and commitment. Marla describes herself as a hippie during this period of time. Her high school years were filled with "enormous turmoil and societal realities" that marked her life with sadness and responsibility. During the Vietnam War, community drug and alcohol use escalated, leaving a wake of warlike casualties in her own rural community. "My brother and I lost count of the number of friends and acquaintances who died in car crashes, in Vietnam, through suicide and even homicide," she says. "The times and the place were a powerful equation that resulted in many tragedies."

In April of 1963, Marla's very close friend, Kristine (Kris) Kalbaugh, was a passenger in a one-car accident that took her life. Marla poignantly describes how Kris inspired and shaped her life. Kris *believed* that one day she would become a U.S. ambassador, and everyone around her believed it too. Marla laughs as she shares, "I didn't even know what an ambassador was." Kris was worldly and confident with big dreams that appeared both real and attainable, Marla says, and she inspired Marla to "see a bigger world and to reach for more than I believed possible."

A close friendship with neighbor Kathy Ito also fueled Marla's connection to the larger world. Kathy was a first-generation Japanese-American. During World War II, her parents had been confined to internment camps in Colorado, where Kathy's siblings were born. Through her close friendship with Kathy from kindergarten through their freshman year in college, Marla was exposed early to Japanese culture and family life, and she also witnessed the prejudice and "otherness" that Kathy and her closest sibling, Millie, endured during their childhood.

Marla's parents also had a tremendous influence on her. Her parents worked hard and focused on the positive. Her mother was one of five siblings born in southeastern Missouri, where they lived in poverty throughout her childhood. Marceline and her brother and sisters were raised by her grandmother. Her father supported the family first as a moonshiner and later as a hobo during the Great Depression. (Marceline's mother was so overwhelmed by the responsibility of caring for five young children that she abandoned the family.) Marceline grew up wandering barefoot in the forests of the Ozarks, wearing neatly sewn flour sacks for clothing. Many days, food was scarce. Marceline and her siblings also endured the bigotry associated with their mixed-race (Native American-French/Scotch-Irish) heritage. And, as a young child, she witnessed the horrific lynching of a black man—a horror that stayed with her throughout her life. Marceline's childhood embedded in her many lessons about social inequities that "connected her life to fighting for social justice," Marla says. As with so many poor people of that era, Marceline's opportunity came about because of a Federal program. At age 18, she boarded a bus to Chicago to join the Cadet Nurse Program at Mt. Sinai Hospital School of Nursing—a major turning point in her life.

Serendipity brought Marla's father and mother together. Everett was in Chicago on a brief furlough from service in the Army during World War II when he found Marceline's wallet in a bar where some of the nursing school girls had gone for a drink. He called her with the discovery and offered to return the wallet on the condition that she would join him for a drink. After almost a year of correspondence, Everett and Marceline married on Christmas Day, 1944.

Much like Marceline, Everett grew up with meager resources. He spent his childhood in Spencer, South Dakota, with a more conventional family structure on a Dust Bowl farm, where he and his three sisters worked with their parents to make a living. As a young man of 17, Everett joined the Civilian Conservation Corps, a federal program aimed at Depression-era unemployed young men. After being discharged from the Army, he decided he would devote his life to medicine. Everett attended medical school at the University of South Dakota and the University of Iowa on the GI Bill. Both

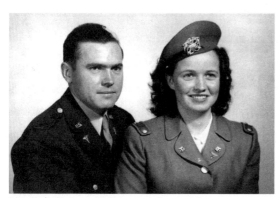

MARLA'S PARENTS, EVERETT LLOYD SALMON AND MARCELINE LOUISE ADAMSON SALMON.

Marceline and Everett had faced adversity and survived challenges, and they grew into compassionate, hopeful adults. Very different in personality and overall approach to life, Marceline and Everett were both strong-willed, intelligent role models who always made room for conflict of ideas.

Her parents, particularly her mother, wanted the Salmon children to "understand the lives of others and develop empathy for them," Marla says. From a very early age, her mother insisted that the children pick berries in the fields with migrant workers and pick up apples and plums with the ground crew. She wanted them to live the experience of others and understand how social inequity feels. "I absolutely fell in love with the migrant workers," Marla says, "and could not understand, nor could anyone ever explain it to me, how any group of people could be treated so horribly." Her father and mother were working side by side building a medical practice in the community, and many of her father's patients were migrant workers. Like so many country doctors of that era, Everett received agricultural goods or farm animals as payment for services, if he received any payment at all.

Both Everett and Marceline were activists who were committed to building a community that took care of all of its people. Together they led in starting a "halfway house" for drug-addicted youth. Everett led efforts to attract young physicians to the area and to improve education in the county. Marceline reached out to others in more personal ways, quietly helping poor and disadvantaged people.

Leadership Lesson Learned

Marla believes that one of nursing's leadership flaws is that leaders often do not show up. With obvious frustration, she posits that "nursing leadership talks about wanting the door open, and then when we have the invitation there is no one to walk through it." She believes, "If we are committed, if we do care, if we do believe that something needs to change, and we want to live by what we believe, then we can't be absent."

Marla remembers her mother as a woman who communicated in short blurbs that packed a powerful message, such as "do the right thing" and "stand up for what you believe." From her mother's wise words, Marla says, grew her own sense of commitment about being where the point of influence is to shape outcomes, not in terms of status where the point of decision is, but where the point of action is.

Marla believes that we create our "coloring book" during the early years of our lives. She explains that in our coloring book, we create the outlines of who we will become. Occasionally, we encounter an experience that is made possible because "at one point we have created space in our imagination for this to become possible." She is convinced that early exposures are extremely important and predictive of leadership outcomes to some extent. Our imagination is fueled by experiences, by what real people around us did or said to create an impression and expand our imagination. Marla concludes that "my imagination of the possible 'me' became who I am—it created my individual coloring book which I continue to color—sometimes within and often outside of the lines."

Her imagination was certainly augmented by growing up in a family of "right-brain thinkers." Her family is very creative, and at times she found they were a little out of synch with the rest of the world. Marla has always loved music—singing and playing instruments—and is a talented artist. Her older brother, Barry, is a musician and composer who teaches communications at The New School, a university in New York City; her sister, Jana, is a poet and journalist; and her younger brother, Jared, studied opera at the Royal College of Music in London where he pursued his singing career.

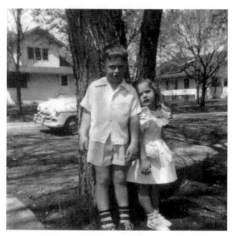

MARLA, AROUND THE AGE OF 3, WITH BROTHER BARRY, ON A VISIT TO SOUTH DAKOTA.

Socially, she was raised with a distinct distaste for cliques and even quit the Girl Scouts because it felt too "we versus they." Marla says she could never understand why someone would create a barrier between groups, rather than examine the entire circle, and notes that there were no gender differences in her neighborhood gang. A self-described tomboy, Marla played all sports, including baseball and powder puff football. Marla believes that her early comfort with "the guys" shaped her "ability to relate to men in a very constructive and collegial way." She appreciated their thinking and approach, which made it easy to be a part of their game and not to feel intimidated.

When Marla was entering the fourth grade, she and her brother Barry were selected for an experimental educational program that they both believed was for kids who had learning problems. She had not been a "conventionally good student" and did not understand her inability to perform at the highest level. The program was a free-learning format where the student selected topics of interest, and teachers constructed opportunities for learning. For example, Marla selected opera and part of the learning experience included a trip to the opera; she also chose space travel and got to meet with a scientist involved in the space program. She remained in this program until junior high school and did not find out until many years later that it was a program for gifted students. Marla laughs at her own intellectual development, speculating that while she is intelligent, it is also

quite likely that she has attention deficit disorder, which she thinks has actually helped her navigate the multiple demands of her life. She also notes that she is "blessed or cursed with a conceptual mind."

Marla is quick to admit that she was never really off track because the "track was never very much a part of who I was." She remembers that she never wanted to become anything but always wanted to do things that mattered—she wanted to make the world better. Her leadership career choices, she says, have been "devoted to things that fundamentally haunt you, such as the shoes

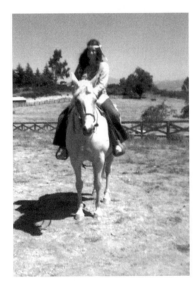

MARLA, HORSEBACK RIDING AT HER FAMILY'S HOME IN NORTHERN CALIFORNIA.

on the beach of Sri Lanka after the tsunami or the faces of the migrant worker children." Her positions as chief nursing officer for the United States, delegate for the World Health Organization, and dean of the School of Nursing at Emory University were not her dreams, but rather have been her vehicles for making a difference in the world.

Her mother also coached the Salmon children to explore life. Marceline would often tell them they needed to leave their small community when

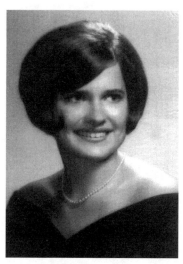

MARLA IN HIGH SCHOOL GRADUATION PHOTO.

they finished high school, noting that girls there "either got pregnant, got married, or got out." As a result, Marla and her siblings were prepared by their parents to leave their small rural community when they reached 18 so they could discover a larger world. They knew home was waiting for them when they had tales of adventure and personal growth to share with the rest of the Salmon clan. There was no fear of leaving because the excitement of going was so attractive—it was part of their life's coloring books.

GROWING THE 'WHY NOT' PHILOSOPHY

In 1967, Marla enrolled in the college of nursing at the University of Portland. She later picked up a double major, the second being in political science. This meant 5 years of long hours and hard work. Her parents paid her tuition, but Marla worked nights as a nursing assistant almost the entire time she was enrolled (a job she had during her high school years as well). She learned to function on very little sleep and gained energy from the experience. Marla was mentored by Vernia Jane Huffman—the dean of the School of Nursing at the University of Portland—who invested in Marla's success from their first encounter.

Marla met Dean Huffman during a pre-college interview, and the dean somehow perceived that Marla's academic record did not reflect her capabilities. Marla believes Dean Huffman became an early engine for the trajectory of her career. It was Dean Huffman who allowed Marla to pursue dual degrees in nursing and political science and helped her navigate the system to make this possible. She also approved Marla taking an extra heavy course load but held her accountable for her academic performance. And, she made it possible for Marla to pursue experiences in the international arena. Dean Huffman was always there to make sure that Marla was maximizing her academic experience. Marla is grateful for that gift, and it has motivated her to do the same for others.

Part of maximizing her experience included spending her sophomore year in Salzburg, Austria. A school friend had convinced her that studying overseas was a great idea. Initially, Marla thought she was applying for Australia, not understanding that she actually would be heading for Europe. Dean Huffman supported the request and in preparation for the travel, Marla studied German.

The German lessons turned out to be very useful, as Marla embedded herself into the culture and became fluent in Austrian German. In her spare time, Marla hitchhiked around Europe and experienced Austria from a local perspective, becoming very close friends with a rural Austrian family. She was captivated by the phenomenal international experience. Her political science and healthcare training were preparing her well for the international healthcare arena, and she was identifying future possibilities.

When Marla returned to Portland, she remained determined to explore international issues. She focused her political science studies in the

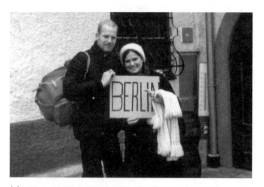

MARLA AND A FELLOW STUDENT HITCH-
HIKING TO BERLIN IN 1968.

international arena and cultivated a particular interest in the Middle East and Latin America. During her senior year, she became interested in the role of the World Health Organization and wrote to seek permission to attend one of its major assemblies. Much to her surprise, the public information officer from WHO, Gino Levy, wrote back, inviting her to observe the upcoming Switzerland session. Marla asked Dean Huffman for special permission to take incompletes in her course work. It meant a more difficult workload for her later, but Marla was convinced this was a once in a lifetime opportunity.

Marla remembers the event clearly. It was May, and she sat in the upper gallery gazing down at the U.S. delegation as world leaders discussed the cholera pandemic. She was amazed by the enormity of the process and the influence of this body of healthcare leaders. This experience became part of Marla's coloring book. Little did she know that 26 years later, she herself would be sitting behind the U.S. delegation sign for the 48th World Health Assembly as the only nurse on the team, staring up at the same gallery in which she had sat as an observer so many years earlier.

In some ways, good fortune reflects a habit of mind—a willingness to entertain different futures.

In her early 20s, Marla was developing a leadership philosophy around "why not," instead of falling prey to the paralysis of the "why" question. "If there is one thing I could inject in every young nurse, it would be the notion that you should approach possibilities with a 'why not' attitude, rather than finding a million reasons for not going forward," she says. "Burdening oneself with too many doubts or 'whys' can become a lifelong habit—a way of keeping one from doing things that are worthwhile. We should not squelch the sense of adventure—it is what makes futures better. A sense of adventure and discovery is a fundamental human characteristic that we see most vividly in children. Each of us should honor this and let it express itself in our-

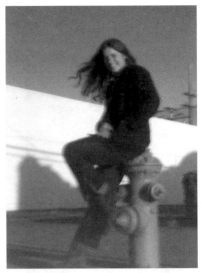

MARLA ON HER 21ST BIRTHDAY, IN SAN FRANCISCO, CALIFORNIA.

selves throughout our lives." Marla learned early on that some of her own greatest discoveries and opportunities resulted from asking the question "why not" and seeking support to reach for what seemed improbable.

Leadership Lesson Learned

Great opportunities may result from asking the question "why not" and seeking support to reach for what seems improbable.

Marla also believes that good fortune plays significantly in one's destiny. "I believe that luck truly is having the state of mind that allows you to recognize opportunity," she says. "If you are not attuned to possibilities and willing to explore them, your own opportunities will pass you by unnoticed. In some ways, good fortune reflects a habit of mind—a willingness to entertain different futures." Her good fortune was not limited to Dean

Huffman but also included Franz Gerbert, her German teacher before her Austria trip. "He knew what was better for me than I did, " she says. Mar-

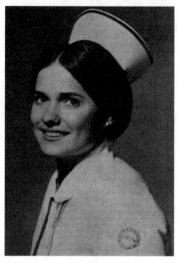

la was nearing graduation, and Franz suggested that she apply for a Fulbright Scholarship. Not knowing what a Fulbright Scholar was, she respectfully ignored the suggestion. He continued to insist that she was qualified and that it would be an important experience for her career. Marla applied at the very last minute, living up to her emerging "why not" philosophy, and was amazed and delighted when she was accepted—making history as one of the first nurses receiving this distinction.

MARLA IN HER NURSING
SCHOOL GRADUATION PHOTO.

FULBRIGHT SCHOLAR EXPERIENCE

In 1972, after working as a migrant health nurse, Marla began her Fulbright Scholar experience at the University of Cologne in Cologne, Germany. Her area of study was national health insurance and public health in Germany, along with the possible application of these concepts and programs to developing nations. The Germans "thought it was very important for people to have healthcare coverage and be recognized as a society in which health and healthcare are a right and an entitlement," Marla says. "They realized very early on—in the late 1800s—that a physically healthy Germany is a financially healthy Germany and took a proactive stance to protect the health of its citizens."

Marla became a student of the German methodology of striking a balance between universal access to healthcare and financial solvency. She learned about the responsibility shared between employers and the German government in meeting the universal healthcare commitment. Marla observed that the notion of a social insurance program came into existence in 1889 when then-Chancellor Otto von Bismarck declared that Germany should provide services for the people that serve Germany. Nearly a century later, Marla was witnessing the processes and outcomes of this cultural commitment. The success in Germany inspired Marla to consider alternatives to the U.S. public health agenda. Little did she know that 20 years later she would be a member of the White House Task Force on Health Care Reform.

During her Fulbright Scholar experience, Marla learned several lessons unrelated to healthcare. She was a lone American, female, and a nurse in a country in which nursing was one of the lowliest occupations. She was living in a German, predominantly male, medical school dormitory. This was at a time when the U.S. involvement in Vietnam was continuing, and Europeans were highly critical of American engagement. "Germans were demonstrating against the U.S. bombing of Vietnam, Cambodia, and Laos at a time when the United States was denying its role there—America was at one of its ugliest moments," Marla says. She learned what it felt like to be an isolated minority, which made the experience "very interesting and very tough in many ways." Marla formed connections with other foreign students, some of whom were political exiles and refugees from other countries. Virtually all her friends were activists, and through them she learned more

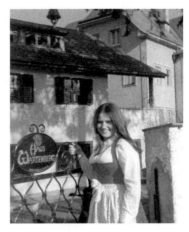

MARLA DRESSED IN SOUTHERN GERMAN/AUSTRIAN ATTIRE DURING HER EUROPEAN YEARS.

about political persecution and injustice and found a new sense of social understanding. She also likely earned a place in the voluminous FBI files on Americans abroad at that time.

As part of her Fulbright experience, Marla also spent time in Kuwait studying its healthcare system. Kuwait had a cultural philosophy of universal access to everything, but the challenge was defining citizens with rights versus non-citizens without rights. A large portion of Kuwait's labor force was imported from Palestine and Jordan, which set the stage for an emerging minority. Marla believes that learning about labor market dynamics of an emerging minority was an important component of her Fulbright experience. Interestingly, the situation in Kuwait mirrored her migrant worker experience and also informed her current involvement in global health workforce debates.

For the first time, she saw herself as a budding intellectual.

The Fulbright Scholar experience provided Marla the chance to see herself in a broader context. For the first time, she saw herself as a budding intellectual. She was able to understand international issues and contextualize nursing and healthcare. Marla applied her political science education to healthcare policy development and had great hope that she could apply some of the knowledge from Germany and Kuwait to U.S. policy development.

Marla believes that being selected as a Fulbright Scholar provided her with numerous leadership opportunities. This exclusive recognition opened many doors in future years and placed her in a world of distinguished leaders. She believes that her selection as a Fulbright Scholar allowed her to move from a baccalaureate degree to doctoral studies at The Johns Hopkins University School of Hygiene and Public Health. On her way to Germany, Marla interviewed with Dr. Alice Gifford for the master's program in public health. Alice convinced her to convert her application to the health policy doctoral program. During that interview, Marla also met Dr. Vicente Navarro, an expert in international health policy, who provided a guided reading program for Marla during her Fulbright experience.

Marla believes her Fulbright Scholar achievement was an important contribution to her acceptance into the doctoral program. She learned the leverage of applying for and being accepted into programs of distinction.

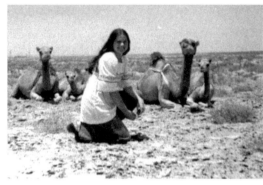

MARLA WITH CAMELS DURING HER STUDIES IN KUWAIT IN 1973.

CODIFYING HER LEADERSHIP

In 1973, Marla returned to the United States to begin her doctoral program. She accepted a position to develop a patient advocacy program in the emergency department (ED) of The Johns Hopkins Hospital (JHH). Her boss was director of the Department of Emergency Medicine, Dr. Donald Gann, a Quaker trauma surgeon with a strong commitment to social justice. Marla found a good match and mentor in Dr. Gann and an opportunity to apply nursing and leadership skills and make a difference in the lives of vulnerable people. Additionally, the hospital was located directly across the street from the School of Hygiene and Public Health, which created a geographically and occupationally seamless world for Marla. "It was through my studies that I grew to understand the policy and organizational aspects of leadership and through my emergency department experience that I actually codified it for myself," she says.

After nearly 1 year as a patient advocate, Marla assumed the nursing director position in the JHH ED at the young age of 24. This was a leadership challenge that pushed her to the limits of her abilities. The JHH ED is located in east Baltimore, which was often a war zone of violence and crime, with a seemingly endless volume of patients. It was not uncommon to have a variety of patients who were in police custody while receiving care. The ED staff had a close working relationship with the Baltimore Police Department, but on occasion they disagreed on methods of patient control.

One defining moment in her leadership development began when Marla observed a situation in a remote hallway in the ED. There, she discovered a group of five police officers beating a small-framed man as he clutched something in his hand. The police erroneously believed he was concealing a weapon and were using all means possible to "take him down." Marla approached the group of officers and had to physically insert herself into the fray to stop the abuse, while demanding the officers' names and badge numbers. In this touchstone moment, she exhibited courage she did not know she possessed. She stepped in and confronted authority figures while facing potential physical harm, because it was the right thing to do.

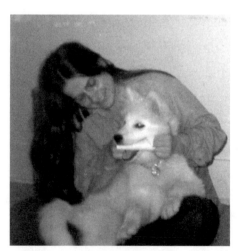

MARLA WITH NIMBRA IN HER APARTMENT IN PORTLAND.

The second defining moment came from the leadership of someone she respected, Bill Albers. Bill was a police officer who occasionally provided security in the JHH ED on his off hours. He was one of the staff favorites because he took the time to get to know everyone and understood the culture of the ED and the Baltimore Police Department. Bill was instrumental in helping Marla develop an understanding with the Baltimore

Police Department that officers would only be allowed in patient care areas if they had official business. Prior to this time, some officers would wander aimlessly and often create additional chaos in an environment that was already teeming with activity. This was a major culture shift and not a popular decision. Bill became a champion of the change. According to Marla, "he characterized the definition of a leader of principle," and she had great admiration for his abilities.

Leadership Lesson Learned

Discovering that she could step in during an abusive and frightening situation was an important gift to her leadership. Marla is clear that you have to pick your battles, "but it is very important that when you encounter things that aren't right, you must weigh in on them. Leadership is learning how to do that effectively."

Marla had established a rule that all policemen must lock their guns in the medicine cabinet prior to entering the patient care area for safety of the staff and patients. After she resigned her ED directorship, this rule was rescinded. Tragically, Bill was later shot with his own gun as he attempted to restrain a psychiatric patient. He died shortly after from his wounds. Nearly 30 years later, Marla has difficulty speaking about the unnecessary loss of a great leader—driving home again the commitment to both courage and creation of a context in which others can be safe and protected.

No matter how inconvenient, irritating, and irrelevant safety guidelines may seem, they have an important purpose. A leader

A leader must have the courage to stick with what is right.

must have the courage to stick with what is right. Another lesson driven home in the emergency department is that ultimately, the boss is responsible—this cannot be handed off.

Marla experienced another life lesson in hospital operations during the first week of her ED directorship. One of the night supervisors discovered a nurse self-medicating with patient narcotics while on shift. When Marla reviewed his personnel file, she discovered numerous personnel actions (blue slips). That was astonishing, because three such actions were grounds for termination. One of his blue-slip warnings was reportedly for holding the ED head nurse in her office at gunpoint for 3 hours. In spite of his abusive record, he remained employed. Marla took responsibility for terminating him for diverting narcotics. Shortly thereafter, the terminated employee was spotted at the holiday party hunting for Marla with vengeance on his mind. She chuckled when remembering she had spent most of that evening in the bathroom to avoid becoming his next hostage or an ED trauma patient herself. From this and other emergency department experiences, Marla learned that other leaders' avoidance of difficult situations does not give you permission to sweep high-risk behaviors under the carpet. Marla advises leaders to prepare for collateral damage if possible, but to maintain the courage to lead for the greater good. Again, the most important consideration is protection of patients, families, and staff.

Despite many difficult situations in the ED, there were also unforgettable humorous moments. One such event was the day of "monkey business." The Blaylock primate research labs were located several floors above the ED. The monkeys mysteriously got loose one weekend and turned on every water faucet, flooding the capacity of the drains. Monkey feces backed up the ED drains, contaminating the entire department. Who would

have guessed that monkey business many floors above could instantaneous-
ly clear out an ED in a matter of minutes?

Another memorable event was when an employee sneaking a cigarette
break sat on the bathroom sink in an isolated area of the ED and snapped
it from the wall, causing flooding of the entire ED. After efforts were underway to correct the situation, Marla and another nurse hopped onto an
empty stretcher and jokingly made rowing motions as the water continued
to rise. On a stretcher nearby, a patient who had been experiencing deliri-
um tremors and hallucinations witnessed their antics and began captaining
his own boat in earnest. For a few moments,
their flotilla sailed on through gales of laughter. Marla is a great believer in humor to dif-
fuse stress and is adamant that "you have got
to find the fun in life."

*The Hopkins exposure
to scholarship taught
her how to think, write,
and debate.*

Her years at Hopkins were transformational, both personally and professionally, Marla says. She met and married David White in a garden on
the JHH grounds. David was an intern at Hopkins working "ridiculous
hours," and Marla was holding a full-time job and working on her dissertation. They welcomed their first child, Jessica, on 2 March 1977.

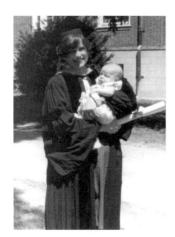
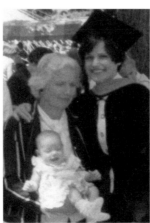

MARLA AT HER 1977
GRADUATION FROM THE
JOHNS HOPKINS UNIVERSITY
SCHOOL OF HYGIENE AND
PUBLIC HEALTH WITH HER
DOCTORATE IN HEALTH
POLICY. WITH HER IN THE
PHOTO ON THE LEFT IS
DAUGHTER JESSICA, BORN 2
MARCH 1977. TO THE LEFT,
SHE AND JESSICA POSE WITH
HER MOTHER MARCELINE.

Marla finished her doctoral dissertation and program requirements in 4 years, frantically balancing her studies, work, and family life. She recounts the many opportunities for leadership development during that time. Among these was her work with fellow students and faculty on the Maryland Health Plan, one of the first state comprehensive health plans. Marla learned that communication is an extremely important part of leadership. She credits her adviser, Dr. Barbara Starfield, for advancing her thinking and communication skills. "Barbara was merciless about producing a well-written, high-quality intellectual product," Marla says. She acknowledges she did not know how to write well prior to her doctoral experience. "Barbara would say I suffered from flowery expression and freight-train sentences," recalls Marla. She believes that clarity in thinking is the key to good writing and has noted that many unskilled writers figure out what they were thinking on the way to the end of a sentence. Marla learned the relationship between precision in writing and critical thinking. The former must precede the latter, she contends. Surrounded by a very bright group of students and professors, she learned how to go toe to toe and hold her own with the best in the business, which was an important part of her leadership development. The Hopkins exposure to scholarship taught her how to "think, research and discover, write, debate, and commit academically," which have all been great assets to her career.

Marla also learned that degrees are important but do not dictate intelligence or capacity. One of her mentors, Sam Shapiro, was a brilliant professor at the School of Hygiene and Public Health, yet he had earned only a bachelor's degree. Sam and another colleague, Dr. Geoffrey Gibson, provided Marla with the opportunity to write her dissertation research project, which became part of a major federal grant that helped to establish the Emergency Medical Service System for Maryland. Professor Shapiro left an indelible impression on Marla through his generosity of spirit, expertise, endorsement of students, and support for their development. He was immensely knowledgeable and his vote of confidence was an important affirmation for Marla. This brilliance without extensive education was consistent with the message of her childhood, as her mother, a diploma-educated nurse, was one of the wisest individuals she knew. She carries the life lesson that "an education is important, but not nearly as important as learning and wisdom."

Marla has learned throughout her development that education happens only when the learner takes responsibility, and that self-education is extremely important. She is concerned that in some doctoral programs, students learn a great deal of information but may not acquire the skill of learning to learn or the passion for discovery. The process of learning to learn allows for autonomous discovery beyond the formal academic setting. According to Marla, self-education is a sort of intellectual "breathing"—taking in information, insight, and knowledge on a continual basis as a sort of life force. It requires a commitment to challenging oneself and a love of discovery. Marla is a naturally curious person who is always seeking a more complete understanding of what is at work, which translates into going beyond the immediate explanation. She states it is essential "to follow the strings beyond the obvious answer to find the more fundamental drivers." When Marla walks into a meeting or decision-making forum, she works to learn all she can in advance—she sees the importance of taking time to observe, ask the relevant questions, and research the background. She also has a strong sense of what she wants to achieve and knows at least part of what her message will be prior to entering the room. Marla sees such forums as important learning opportunities, noting that observation and listening are wonderful vehicles for self-development.

Joining Academe

In August 1978, Marla accepted an assistant professor position in the School of Public Health at the University of Minnesota, teaching in an MPH public health nursing program and a nursing and patient care administration joint MSN/MHA program. She had gone through a lifetime of experiences at Johns Hopkins University and was ready to apply her degree in public health. Her husband had secured a residency at the University of Minnesota. Their son, Matthew, was born 19 July 1979, within a year of their arrival in Minnesota. When Matt was about a year old, Marla and David divorced after 6 years of marriage.

Work was both an anchor and challenge for Marla as she continued to grow and also grapple with her life circumstances. In 1980, Marla was asked to head the public health nursing program. She moved into this role during a particularly challenging time for both the university and the state of Minnesota. In 1980, the University of Minnesota entered into a consent decree with the federal courts to settle a sex discrimination lawsuit filed by faculty member Shyamala Rajender. The consent decree provided a long-term mechanism for reviewing charges of sex discrimination within the university, addressing more than 300 such complaints. Also during that time, the state was experiencing financial difficulties, and approximately 50% of Marla's budget at the School of Public Health was cut. As director of the Public Health Nursing Program, it was her responsibility to manage the impact of this massive budget cut. Her department had a disproportionately larger cut because there were fewer tenured faculty members—this meant that most of the public health nursing faculty could be discontinued, while tenured faculty salaries could not be modified in accordance with their status. The ultimate result of this circumstance was that several faculty members filed a complaint under the consent decree, claiming that tenure had been granted mostly to men and not women, leaving them vulnerable to losing their employment. Marla was a respondent in this case but fully understood their claim.

Shortly thereafter, a new dean arrived and Marla decided to step down from her director's position. She had recently been selected as a W.K. Kellogg national fellow and was devoting considerable time to her project. Almost immediately after Marla communicated her decision to return to her faculty role as an associate professor, the dean decided to reduce her salary. Marla had an agreement with the previous leadership that if she served her term and chose to step down, her salary would not be reduced. Additionally, in the history of the school, salary reduction after service had not been the practice. The new dean was not interested in her previous agreement but asked her to produce evidence that other salaries were untouched after stepping down. When she produced the evidence, he refused to change her salary back to its previous level and ignored the information she provided that detailed the consistent experience of nonreductions for male program directors and other key leaders. In short, Marla discovered that without exception, the salaries of men remained the same, and even increased, after they stepped down.

After a great deal of thought and advice from trusted colleagues, Marla concluded that while the salary reduction was relatively small, the principle was a major concern for her. The salary had become secondary to the overarching ethical considerations. With great reluctance, Marla filed a sex discrimination action against the University of Minnesota and the dean. This was a difficult decision, but the right thing to do for her. As she moved through this process, Marla sought the counsel of Patricia Mullen, then-director of equal opportunity and affirmative action for the university, who gave her some excellent advice. Marla recalls that Pat cautioned her to

It was so wrong on so many counts and was simply another symptom of a deep, underlying problem that needed to be addressed.

think very carefully about the choice to move forward on a complaint of this nature and to be very clear why she was choosing this path, because inevitably it would become personal and it would feel personal. Pat warned her that whether a person won or lost, there was a very high probability that he or she would become embittered by a process that was difficult at best. Marla recalls that Pat also advised her to find an outside coach who did not know her very well to serve as an anchor and compass through the process, helping to keep the process aligned with the real intent and meaning of the action. She went on to advise that the coach would help keep Marla out of the "hate game" that inevitably occurs.

Marla clearly understood that she could be wrecking her career, but this was a battle she could not back down from because "it was so wrong on so many counts and was simply another symptom of a deep, underlying problem that needed to be addressed." Ultimately, the case went before a review panel, where it was determined that Marla's allegations were valid. The panel found in Marla's favor and granted her the relief she sought—that the university specifically investigate the situation for women in the School of Public Health and help to develop policies that would prevent future discrimination. The panelists also restored Marla's salary and back pay.

When Marla recounts this situation, she becomes deeply reflective and somewhat amazed at this period of her life. "I had to come to grips with my own deep assumptions about success and failure that I had previously placed heavily on myself," she says. She learned that sometimes no matter how hard one works or how bright or attractive he or she may be, the harsh forces of discrimination, negligence, and arrogance can prevail. While she more clearly perceived injustice, she also became more forgiving of her own failures, learning to understand that many things beyond self-determination were at play. Marla learned to fight for herself. She had always advocated for others with ease, but she says this was the first time she had to acknowledge she was important enough to herself to say this is just not okay. This was a major turning point in her development.

Another major turning point in her life was the day she decided to buy a puppy. After 4 years of juggling single parenthood with the dating scene, Marla decided that it might be easier if she replaced male companionship with owning a dog. She and her children went to a friend's house to see the newborn golden retriever puppies. The last thing she imagined was that she would meet her future husband—Jerry Anderson—who was her friend's housemate. The outcome of their chance meeting was a lovely dog, whom they aptly named Karma, and a marriage that is now in its third decade. Jerry, an attorney working for the Minnesota Attorney General's Office when they met, had a fairly idyllic bachelor's existence before meeting Marla, Jessica, and Matthew. The transition in his life was foreshadowed by an unforgettable event that took place on the night he moved into Marla's home. That evening, a major tornado hit their community, destroying part of their roof and flattening many homes beyond. Their first major project together was the recovery effort, including putting tar paper on the roof that night and the following day. She laughs and says "It wasn't easy from day one, but we have learned that we work well together—Jerry is my hero." Jerry stood by Marla as she moved through her sex discrimination case against the University of Minnesota. He also gave her the freedom to search for a new career opportunity, even if it meant looking out of state. The karma around this relationship has always been right, and the family they became is a treasure to Marla. Interestingly, Jessica and Matthew have followed their parents' career trajectories—Jessica is a third-generation nurse and Matthew a third-generation attorney. Evidently, their family shop talk took hold.

In the spring of 1986, Marla was pursued by the University of North Carolina at Chapel Hill to develop the doctor of public health program and to take the school's public health nursing program to a new level of performance. Marla was completely forthright with the dean of the School of Public Health, Dr. Michel Ibrahim, and shared her University of Minnesota experiences with him. Marla was clear that her history at Minnesota could be viewed as a liability for Michel, but she also believed that this was an important part of who she was as a person and not something to hide.

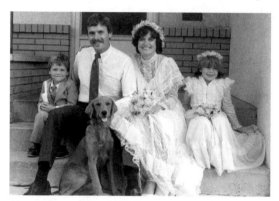

MARLA AND JERRY ANDERSON MARRIED ON 1 AUGUST 1984. FROM LEFT TO RIGHT, MARLA'S SON MATTHEW, JERRY, MARLA, AND MARLA'S DAUGHTER JESSICA. IN FRONT OF THEM ALL SITS KARMA, THE GOLDEN RETRIEVER WHO FORTUITOUSLY BROUGHT THEM ALL TOGETHER.

Marla also knew that taking the position at Chapel Hill was a risk for her—a few years earlier, Michel had attempted to close the Public Health Nursing Program because he had not seen it as academically strong. Marla was intrigued and Jerry was willing to go along; Michel hired her before he knew the outcome of her case.

MOVING ON TO CHAPEL HILL—THE GIFT OF A GOOD BOSS

In May 1986, Marla became an associate professor at the University of North Carolina at Chapel Hill. This was a career opportunity where Marla thought she could "build a legacy for public health nursing at Chapel Hill." She sat down with Michel to arrive at a clear understanding of what success would look like, to avoid changing expectations. They agreed that the public health nursing program would need to integrate with other schools and develop a sense of interdisciplinary collaboration. The goal was to educate first-class public health nurses who were highly effective and professional and to advance research in the area of public health nursing.

Marla knew the quality of the program was under scrutiny, but she did not know that she was actually a target of external forces. A powerful state public health nursing leader was adamantly opposed to Marla's selection for the position. Marla elected to take the high road and act as if there was no problem. Slowly, the rest of the senior leaders in the region and the state began to engage in building the program. The program's success isolated the one leader who was negative. The message became clear, Marla says, that "the train was leaving the station, and it was becoming crowded with people who believed in the vision."

Another lesson learned was to choose your boss carefully. "If you are considering a new position, and it is extremely attractive, but you don't have a sense of connection and agreement with the vision of the organization, then don't bother," Marla says. She knew she was on the same page with her boss, Michel, from the beginning when he interviewed her at the University of Minnesota. Other signals that she had chosen the right boss were his forthcoming nature and the comfort she felt in their working relationship. Common ground was established on the direction of the program at the interview stage. She cautions that, "Just like we ought to be careful who we marry and who we are involved with, we should be careful who we work for, because it is practically impossible to succeed if you have made the wrong choice." Your reputation may depend on making the best possible choice.

Marla defines a good boss as a person who will be challenging, have high expectations, be a good collaborator, and understand his or her role as creating a context for success. She believes that good bosses develop and mentor those who report to them. Michel, who had demonstrated great support for the program, was all of this to Marla at Chapel Hill. Marla had chosen her boss well and learned how important that choice is to success.

When Marla is the boss looking for a team member, one important metric for her is how the prospective employee responds to the question, "Do you have any questions for me?" She says it is incredibly instructive to see an applicant's interest, acumen, and maturity through the questions the person asks about the position and the organization. Marla believes their questions indicate what is important to them and create an understanding of their potential as an employee.

Marla finished her 3-year Kellogg National Leadership Fellowship Program while at Chapel Hill. Her fellowship focused on women's leadership development, with a strong global emphasis. Marla sought to understand possible differences in the ways women lead and if women can—and how women can—have it all. Meaning, can they have a work-life balance and an overall sense of fulfillment. She concluded that there was no one pattern of choices that led to fulfillment, but there appeared to be two main life themes associated with this sense of well-being. The first was having something in life that was just yours that you had achieved and that you were proud of. Whether this achievement was running a megacorporation or canning pickles and winning a State Fair award, the magnitude didn't matter. The second ingredient was lasting and loving relationships. Marla discovered that fulfillment and balance in lives did not occur without people who were with you through thick and thin and supported you through the worst of times. Marla also concluded that you *can* have it all, but not necessarily all at once or in neat order.

The concept of lasting and loving relationships is something that Marla can readily relate to. Her family is her touchstone and her "humility check." When asked, Marla will say that the thing she is most proud of is her family. She talks about the many lessons she has learned from her family and her gratitude to Jerry for always being there for them. The difference that Jerry has made in Marla's life has led her to believe that everyone should take a course on choosing one's life partner and managing one's personal finances. As one might imagine, Marla's family life is often unconventional. One of the favorite family activities was studying tae kwan do and entering competitions together. They still joke about how the children quickly learned not to mess with mom, as she earned a second-degree black belt (though she admits to being the soft touch in the family). She has always been grateful for the family's flexibility, as she moved them around the country while she sought to do the good that she could throughout her career. Marla recognizes that her career truly belongs to her whole family, and that each has made sacrifices along the way.

She had finally found a home in Chapel Hill. In 5 short years, Marla had made great progress. The Public Health Nursing Program was flourishing, and Michel and the community leaders were pleased with the quality of the graduates. Marla's own reputation

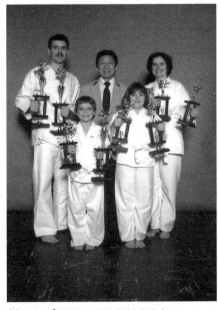

MARLA, JERRY, AND THE KIDS—
MATTHEW AND JESSICA—SHOW OFF
THEIR TAE KWON DO TROPHIES AT
THEIR FIRST TOURNAMENT IN 1987.

nationally as a leader in nursing and public health had also grown. In 1991, she was promoted to full professor and believed that she had it all.

That same year, Marla received a phone call from Naomi Josephs of the U.S. Department of Health and Human Services, inquiring if she had seen the advertisement for director of the Division of Nursing. Naomi told Marla that her name had come up several times as a potential candidate. Marla knew of the opening but had not considered herself for the position. Naomi encouraged her to think about it and told her the deadline was fast approaching. Marla saw the position as an exceptional opportunity in terms of having an impact. However, she was not sure she was the right person, because she did not have a traditional nursing background—her career had been in public health. Following Naomi's encouragement, Marla did think about the position, but that was the extent of her energy on the subject. On the morning of the application deadline, Naomi called again, asking her to submit her application. The postmark deadline was 5 p.m., and Marla arrived at the post office at 4:55 p.m. with the application in hand and the wheels turning in her head about how she might be able to live out her commitment to the public's health and nursing's contribution at a national policy level.

Michel supported her application to the Division of Nursing and refused to accept her resignation if she was selected. He agreed to put her on a 2-year leave to the U.S. Department of Health and Human Services, so that Marla would consider returning to Chapel Hill.

DIRECTOR OF THE DIVISION OF NURSING AND CHIEF NURSE OF THE US

Marla went into her interview for the position as director of the Division of Nursing for the Department of Health and Human Services with a good sense of who she was and what she could do. Marla understood what the agency's role was, but she had to articulate what she brought to the table. She knew that her competition would have a strong traditional nursing track record, and she would have to be clear about what she could contribute to public health and public policy development with her background as a political science major and Fulbright scholar.

Interestingly, one of the interview panelists was Denise Geolot, then-acting director of the Division of Nursing. Marla had interviewed Denise for a position at the JHH ED nearly 20 years earlier. Denise became Marla's deputy when she received the position, and they had a remarkable working relationship. Denise describes Marla as "possessing highly effective interpersonal skill that moved the group to rally around the common ground." This is not an easy feat in Washington, DC. Additionally, Denise was amazed by Marla's work ethic, stating that "Marla is one of the most productive people I have ever seen and was actively involved in all aspects of the project." She remembers that Marla was a "forward and big thinker" and "in the 1980s was one of the first nurse leaders to express concern about the aging workforce. … She could see the problem coming" when no one else was talking about it. According to Denise, Marla's leadership hallmarks were her unflappable nature and exquisite preparedness. Marla developed a reputation for focusing the conversation on public policy to emphasize improving public health.

Marla again demonstrated her ability to work across disciplines and with leaders outside her own field. She established a positive relationship from the onset with her boss, Dr. Fitzhugh Mullan, which became an important partnership throughout her years there. "Fitz" was supportive of Marla and saw the need for advancing nursing as part of an overall strategy for meeting the needs of all people. He and Marla shared a strong commitment to serving those in greatest need, particularly the underserved and those with the least access to care.

When Marla assumed the position of director of the Division of Nursing, her first order of business was to conceptually understand the organization and define how she could optimize its role. At that time, the division was perceived as primarily a funder of projects located in nursing schools. Marla rallied the team to conceptualize what the division could be.

Working closely with Denise Geolot and other senior leaders, Marla developed a clear vision describing the four key ways in which the Division of Nursing shaped the nation's capacity to deliver nursing services:

Analysis and planning—providing data, analysis, projections, and planning necessary to support ongoing sufficiency of the nation's nursing work force, particularly with respect to supply, distribution, diversity, quality, requirements, need, and utilization. The Quadrennial National Sample Survey of Registered Nurses forms the overall data foundation for this work.

Innovation, demonstration and evaluation: This function relates to seeding, supporting, and evaluating demonstration projects and other initiatives through which important insights and lessons can be learned with respect to advancing nursing education and practice. Examples include the initial funding for the early development of the nurse practitioner role and the creation of intensive care units.

Overall capacity building: This function relates to funding that is specifically aimed at developing the nation's ability to produce nurses and to enhance the impact of their practice in an ongoing fashion. Examples include funding for educational programs, scholarships, and traineeships; development of the pipeline to prepare minority and disadvantaged young people to enter nursing careers; and recruitment and retention programs for registered nurses.

Technical assistance and consultation: Providing guidance and expert consultation to key constituents, including the nursing community, the broader public, the Department of Health and Human Services, Congress, and other nations and international agencies. The division serves in a key advisory and interpretive role in this regard. Its ongoing support for the National Advisory Council on Nursing Education and Practice is another way in which the division lives out this function.

The conceptual framework both guided the division in its work and helped to explain its unique function and market its important work internally and externally. Along with consistent, strategic leadership and positioning of the division, a much greater awareness and appreciation of the Division of Nursing's significant contributions came to light.

In 1992, the administrator for the Health Resources and Services Administration (HRSA) created a new position for a chief nurse of that agency. He wanted an adviser on nursing issues that would cross the entire agency, not just the Division of Nursing. Marla was appointed to this position in addition to her responsibilities as director of the division. In 1993, she was invited to become a member of the White House Task Force on Health Care Reform. Joining her boss, "Fitz" Mullan, and colleague Dr. Linda Aiken, Marla focused on the health workforce as part of healthcare reform. Marla and Linda were among a very small group of nurses included in the work of proposing a health system that assured access and quality while controlling cost. Her memories of Germany and Kuwait came flooding back as she engaged again in questions that were relevant to her Fulbright experience.

Although the concept of universal access to healthcare did not become operational, this was a good time for the advancement of nursing. Accord-

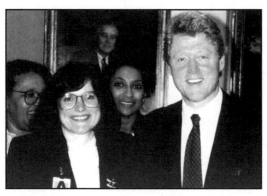

MARLA WITH FORMER PRESIDENT BILL CLINTON. SHE HELD THE POSITION OF CHIEF NURSE OF THE UNITED STATES IN HER 1991-97 ROLE AS DIRECTOR OF THE DIVISION OF NURSING FOR THE DEPARTMENT OF HEALTH AND HUMAN SERVICES. SHE WAS ALSO A MEMBER OF THE WHITE HOUSE TASK FORCE ON HEALTH CARE REFORM IN 1993 AND CHAIRED THE NATIONAL ADVISORY COUNCIL ON NURSE EDUCATION AND PRACTICE FROM 1991-97.

ing to Marla, the value of nursing was front and center, and what came from this was a "pro-nursing stance at the highest levels." She credits the initial stance of the administration to the leadership of Virginia "Ginna" Trotter-Betts, who was ANA president at the time and a friend and colleague of Vice President Al Gore. Ginna's relationship with the vice president and President Clinton's mother having been a nurse were important in creating a high-profile status in the government. In many ways, Ginna's leadership and ANA's support for the administration opened doors for nursing to have an impact. And, as one might imagine, Marla and Linda were prepared to accept the invitation and walk right through that door. Their considerable behind-the-scenes strategy and expertise fashioned important progress both within and beyond the actual Healthcare Reform bill. They were instrumental in helping nursing keep its "political eye" on the ball and speak with one voice as often as possible. They co-authored an important article that helped to shape nursing's political action and define the agenda in Washington and beyond.

During this time, the Division of Nursing also sponsored the Institute of Medicine study and subsequent report (1996) on nurse staffing levels and quality outcomes. This seminal report became foundational to virtually all of the subsequent development of nurse-sensitive quality measures and staffing initiatives. This was a very exciting and almost explosive time in nursing, and Marla was at the center of many of these important discussions and strategic plans for the future of nursing. In 1996, Marla's standing in and beyond nursing was recognized through her election to the Institute of Medicine.

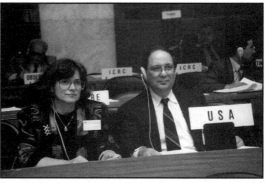

IN 1995, MARLA WAS A MEMBER OF THE UNITED STATES DELEGATION FOR THE 48TH WORLD HEALTH ASSEMBLY OF THE WORLD HEALTH ORGANIZATION (WHO). HERE SHE SITS NEXT TO CIRO SUMAYA DURING THE ASSEMBLY HELD AT THE PALACE OF NATIONS IN GENEVA, SWITZERLAND.

This was also a time in which Marla's leadership impact expanded internationally and the division's reach extended beyond U.S. borders. Marla was successful in her efforts to have nursing representation in the U.S. Delegation to the World Health Assembly, and she was asked to serve in that role. In addition, Marla was nominated by the United States government to serve as chair of the World Health Organization's Global Advisory Group for Nursing and Midwifery. She served with distinction for 3 years, beginning in 1997. In this capacity, she led in advising the director general of WHO and is credited with preventing the Global Advisory Group from being discontinued during a major leadership transition in her second and third year of service.

Marla's concern for the wellbeing of vulnerable people worldwide was consistently reflected in her work to serve those in greatest need in the U.S. Among these were people who suffered health disparities, particularly those identified as "minorities." She recognized that the demographics of the U.S.

were changing dramatically and that these individuals really constituted the emerging majority. Marla also recognized that nursing neither reflected the ethnic composition of the overall population nor had adequately attended to their health issues. For these reasons, Marla led in the development of three historic national congresses called *Caring for the Emerging Majority,* which brought together nursing leaders and collaborators from across ethnic groups for the first time. These meetings occurred over a period of four years and had concrete results that ranged from local, community actions to changing national policies and programs in ways that would reach those in greatest needs. The collaborations set in motion during those meetings continue today and have had lasting and significant impact.

In 1997, as she entered her 7th year at HRSA, Marla believed it was time to consider the next step of her career. The University of North Carolina at Chapel Hill had told her that the 2-year leave, which was extended for an additional 5 years, was about to expire and she needed to decide whether or not she would return. Additionally, after 7 years in a high-profile position in the federal government, it was time for a change. President Clinton was at the end of his second term, and it seemed like a good time to think about other options. In 1997, Marla joined the University of Pennsylvania School of Nursing. She saw this as a good place for her first employment as a nursing faculty member, as opposed to her prior experience in public health. There, she served as the graduate dean and a professor of nursing. Marla was eager to collaborate further with Linda Aiken and to learn from and contribute to the work underway there. And, Penn's international nursing mission was very consistent with Marla's leadership and career development.

Marla's 2 years at Penn were important to her leadership development, as she learned a great deal about nursing education and the roles of private universities in the broader society. This was also a time of stress and loss for her personally. In January of 1997, her mother was diagnosed with lymphoma of the brain, and she died 18 months later after a valiant struggle. During that time, Marla's daughter, Jessica, gave birth to her first child, Parris Davis, who met his great-grandmother Marceline for the first and last time during Christmas of 1997.

Experiencing her grandmother's illness and death launched Jessica's aspirations to become a nurse. In 2005, she graduated from the University of Maryland School of Nursing, adding a third generation of nurses to the family.

In 1999, Marla received a call from a search firm for the deanship at Emory University School of Nursing. She wasn't interested. Over the course of several phone calls, recruiter Paula Caribelli (who later became a dear friend) convinced her that Emory was seeking a visionary leader and "builder" with credentials in public health, policy, leadership, and nursing. Funny, this sounded just like her credentials! Reverting to her philosophy of "why not," Marla decided she would talk to them, though she did not believe anything would come of it.

EMORY UNIVERSITY—LILLIAN CARTER CENTER OF INTERNATIONAL NURSING

The chair of the search committee was Dr. James Curren, dean of the School of Public Health. "He did a great job of showing me where Emory was and where it was going," Marla says, "and he epitomized the kind of people that I particularly like—a person with values and commitment and a tireless worker for change." Her impression from the numerous interview encounters was that the School of Nursing had strong organizational values and open collaboration across disciplines. The school also had a remarkable community of close partners—CARE, CDC, The Carter Center, and the American Heart Association. Marla recalls that she was also attracted to the very strong sense that Emory was a place that was fundamentally committed to doing the right thing.

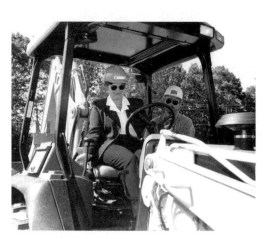

MARLA OPERATES THE BULLDOZER AT THE GROUNDBREAKING FOR THE NEW NELL HODGSON WOODRUFF SCHOOL OF NURSING AT EMORY UNIVERSITY IN ATLANTA, GEORGIA.

Ultimately, Marla was struck by the incredible potential of the Nell Hodgson Woodruff School of Nursing, particularly given its context and the leadership support for development of the school. Her discussions with Dr. Michael Johns, who ultimately became her boss, helped her understand that there was a real appreciation for nursing within the health sciences and a strong commitment to inter-disciplinary collaboration. Marla was also inspired by the remarkable vision and energy that she observed in Michael and her future colleagues within and beyond the health sciences. In the final analysis, it was the "fit" and the real potential for making a difference in the world through nursing that drew Marla to the position. Again, with the support of her family, she accepted the position.

When Marla arrived at Emory University School of Nursing in 1999, she quickly recognized that the school's future should reflect a development strategy in which "the focus should be on the unique opportunities to do those things that matter and that cannot be done anywhere else." Marla believed that one of these opportunities was working with The Carter Center, which is part of Emory University, on international health.

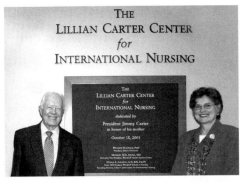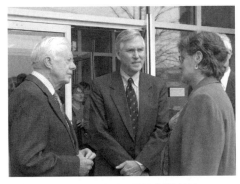

MARLA AND FORMER PRESIDENT JIMMY CARTER, AT THE OPENING OF THE LILLIAN CARTER CENTER FOR INTERNATIONAL NURSING (LCCIN) (LEFT). THE LCCIN IS LOCATED ON THE EMORY UNIVERSITY CAMPUS IN ATLANTA, GEORGIA. IN THE PHOTO ON THE RIGHT ARE PRESIDENT CARTER (LEFT), AND JOHN HARDMAN (CENTER), EXECUTIVE DIRECTOR OF THE CARTER CENTER—ALSO HOUSED ON THE EMORY UNIVERSITY CAMPUS WHERE THE STAFF "WAGE PEACE, FIGHT DISEASE, AND BUILD HOPE"—WITH MARLA AT THE OPENING OF THE LCCIN.

Shortly after her arrival, Marla had lunch with former U.S. President Jimmy Carter, whom she describes as a brilliant, values-driven leader. She shared with him her hope that the school could develop a center for international nursing that would honor his mother's memory. Lillian Carter was a remarkable woman and nurse who volunteered for Peace Corps service in India. The ultimate result of their discussion was that Marla would lead in the development of the Lillian Carter Center for International Nursing (LCCIN) and that its mission would be "the improvement of the health of vulnerable people worldwide through nursing education, research, practice, and policy." On 18 October 2001, Jimmy Carter dedicated the Lillian Carter Center during its first Global Health Partners Forum. In attendance were Archbishop Desmond Tutu; government chief nurses and national nursing organization leaders from 65 countries; and the senior leadership of the World Health Organization, International Council of Nurses, and Commonwealth Ministers Steering Committee for Nursing and Midwifery. The founding director of the Lillian Carter Center, Marla has been instrumental in moving its mission forward. The achievements of the center have been remarkable, as evidenced by its third Global Health Partners Forum, in which the most senior nursing and medical government leaders from 106 countries participated in meetings in Atlanta at The Carter Center and the Centers for Disease Control and Prevention.

The Lillian Carter Center itself reflects the notion that doing what it can do uniquely well is what matters. It has four distinct functions. The first function is to assume the role of "the neutral convener" to bring global leaders together around key issues. The Global Government Health Partners Forums are examples of this convening function. These forums bring together senior leaders from within and beyond governments to focus on health issues of mutual concern. Themes for discussions have included biological threats, avian influenza, and the global health worker shortage.

The second function is developing leadership among government chief nursing officers and others. One example of this is the unique role that LCCIN plays as secretariat for the Government Chief Nursing Officers' Network, which was established at the request of CNOs during their first meeting at the Global Health Partners Forum in 2001. The center's third overall function relates to fostering academic and service-learning exchange and partnerships. Several faculty and student experiences have been developed that involve partners in other countries and programs. The fourth center function is to provide support for the development and dissemination of knowledge through research and technical assistance. An example of this work is the Kenya Nursing Workforce Project, which is funded by the Centers for Disease Control and USAID. This project involves the development of a comprehensive nursing workforce analytic system and its application to policy and education in Kenya. Ultimately, the project will also inform the development of similar systems worldwide. All of these functions are aimed at advancing the contributions of nurses to the health of vulnerable people worldwide.

At the 2005 International Council of Nurses conference, Frances Hughes from New Zealand recognized the influence of the Lillian Carter Center as a "best practice in international nursing." Marla says with a smile, "We have come a long way in 7 short years with many great things to come."

During those 7 years, the faculty, staff, and students of the Nell Hodgson Woodruff School of Nursing have advanced the school's rankings, tripled both its research and educational extramural funding, and established important interdisciplinary collaborations. The recent addition of Dr. Sue K. Donaldson to the faculty as a university distinguished professor is one important indication of the school's progress. Sue was recruited as a professor in both nursing and medicine whose unique leadership role is to advance the development of nursing and interdisciplinary science.

On Leadership

Marla's definition of leadership is "being able to help develop and nurture a vision that engages and inspires others—one to which they can contribute and through which they can see a better future. Leadership creates the context in which people actually can contribute and grow. It is about making the world better and creating lasting, meaningful change—this only happens through the commitment and work of people." Marla is quick to say that her leadership is really the leadership of those with whom she has worked, and that they deserve the bulk of the credit. "Leadership is also about being able to navigate within and beyond the organization to engage the outside to support the enterprise and to engage the inside to advance the enterprise," she adds. She further states that "leadership is legacy—it is ensuring that the enterprise goes beyond and is composed of more than the individual. Leadership is making a difference and causing a difference to be made."

Leaders must also have the wisdom to know when they are no longer making a difference. Marla believes that "if you are a reflective person, the signs are obvious when your leadership is not working ... and it is a question of when the not working is a permanent versus a temporary state." She believes that there are "developmental pauses in any organization when you need to stop, integrate, assimilate, and regenerate" before forward movement can occur again—this would be a temporary state of leadership lag.

Marla believes there is a tipping point when the leader is no longer adding value. Her observation is that there is a natural lifespan of leadership whereby you must "re-create yourself or in some way change the organization to continue to remain effective and successful." She believes it is "possible for the system to learn how to stop you from being effective; to make a major change requires a disruptive innovation"—this could lead to a more permanent state of ineffective leadership.

A good leader is someone who is always processing the signals—from the inside and outside—about the state of affairs surrounding the effectiveness of one's leadership. Marla is certain that "if you lose your internal credibility, it doesn't matter much what you do on the outside." To validate the signals, Marla recommends utilizing your "trusted internal deputies" who can tell you what you need to hear, not what they think you want to hear, without fear of reprisal. This garnered trust is predicated on the mutual understanding that

This is leadership self-knowledge—knowing who you are, what your innate and learned abilities are, and what revitalizes your leadership energy.

the feedback is distinctly a work issue, not a personality issue. She says that leaders who lack this kind of relationship "can erode their own sense of competence."

Marla is constantly reading the signals of her own leadership. Because she has moved several times in her career—literally and figuratively—and created new pathways for her leadership, she has confidence that it is always possible to leave. To Marla, it is freeing to read the signals because the notion of leaving is comforting, if the time is right. If a leader believes she or he is trapped and there is no way out, then reading the signals can become very painful and nonproductive. Marla often writes a reminder to herself that serves as a compass for her development. Her current one reads:

> *Why am I here?*
> *To help build the School of Nursing that this one can be in ways that no other can*
>> *Scholarship, leadership, social responsibility*
>> *Lives up to its responsibility to use the precious resources*
>> *Give back*
> *To give nursing another dimension of its value to people, particularly vulnerable people*
> *To learn new lessons in my own leadership*
>> *—Learning to really move nursing*
>> *—Health sciences system*
>> *—Private university*
>> *—Corporate social responsibility*
> *To advance global health through nursing*
> *To cultivate some community roots*
> *To move into the next stage of my own self-development*
>
> *When to leave ... when it doesn't work and won't work*
> *When I and those I love move into the crosshairs in a way that diminishes all of us*
> *When there are better ways to do what I can do...*
> *When it isn't fun anymore...*

This is her professional and personal roadmap—her leadership measurement and outcomes. Marla does not believe in developing a personal 5-year plan for her own leadership development. She believes that such a plan causes you to work toward a job instead of toward commitments. Marla sees her commitments in terms of "this 'little framework' in my head that is dedicated to what I care about, what I want to do, what I find rewarding, what I want to learn, and how this fits with my family." This is leadership self-knowledge—knowing who you are, what your innate and learned abilities are, and what revitalizes your leadership energy.

In contrast to a linear view, Marla is a relational thinker who is anchored in values and commitment. She sees things in "terms of contingencies and the world as a very interesting moving system." Her perspective is big-picture and forward-thinking by nature. She learned that her thinking was different in high school. She would walk down the street with friends, and they would report an entirely different landscape than she saw. She *can* be linear and methodical. However, that is not her leadership choice, but rather her learned administrative capacity. This seeming contradiction is apparent in her disavowal of 5-year plans for herself on one hand, and her view that strategic planning is fundamentally important for organizational development on the other.

Marla believes that a leader must strike a balance between leadership choice and the capacity to be effective. She identifies her style of leadership as that of a "builder." She loves a worthwhile challenge and is most comfortable in the moving-forward stage of leadership. There are times when an organization has reached a "saturation point" that requires a "maintainer" leader; however, Marla is not a leader who likes performing the maintenance leadership role for long periods. What revitalizes her leadership energy is making a difference for nursing and those that nurses serve—and the connection that she has with her family.

Marla believes that effective leadership comes with the understanding that "you don't have to carry the water all the time." It is important to work closely with others so there are many people who carry the water. Marla reminds others that, "If you are the only one carrying the water, at some point you are going to trip or someone is going to stick their foot out, and the plan may be lost." The team approach is essential for sustaining the vision and outcomes. She describes vision as being able to describe a future that is fundamentally better than the current situation; however, this future actually draws from and builds on the current situation. Marla calls vision the coloring book for an organization.

Operationalizing vision is the responsibility of the leader. Conflict often occurs as the vision is interpreted and then operationalized. Marla declares that she is a common-ground leader rather than a consensus leader. She says she does not believe in consensus leadership because she does not think it is possible. In achieving consensus, "You wear people down in the process and you lose what people have to offer that may be different," she says. Marla leads by finding the common ground that lies within group members that hold differing perspectives, rather than by creating convergence. In convergence leadership, the common ground is the point of convergence where conflict is minimized and agreement is maximized. For example, she believes the common ground for nursing and medicine right now is not established around advanced practice or reimbursement but is found in the professional bedrock of quality and safety of care. According to Marla, "Working from the vantage point of quality of care and safety, in a partnered way, is the common ground

The bridge you burn is the one you will need to cross later.

between the disciplines where the differences are easier to manage." Marla also notes that when one truly finds common ground, one is also honoring differences. When one honors differences, one also recognizes that diversity creates opportunities otherwise unseen.

The art of leadership is managing differences to a successful conclusion. She declares that, "The bridge you burn is the one you will need to cross later." The best leadership choice in avoiding bridge burning is to treat others with civility. She means civility in the most basic sense of the word—not just being polite, but treating others with respect. Marla's method for achieving civility is engaging, understanding, and appreciating differences. "Reciprocity starts with you," Marla says. "Extend yourself first and don't wait for others." Early in her life, Marla was encouraged to take the high road, even though that sometimes means taking the tough road. Numerous times in her career, Marla has been reintroduced to people whom she had known from another period in her life. She has been grateful for the time she invested in maintaining civility and taking the high road when differences have occurred, because a history of respect and trust has already been established.

Marla commonly avoids conflict through the effective use of strategy. Being strategic means coming prepared, having the proper people aligned, and understanding what you need to achieve from the encounter. She believes it is important to "know in advance what you would consider success, because once you are in the situation the stakes escalate." Linda Aiken describes Marla as a "great strategist who knows how to mobilize resources for nursing." According to Linda, when Marla was appointed chief nurse of the United States, she insisted that the position hold a seat on the U.S. delegation for the WHO. Historically, nursing had not been represented in the delegation. This was a great success for nursing.

For Marla, the success is "not that nursing has a role in the WHO process, but that nursing has an opportunity to contribute." She rejects the notion of role. Marla views a role as "a name we call ourselves" that tends to be mechanical and limiting in nature. She saw herself as a member of the U.S. Delegation of the WHO, and this meant she needed to be an effective member who understood the issues being addressed. Her starting point was to understand what this country expects of the membership and what makes a member of the delegation effective. From there, she asked what her function was in that context. As an effective member, Marla played many roles, only one of which was chief nursing officer of the United States. As with most matters, Marla sees the notion of role in a bigger context than many other leaders.

> *Boards are fundamentally about governance—assuring that the organization is functioning as it should and representing the interests of the public and share- or stakeholders*

In recent years, nurse leaders have been invited to join corporate boards. Marla counsels that "nurses need to understand what it takes to be a good board member rather than a good nurse leader sitting on the board." She analogizes this situation to "being a baseball player and being invited to a football field and playing baseball." Marla believes that a good board member is like an athlete who can express that athleticism in a variety of ways. She also warns that nurses need to be careful when accepting a board position. "Boards are fundamentally about governance—assuring that the organization is functioning as it should and representing the interests of the public and share- or stakeholders," she says. Boards are not concerned with daily management of an organization. Governance leadership is more foreign to nurses than daily operations. This is a stance she has worked to develop in her own role on the Board of Trustees of the Robert Wood Johnson Foundation.

Marla advises nurses who want to be on a board to think about which boards they would be qualified for and interested in serving on, and to be sure they understand the responsibility of service. Today, as a result of corporate debacles such as the Enron Corporation, board members are held to a higher level of responsibility and accountability. She encourages nurses to consider board appointments, but she reminds them to be careful and know what you are doing. Ask plenty of questions.

When asked what she admires most in leaders, Marla is quick to identify three qualities: "leaders who leave the campground cleaner than they found it; leaders who have the ability to match potential with opportunity; and leaders who possess vision of what is possible and what can make it possible." Marla is certainly all that she admires in others.

Summary

Marla is a nurse leader who has sat at some of the most influential health-care tables in the world and has never forgotten what and who she represents—quality patient care and underprivileged populations. Her message, generated by a deep social conscience, reminds us that, "In nursing when the shift is over, when the contact is done, or worse yet, when you are in the process of providing patient care, you don't realize that there are people out there with absolutely no access to services." She did not plan a career of leadership greatness, but her drive to make a difference placed her on a road of public health nursing that touched the world. She would tell you that serendipity created her opportunities; however, it is obvious that her brilliance, big-picture thinking, integrity, interpersonal skills, and focus—not chance—were the main ingredients of her leadership success.

When you examine Marla's individual coloring book, it is easy to become overwhelmed by the depth and breadth of her leadership image. Marla wants nurses to know that leadership is a choice and, as her husband would say, "the world is run by those who show up." Believe that you can make the world a better place, commit to making a difference, and keep asking "why not?"!

REFERENCES

Larson, S.M. (1999, January 21). Suit set to challenge U Rajender decree. *The Minnesota Daily Online*. Retrieved February 19, 2007, from http://www.mndaily.com/daily/1999/01/21/news/ian/

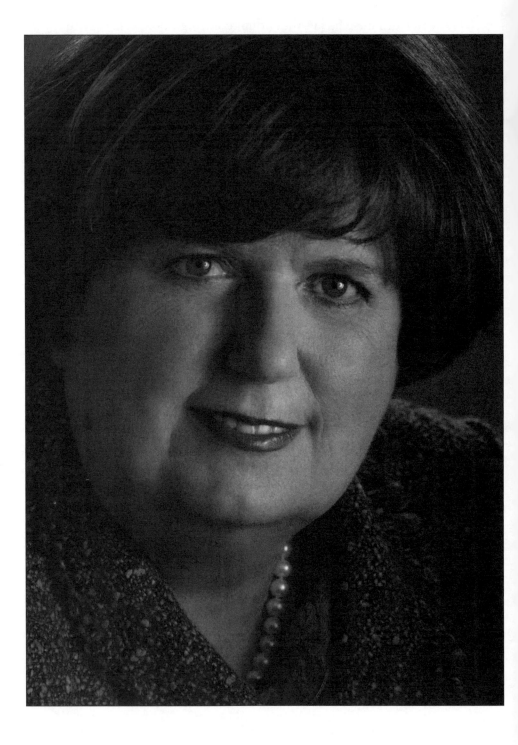

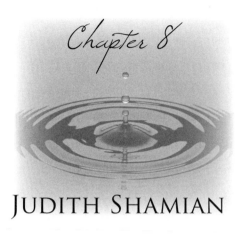

Chapter 8

JUDITH SHAMIAN

"Nurses complain about all that is wrong with the nursing profession or heathcare, but we are not going to change anything if we don't break out and influence the agenda from the outside."

—Judith Shamian

Judith Shamian, RN, PhD, was born in Debrecen, Hungary, in 1950. An only child, her parents were in their early 40s when she was born. Her father's first family—a wife and seven children—all perished in the Holocaust. The marriage to Judith's father was the first for her mother. Both, however, were Holocaust survivors. Judith herself remembers living through her first war at the young age of 6, when the Hungarian Revolution broke out in 1956. She remembers watching the Russian tanks roll through her city. Many of the Jewish families who stayed in Hungary after the Holocaust left the country during the Hungarian Revolution through any means they could find. The majority of families left through illegal methods, such as crossing the border to Austria and then traveling to North America, Europe, or Israel from there. Judith's family was no different. "We tried to escape from Hungary numerous times by paying off the train conductors, but were caught on every attempt," she says.

It was during this time of chaos that Judith came to realize her family was different. She was beginning to understand the significance of living in a country where her family was Jewish and the majority of other families were not. These early life experiences largely influenced the values she held and helped to shape the nurse leader she was destined to become. Having lived through the Six Day War, the Yom Kippur War, and the Hungarian Revolution, Shamian grew up with an appreciation for life and a strong desire to survive.

> *"I remember as a child riding in the ambulance with her to the hospital and how we came to know the ambulance attendants quite well."*

EARLY BEGINNINGS

Judith grew up within the USSR-style communist government, but she lived in a religious Jewish household where all the holidays and Sabbaths were fully observed. Out of sheer necessity, she grew up with the skills of a nurse. Her mother was seriously and permanently injured by a bomb explosion during World War II (WWII). A large brick wall collapsed, killing Judith's uncle and leaving her mother with massive internal injuries. She was hospitalized with a collapsed lung and several broken bones.

"During the end of WWII, there were major raids on the city, and the hospital patients were taken to shelters," Judith says. "But they could not move my mother because her condition was so critical she would have died." Her mother had chronic respiratory disease and neurological disabilities that were similar to epilepsy. Because Judith's father traveled with his job, she was left home to take care of her mother. Her mother had seizure-like attacks that varied in frequency. At times, her condition would be stable, but at its worst state, the condition could produce seizures with such intensity and frequency that hospitalization was required.

"I remember as a child riding in the ambulance with her to the hospital and how we came to know the ambulance attendants quite well," Judith says. When she felt her mother was not receiving care as quickly as she should, she approached the nurses and insisted they do more.

Judith's mother had a pampered childhood, so she found herself ill-prepared to face the concentration camps. Thus, she wanted Judith to grow up strong and independent, capable of dealing with any situation.

Even with her mother's chronic health issues, Judith's family was more fortunate than many other families in her community. Her aunts in Canada sent polio vaccine to Hungary for their young niece, giving her a health advantage many of her friends did not have at the time. Her father was employed as a top executive in the city of Mako at a large communist factory that catered to Jewish employees. He was second in

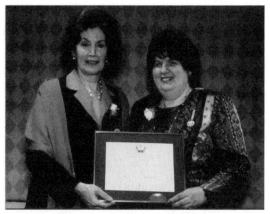

THE HONOURABLE LUCIE PEPIN PRESENTS DR. SHAMIAN WITH THE GOLDEN JUBILEE MEDAL, 2002. THESE AWARDS WERE GIVEN TO CANADIANS WHO HAD MADE OUTSTANDING OR EXEMPLARY CONTRIBUTIONS TO THEIR COMMUNITIES OR TO CANADA AS A WHOLE ON THE OCCASION OF THE 50TH ANNIVERSARY OF THE ACCESSION OF HER MAJESTY QUEEN ELIZABETH II TO THE THRONE.

charge at the factory, an unusually prominent position for a Jew to hold at the time. The factory was set up primarily for Jewish workers, as it facilitated their keeping the Sabbath and Jewish holidays. Numerous divisions within the factory manufactured various products, including toys, small home appliances, and clothing. Judith's father, the buyer for the factory, traveled to the capital city of Budapest every week to purchase supplies. He would return home on Thursday night.

"Actually, some of the best memories growing up were that every summer he took me for a week with him to Budapest," Judith says. "That was my big outing in the big city, allowing me to stay at hotels and eat out in restaurants."

Judith attended a private Jewish nursery school and kindergarten, so she did not realize anything was different or significant about her religious upbringing during her early years. When it was time to attend elementary school, her parents enrolled her in a state-run school. It was the first time she realized her family was different, as she could not attend school activities scheduled on Saturday, which was her Sabbath. Between her state schooling and the outbreak of the Hungarian Revolution, Judith recognized her family held a different belief system. Judith's formerly uneventful life would change drastically with the start of the Hungarian Revolution.

Judith was only 6 years old during the height of the Hungarian Revolution. She was with her parents visiting family in Romania when war broke out. "I remember standing on the street and seeing tanks speed down the street, which was pretty scary for a 6-year-old," she says. Society as she knew it became chaos, for her close friends and neighbors were trying to escape while the Russians were invading the country. Her family was no different in trying to flee for safety. She still remembers the traumatic episodes when her family tried to escape to Austria. They were caught on each attempt.

"The basic process was that if you could bribe a train conductor, he would let you on board the cargo train. Once on the train, you would crouch down, so as not to be seen through the windows," Judith says. As the train came to the point closest to the Austrian border, families would jump off and try to walk the last kilometer or so. Since many of the Hungarian citizens had already fled the country, the Hungarian patrol had soldiers and patrol dogs out to catch whoever else might try to escape. In three attempts to flee Hungary, her family was captured each time and put in remote barracks surrounded by fenced wires that confined the other captured families. They would stay until their paperwork cleared and then would be sent back home.

It was not until 1960, when Judith was 10 years old, that her family received official papers granting permission to leave Hungary. Judith's parents decided to settle in Israel because they wanted her to grow up Jewish and fully embrace all the religion has to offer. They boarded a train to Italy. From Italy, they took a boat to Israel. Judith came to love her new life in Israel and no longer felt different because of her belief system.

> She was old enough to have friends who served in the Israeli army and lost their lives. It was the first time Judith learned to fear for her survival.

NURSING SCHOOL IN ISRAEL

Growing up in Israel, Judith made many new friends and had access to quality schools. As she had so much exposure in her childhood to hospitals and illness, she decided early in life to enter the nursing profession. The high school she attended was built and run by a group that, in 1948, had

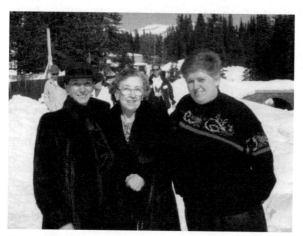

FROM LEFT TO RIGHT—DR. ROZELLA SCHLOTFELDT, FORMER DEAN OF CASE WESTERN RESERVE SCHOOL OF NURSING, JACQUELINE FAWCETT, RENOWNED NURSE RESEARCHER AND SCHOLAR, AND JUDITH AT LAKE LOUISE, ALBERTA, NURSING THEORY CONFERENCE.

had to leave areas outside of Jerusalem that had been taken over by Jordan. "As such, I had extremely Zionistic, well-informed teachers who instilled in us a great love of Israel," Judith says.

Before she came of age for college, Judith experienced her second war from an even closer perspective and observed firsthand the permanent effects war has on those who survive. In 1967, the Six Day War broke out. Even though this war was over in almost the blink of an eye, it left a different impression on Judith than the Hungarian Revolution. The first day the war broke out, she and her classmates were forced to walk home an hour's drive away. Since there was no other transportation, it took her 6 to 7 hours to walk to her town. When she arrived, the entire town appeared deserted. Windows were covered with dark curtains, and no one was in the streets. It was an eerie and haunting feeling for her, giving her a sense of doom. She was old enough to have friends who served in the Israeli army and lost their lives. It was the first time Judith learned to fear for her survival.

The next year, at 18 years of age, Judith enrolled in a religious, hospital-based nursing program. In Israel, nursing is viewed as a very noble profession, and the norm is to have children from upper-middle-class families attend nursing school.

During the second year of her program, Judith met her future husband, Chanoch Shamian. Judith and Chanoch married in 1971. Her parents helped plan the large wedding celebration. Being married while still in nursing school, however, was a major issue. She was one of the first married nursing students attending the religious school. It created

"I was so young to be overseeing the care of the burned, wounded, emotionally distraught soldiers. ... It left a lasting impact on me."

a fair amount of tension for her, primarily with one particular supervisor who was fairly abusive to her. The full nursing program was 3 years of didactic studies and clinicals and then a full year of residency. For her residency choice, she worked at Shaare Zedek Hospital in the emergency room (ER) where, upon graduation, she was hired.

THE NURSE LEADER EMERGES

Life drastically changed once again for Judith when the Yom Kippur War, also known as the Arab-Israeli War, broke out in 1973. She remembers how deserted Jerusalem seemed with all the men serving in the Israeli army. As she now had two children and a husband in the military reserves, the stress was much greater. She was raising the children while working part time. "I chose to work primarily night shift, so I could be home with our two girls during the day, as my husband would be home at night," she says.

Only 23 years old, Judith was a wife and mother, as well as a nurse in charge of night shifts in the ER. It was a lot of responsibility in the midst of a war. "I was so young to be overseeing the care of the burned, wounded, emotionally distraught soldiers. ... It left a lasting impact on me," she says. But she was confident in her nursing skills and enjoyed her work.

Judith's second child had a number of upper respiratory problems during her first year of life, which meant many nights Judith would have to call off her night shift at work to care for her daughter. The very same nursing supervisor who disliked Judith's rebellious ways in school demanded she be transferred from the ER to a medical floor.

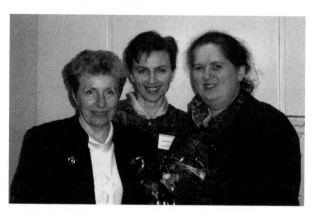

JUDITH, RIGHT, WITH MEMBERS OF THE NEWLY ESTABLISHED NURSING ASSOCIATION IN POLAND.

"I remember trying to fight it, speaking to the CEO of the hospital, which nurses never did back then, but nobody would be willing to take on this particular supervisor," Judith says. "They could see my point, but would not cross her."

Judith decided to leave the hospital and work as a kibbutz nurse (community health nurse). She loved her work in the kibbutz and worked alongside a more senior nurse who acted as her mentor. "This type of nursing required an ability to build systems and relationships, yet work independently," she says.

The position offered outstanding lessons in leadership, and it taught her the importance of family and community care. As a kibbutz nurse, she honed diagnostic skills, as the physician came in only twice a week. It strengthened her ability and confidence in decision making and problem solving, and gave her the opportunity to work with the kibbutz leader to manage the care of a 500-member community. This experience helped solidify her thinking about the role of nurses in building healthy communities.

MOVING FROM ISRAEL TO CANADA

"There is really no logic as to our decision to move the family to Canada," Judith says. "I knew while working in the ER that I was restless but perhaps did not know why." While growing up in Israel, Judith recalls what excitement the dream of moving to North America held for her. She had two aunts who immigrated to Canada in 1956, so her family could qualify and receive the necessary sponsorship to immigrate. Before they knew it, their paperwork had cleared and literally, the day before the papers expired, they left Israel.

Judith stopped nursing for 2 years while she attempted to heal and remembers asking herself the pointed question "Is my life over?" because she could not imagine doing anything else but nursing.

Interestingly, the trip to Montreal, Canada, was intended to be for a short while. "We never closed down our home when we moved, because the plan was to return within the year," Judith says. Years later, when the family returned to their apartment in Israel for a visit, the cupboards still had sugar, salt, and other items left in their original state. They had emptied the refrigerator, but everything else was left in such a way that anyone might suppose the owners would return at any time.

Although Judith loved her clinical work, she wanted to expand her nursing career. She even thought about branching out into technology and integrating that knowledge into the healthcare arena. She was ecstatic

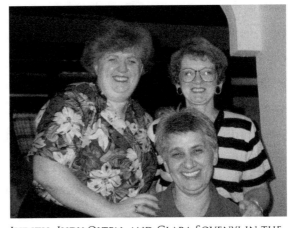

JUDITH, JUDY OLTEN, AND CLARA SOVENYI IN THE 1990S

to be a mother, but still craved to climb the career ladder. Prior to leaving Israel, she had interviewed for and accepted a position in Canada as a staff nurse in a neurosurgery unit at Sir Mortimer B. Davis Jewish General Hospital in Montreal. Shortly thereafter, she accepted a position as an intravenous nurse within the same facility.

During Judith's work in neurosurgery units, she suffered a back injury. Around this same time, Judith realized she was pregnant with her third child. She postponed back surgery for 9 months, until her daughter was born. However, shortly thereafter she knew surgery was needed. Following major back surgery, she was told she could never do bedside nursing again. She was encouraged to seek work in a physician's office.

"I will never forget that meeting, as it was devastating to hear the news," she says. Judith stopped nursing for 2 years while she attempted to heal and remembers asking herself the pointed question "Is my life over?" because she could not imagine doing anything else but nursing. But Judith was tenacious. "I picked myself up and dusted myself off, looking for the next window of opportunity."

One of the opportunities was a position with an intravenous (IV) team at Jewish General in Montreal, Quebec. The IV position led to education that changed her future career focus. "As part of my job, I floated throughout the various units of the hospital drawing blood on patients," Judith says. "While in the intensive care unit (ICU) one day, I asked a physician why we were not drawing blood from the heparin lock." The ICU patients were bruised from all the needle punctures needed to get laboratory reports on their status.

A good leader asks the right questions. In this situation, it puzzled Judith enough to ask a question when the answer appeared so very obvious. The medical director of ICU told Judith they couldn't use heparin locks for blood draws because heparin, used to keep the lines open, was mixed with the blood and there wasn't enough information in the literature to prove the heparin wouldn't interfere with the lab results. He then asked her if she wanted to research the topic. She didn't know the first thing about research but was lucky enough to have stumbled upon a teacher right there and then, as the medical director turned out to be a terrific instructor and taught her all about the work of research. They collected data for several months and then wrote a paper. Judith and her physician mentor presented the outcomes in what was the first speech on this topic at the International Critical Care Conference in San Antonio, Texas. Shortly after that conference, practice changed, and blood draws could then be taken from arterial lines. Judith witnessed firsthand the power of research in changing clinical practice.

My instructors recognized qualities within me that I did not know I had. Their encouragement and support helped me stretch professionally to new heights.

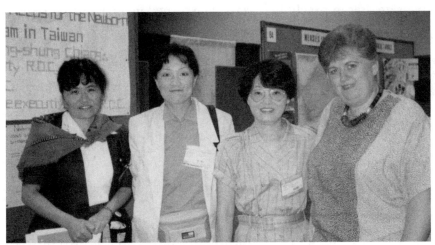

INTERNATIONAL CRITICAL CARE CONFERENCE, SAN ANTONIO, TEXAS, 1988. DELEGATES FROM TAIWAN AND JUDITH.

Judith befriended some colleagues in the hospital who were attending Concordia University. The nursing baccalaureate program at Concordia appeared to Judith. In the fall of 1976, just a year after her arrival and while she was still mastering the English language, she began to juggle work, family, and school. "It was very traumatic because I had no sense of what universities were about and was not familiar with the North American educational system," she says.

As a relatively young nurse (30 years old) attempting to step into key leadership roles, Judith was turned down the first several times she applied.

It wasn't long before instructors began to see just how special Judith was. "My instructors recognized qualities within me that I did not know I had. Their encouragement and support helped me stretch professionally to new heights," she says.

Judith remembers she was required to write an academic paper during her first semester in psychology class. She turned in a paper that resembled a composition or essay, with no references. The professor pulled her aside and praised her for all the good ideas she had, but told her the importance of research and references in an academic paper. She was also taking statistics that semester. The subject did not come easy to her, but the professor saw qualities in Judith that she did not know she had and offered her a job as a teaching assistant in statistics. She accepted, and it was from this position that her career started to change, and doors to new opportunities opened for her.

However, she did not rise to the top overnight. As a relatively young nurse (30 years old) attempting to step into key leadership roles, Judith was turned down the first several times she applied. With perseverance, however, she received a promotion to a director-level position at Sir Mortimer B. Davis Jewish General Hospital. This made her the youngest among her senior-ranking contemporaries in the hospital. Even with the earlier rejection, she never became discouraged or thought about quitting because she was passed over for other candidates. Judith knew she was very capable, and the time would come when her talents would be recognized—and it did.

Judith credits the majority of successes and great opportunities along her career path to leaders who saw potential in her. "I was only '4 years off the boat' as an immigrant, with minimal language capacity and a bachelor's degree, when Mary Barrett offered me an amazing position," Judith says. Mary was a nurse in her 50s, with no husband or children, who had the time to mentor a young nurse. "She had a strong presence and hired me into a position that others would have overlooked me for and never taken the risk. Years later, I asked her what she saw in this young 30-year-old,

and she replied that she paid attention to me in the medical library one day while I was doing coursework and she was working on research." Judith had offered Mary her research assistance. After that, Mary continued to observe Judith's work and recognized great potential.

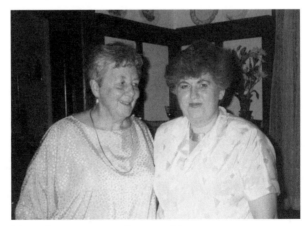

MARY BARRETT AND JUDITH. MARY WAS THE DIRECTOR OF NURSING UNDER WHICH JUDITH HELD HER FIRST MANAGEMENT POSITION

GRADUATE NURSING SCHOOL

Judith was offered a position as a nursing coordinator (equivalent to a nursing director in today's hospitals) in special services and research. While working in this position, she went back to school during the summer to obtain a master's degree in public health, focusing on international health and education, from New York University (NYU). She maintained the pace of working for 9 months, while taking a leave for school during the summer, for 2 years.

As she reflects upon all the research experience she has today, Judith credits mentors such as Marian Hamburg from NYU and Joyce Fitzpatrick, the dean from Case Western University, with planting the seeds for her future research career. The research position also put her in line for the academic arena, as she was offered to teach a graduate research course at the University of Toronto.

Even before she finished her master's in public health, Judith knew she wanted to pursue her doctoral degree. She was very deliberate in choosing where she would go for her doctorate. Her family lived in Montreal but did not speak French, the official language of Quebec. In addition, she was not pleased with the Jewish education her daughters were receiving. "We seriously looked at moving to the U.S., but I just could not bring myself to move to the American healthcare system, so we decided to stay in Canada," she says. In Canada, healthcare is available to all citizens and not just for those who can afford private insurance. "This philosophy of healthcare for all is core to my values. ... I could not live in a country that did not ensure equal access to all citizens. Even though

> *The idea that healthcare is a commodity rather than a social human right ... I just could not stomach that set of values.*

the educational system in the U.S. is superb, I have a value conflict with the design and delivery of the U.S. healthcare system. The idea that healthcare is a commodity rather than a social human right ... I just could not stomach that set of values." Judith remembers debating this issue with her colleagues at Case Western University

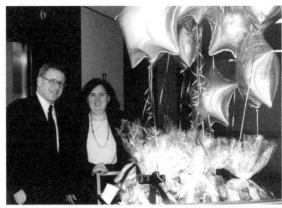

JUDITH, RIGHT, WITH JOE MAPPA, PRESIDENT AND CEO OF MT. SINAI HOSPITAL, TORONTO, PREPARING TO DISTRIBUTE NURSE WEEK GIFTS IN 1998. JUDITH WAS VICE PRESIDENT OF NURSING AT THE TIME.

and discussing how Americans do not actually *get* healthcare and risk being pushed out of hospitals prematurely, as if the care is related to the size of their wallet. "I don't want to be part of a system that is incongruent with my basic value and ethical system," she says. Judith recognizes the challenges within the Canadian healthcare system, but they make her work harder because she wants to be a part of it.

Once her family decided to stay in Canada, the only other place for them to live was Toronto. "Toronto had the type of religious education we were looking for for our daughters, so it was a good fit all the way around," she says. Judith started her PhD at Case Western University while living in Montreal and finished it after the family moved to Toronto. Judith knew she wanted her PhD to be in nursing, because she felt her nursing needed to be strengthened. She had carefully chosen this

Knowing when the time has come to leave an organization is something every leader should know. As important as it is to work through changes, it is equally as important to know when to get off the bus.

program because it had summer programs in leadership, which allowed her to work the majority of the year and earn money to pay tuition costs. After the first summer, Judith decided to switch to the full-time program stream. Even though she knew it would be more grueling, she believed it would provide her with a better education.

In 1986, Judith was offered a position as director of nursing research at Sunnybrook Medical Centre, in addition to teaching graduate level research at the University of Toronto. At that time, the director of nursing research was one of the first full-time positions in Canada within a medical hospital. Judith worked under the innovative leadership of Barbara Burk, who was vice president of nursing.

After Judith had been with Sunnybrook Medical Centre for 3 years, Burk left the organization. Judith applied for the newly opened vice president of nursing position. Even with her management experience, she was passed over for a woman who was recruited from outside the organization. The candidate had a very different leadership style, which Judith realized would clash with her own. "I knew that she and I would struggle along over time, as our styles were very different, so I started to look for employment elsewhere," she says. "Knowing when the time has come to leave an organization is something every leader should know. As important as it is to work through changes, it is equally as important to know when 'to get off the bus.'"

Judith took over at Sinai during an era of cutbacks, layoffs, and widespread malaise in the nursing ranks, but she managed to create an environment where nurses felt valued (Chatelaine, 1997).

Judith landed an interview at Mount Sinai Hospital in Toronto. The job was executive vice president of nursing, and Judith knew she would accept this "dream" nurse executive position. Even though Sinai had a great reputation, the nursing services needed to be modernized, and that would be one of Judith's first challenges.

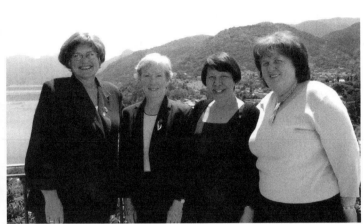

FROM LEFT TO RIGHT: MARLA SALMON, LINDA AIKEN, JEAN YAN, AND JUDITH IN BELLAGIO, ITALY, FOR THE HEALTH WORK-FORCE MEETING.

At Sinai, Judith learned the lesson of stepping into "big" shoes by replacing an individual who was well-respected. Instead of being overwhelmed by the challenge, she viewed it as an opportunity to use her strengths as a leader to take Mount Sinai Hospital to the next level. The teaching hospital culture was flexible and open-minded to her style of leadership. "There had been some detrimental decisions in healthcare in the 1990s that were taken on by teaching hospitals because of budget cuts," she says. Judith took over at Sinai during an era of cutbacks, layoffs, and widespread malaise in the nursing ranks, but she managed to create an environment where nurses felt valued (Chatelaine, 1997). Mount Sinai was the only hospital in Canada that had an all-RN staff and kept the nursing structure, both of which are a credit to Judith's dedicated leadership as vice president of nursing.

During a time when criticism of hospital administrators was deafening, she was getting praised.

The first decision Judith credits to turning the nursing community around at Sinai was implementing a registered-nurse-only policy. "I took the idea to our board that the organization should replace all our licensed practical nurses, based on the evidence that with patients' shorter lengths of stay and higher acuity levels, we needed the most highly educated and trained nurses," she says. The trend had been to allow lesser skilled personnel such as cafeteria workers and housekeepers to attend several weeks of training so they could be taught how to feed and bathe patients. Judith argued that when registered nurses give a sponge bath, they do more than rub soap and water over a patient. They are assessing the patient's skin integrity, hydration, mental acuity, movement of joints and muscles, and conditions of surgical incisions, in addition to providing education to the patient. She presented the case by tying the evidence to investment of organizational dollars, which is what the board members could best identify with in making their decision. "I told them hiring a licensed practical nurse was $10,000-$15,000 less than hiring a registered nurse, but if you add in the evidence related to patient care, the investment pays for itself quickly," she says. In a 1997 interview published in *Chatelaine* (a Canadian women's magazine), one of her employees stated, "If Judith loses, we all lose." During a time when criticism of hospital administrators was deafening, she was getting praised.

Other hospital administrators pressured both Judith and her CEO about their decision, because it had tremendous implications for their workforce and budget. She was elevating the standard of care, and the competition did not like it. Judith implemented the nursing decisions she believed to be right and was ready to be fired if her own organization caved under the pressure. Judith's

She was elevating the standard of care, and the competition did not like it.

style was to ask the CEO what portion of the budget was for nursing personnel, then she wanted him to let her decide how to spend that money. The CEO and board of directors allowed her that control and power.

> *"I knew that whoever held the money held the power, and it was the key to negotiating."*

Her decision to change to a registered-nurse-only model of care within the hospital gained national prominence. She could not accept the trend toward "de-skilling" of nursing personnel with less qualified individuals, so she proposed the opposite. "Some hospitals did not want nursing personnel to identify their professional status to patients, so the lesser skill mix could remain a hidden secret," she says. Judith made sure at Sinai that the only individuals giving nursing services at the bedside were registered nurses.

Five years after implementing this change, she remembers that their budget expenses for the more highly educated personnel were not the lowest in the country, but not the highest either. They fell in the middle of national averages for hospital nursing expenses. "Our patient outcomes were terrific, and it was during the time Linda Aiken and I worked on the Magnet data," Judith says. Sinai had the highest retention scores for nurses and the highest nurses' satisfaction scores.

Another trend during the 1990s in hospitals was moving toward a program management model, which meant nurse executives were no longer in charge of the resources and budgets for nursing areas. Instead of nurse executives overseeing these responsibilities, other health care personnel were tasked with this charge. The explicit argument was that this would produce better patient outcomes. From the inside, it felt like physicians did not want nurses making decisions related to the budget. This was the second leadership change Judith referenced. "I knew that whoever held the money held the power, and it was the key to negotiating," she says. Unlike nearly every other Canadian hospital system, Judith was given control over her own budget. Her CEO took much heat, because allowing Judith to hold the key to the budget put pressure on how competitive organizations structured their systems. "My CEO would say that other administrators approached him complaining that 'Shamian does this and Shamian does that.'" Other CEOs were getting pressure from their nurse executives to institute some of the same changes. Few organizations, however, followed. "Sinai was like a gift from heaven for me, because it was my own testing ground for implementing what I believed was right for both nurses and patients," Judith says.

During her 10-year term at Sinai, Judith readily admits she developed an appetite for being a change agent. She honed her skills during the worst and the best of her time there. When she arrived at Sinai, she was determined to build a professional environment. It did not come without its lessons in leadership. Her professional environment vision did not allow room for shared decision-making and power among all members of staff. She did hold town hall meetings to hear concerns and new ideas, and she always kept her office door open for employees or physicians. It was an environment that allowed "heart-to-heart," honest discussions through a time of downsizing.

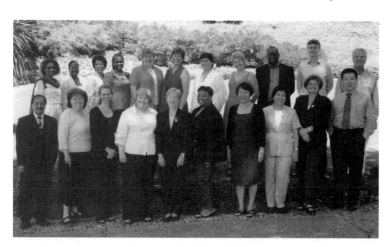

BELLAGIO, ITALY, HEALTH WORK-FORCE MEETING ATTENDEES. JUDITH IS SECOND FROM LEFT IN THE FRONT ROW.

Judith had a very strong leadership team with diverse talents. She was determined to not just have a collection of stars, but to have an amazing team that together would move mountains. Many of these team members today hold major leadership positions throughout Canada.

Not everyone uses power wisely.

However, as good as this may sound, Judith remembers a group of union labor and delivery room nurses who threatened to get the hospital blacklisted by the university. "To be blacklisted means that the union board of directors passes a motion stating the medical center is a 'bad' employer and basically, the whole country knows it," she says. To Judith, this would have been the worst slap in the face, considering the intense work she had done and the progress being made. "We were thinking there was no healthcare organization like us in the country, because of our national reputation for excellence." It was a personal pain like no other Judith had experienced in her career, brought on by a small group of nurses who were bent on creating destruction. Justice was served, however, when the union dismissed the charges as having no merit.

The situation still pains Judith, as she came to realize what horrible things can result when there is an abuse of power. "We have seen this in history, and it is no different in organizations," she says. Not everyone uses power wisely, and as much as you can do with the best intention of caring, it will not be enough for some. "We talk about nurses being deprived at times or disadvantaged, but this group took advantage by using the union to instill fear."

After 10 years of service in acute care, Judith came to realize how difficult it was on her soul. She was the best paid nurse executive in the country and had the support and power to make the necessary changes for nursing. She was a nurse executive at a hospital that was actually involved in research. It was all pretty heady stuff, but she knew there were other things she wanted to do. On a weekly basis, she would get calls about other opportunities.

It was not too long before she heard of a position opening in the Canadian government for an executive director for the Office of Nursing Policy, Health Policy and Communications Branch of Health Canada. Basically, the position was equivalent to what some recognize as the chief nurse of Canada. Judith had the privilege to be the first person in this position and office. It allowed her to test her ability to build something from nothing. It was a complete change from hospital administration. Her colleagues could not understand why she would make such a career move. "To move from a dream job and take a cut in salary did not make sense to some, but I knew it was right for me," she says.

Judith was always very interested in healthcare policy, so this gave her a front row seat in influencing change. Nurses from around the country applied for the position, but Judith was the chosen candidate. She was honored, yet sad to leave Mount Sinai Hospital. It had been wonderful, but she also recognized it was time to move on to a new career adventure and take a risk. "I had developed enough of a reputation to be able to compete successfully to work for the benefit of healthcare and nursing across Canada, rather than in one institution or even in one province," she says.

As Canada's chief nurse, she sharpened her skills in directing and shaping public policy. "Nurses complain about all that is wrong with the nursing profession or healthcare, but we are not going to change anything if we don't break out and influence the agenda from the outside," she says. Judith has figured out how to do this, how to share it with others, and how to teach those wanting to learn. Her role of mentoring others to influence change is an enormous contribution that still continues to pay dividends.

The Office of Nursing Policy gives nursing issues a more prominent position at Health Canada and brings the perspectives of nurses to the department's policy work and decision-making. Through the Office of Nursing Policy, decisions made by the Minister of Health were seen through a different lens. By the late 1990s, soaring levels of overtime, workplace injury, illness, and absenteeism had combined with the aging of the nursing workforce to bring the nation's nurses to a point of crisis. These issues only highlighted the crucial role nurses play in the healthcare system.

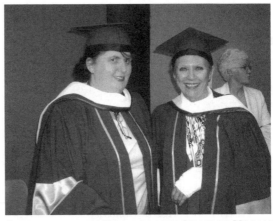

JUDITH AND THE HONOURABLE SENATOR VIVIAN POY, RECEIVING AN HONOURARY DOCTORATE (LLD) FROM THE UNIVERSITY OF LETHBRIDGE, LETHBRIDGE, ALBERTA.

WORLD HEALTH ORGANIZATION

Having lived in Hungary, Israel, and Canada, Judith had experiences and national and international opinions on healthcare and nursing. Her master's program at New York University, which focused on international health, required students to travel every summer. She went to Puerto Rico one year and Australia the following year. Throughout her career, there were mentors or leaders who helped to open doors that, in turn, allowed additional opportunities for her. "Because I am eager and hard-working, other leaders knew it was worth their time to invest in me—they saw potential," she says.

> *Because I am eager and hard-working, other leaders knew it was worth their time to invest in me—they saw potential.*

One such mentor was Marian Hamburg, director of the graduate program at New York University. She introduced Judith to the international world. "I remember going with Marian to my first American Public Health Association meeting in Detroit with over 10,000 people," she says. Marian introduced Judith to others in the international world of public health. It was through Marian's network that Judith was asked to be on the board of the International Union of Health Education (IUHE), a Paris-based organization. "That is what introduced me professionally to Paris, France, and the international network of health professionals," she says. The interesting point is that when Judith first started working in the international arena, it was not related to nursing, but rather to public health education. She built her original network through IUHE and later used that to cross over into international nursing. Throughout her career, Judith built partnerships within and outside of nursing. This helped Judith to continually build a broad view on healthcare.

In 1985, Judith received a call from the World Health Organization (WHO) office in Europe, asking if she could help them with some focused work in Hungary. At the time, the chief nurse of WHO, Miriam Hirschfield of Geneva, Switzerland, was a professional friend of Judith's. She excitedly accepted the assignment of teaching a workshop in Hungary. It was the first time she had returned to her native country since she left with her family at age 10. "My Hungarian is the Hungarian of a 10-year-old child, but at that time, not like today, very few spoke English in Hungary, so they were grateful for somebody even with my Hungarian," she says. Judith remembers they laughed good-heartedly at her every second sentence, but they could connect with her.

Working with the WHO opened doors for Judith's research work. Around this same year, while Judith was attending a conference in Edmonton, a woman dressed in African attire walked off the elevator. Not

knowing who she was, Judith asked her if she would like company for breakfast. This started a lifelong friendship with Dr. Serara S. Kupe, whom Judith considers the Florence Nightingale of Africa. "I received funding to do some research work with her in Botswana, which was one of the most memorable moments in my nursing career," she says. Together they brought the first computer to the university's school of nursing in Gabarone, the capital of Botswana.

The power of one's network is a lesson she has learned throughout her international journey. Marian Hamburg had introduced her to the IUHE. She then reached out to a stranger at a conference and made the connection to Botswana, and she had her own personal connections in Israel, Geneva, and Hungary. All the dots on the paper connected to create the international picture, which blossomed based on her research, leadership, and reputation. Through her work with the WHO, Judith also became involved with the Global Advisory Group (GAG) on Nursing and Midwifery. This group advises the WHO director general on nursing issues. Judith also worked as a consultant to GRASP, a workload measurement system based in the United States. Judith's international work that fell outside her full-time job focused on supporting the WHO chief nursing office. She built the WHO Collaborating Centre at Mount Sinai and continues to work closely with WHO nursing executives.

THE HEALTHCARE SYSTEM IN CANADA

Healthcare reform began in Canada after World War II, in the wake of widespread social reforms across Europe. The United Kingdom had a comprehensive government health insurance plan as early as 1948. Canada was a little slower. By 1957, the country had a nationwide plan insuring Canadians against the cost of hospitalization. In 1968, new federal legislation was passed, extending coverage to physicians' services. The new legislation was intended to eliminate economic and regional barriers to access to healthcare. Legislation was passed in 1984 that requires all provinces to provide health plans to their residents that covers all "medically necessary and medically required" services. Private billing and user fees are prohibited. In other words, the Canadian health system currently guarantees the provision of universal, portable, accessible, and comprehensive health services.

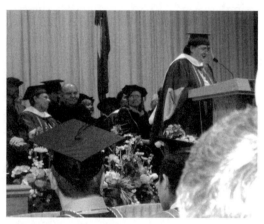

ADDRESSING THE GRADUATES.

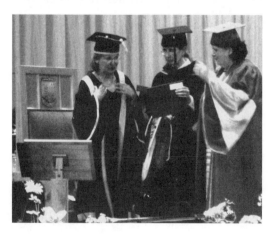

One of the exciting trends in nursing throughout Canada is the standard of baccalaureate education for all nurses, as well as the degree of their participation in the Canadian Nurses Association. Nurses are members of the self-governed regulatory association for their province. By virtue of this membership, nurses belong to the Canadian Nurses Association. Quebec is an exception to this standard. Most nurses in Canada are unionized.

Judith watches as the trend in Canada is for nurses and physicians to be enticed by high-paying offers and incentives to take cases in the private system. Consequently, patients requiring surgery in the public system are pushed further back on a waiting list. Some provinces and political parties are strong supporters of private healthcare, "but the citizens of Canada are not," she says.

In Canada, even at the small community hospital level, nursing professionals of all levels can interface with research projects.

When asked what the differences are between nursing in Canada and other countries, Judith replied, "In Canada there is a smoother and easier walk over the bridge of research, policy and practice. In the United States, for instance, some of the best nursing research is taking place, but in the large picture, it is done by the top 5-10% of nursing researchers. In Canada, even at the small community hospital level, nursing professionals of all levels can interface with research projects." The federal government established a Health Services Research Foundation that has helped develop some exclusive mechanisms by which researchers must engage decision makers in projects to qualify for grants, which it has cultivated a culture of evidence-based practice across the country.

In addition to a comfortable bridge between academics and practice in Canada, Judith views the nursing leadership within the country as a strong collaborative force that is less likely to be influenced by politicians who may try to "divide and conquer." The country's nursing leaders are also active in international work.

21st-Century Nursing

Judith has been honored over the years with many awards. She is most proud of several key recognitions. She received the Jubilee Medal during the 50th anniversary of Queen Elizabeth II, a medal awarded only to Canadians who have made significant contributions to the country. Judith was recognized for her years of work and contributions to the Canadian healthcare system. In addition, receiving the Alumni of the Year award from Case Western was very meaningful to Judith. She has also been given two Canadian honorary doctorates, one from Lethbridge University in Alberta and the other from Ryerson University in Toronto, Ontario.

She is most proud of being the first Canadian PhD-prepared nurse to play an executive role in a service setting. She modeled a philosophy different from the norm at the time. "I never stopped having research as part of what I did, so I modeled the role of an executive director and vice president, with a staff of over 1,000 and a budget of more than $50 million, still exercising my academic responsibilities," she says. The other area Judith cites with great pride is her ability to develop a strong relationship between Mount Sinai Hospital and the university, as she introduced evidence-based management. At the time, it set leadership apart.

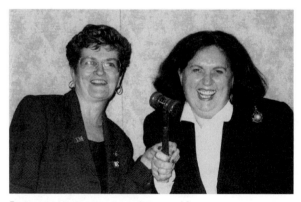

President of the registered Nursing Association of Ontario.

One powerful lesson Judith learned in shaping and influencing health policy is to frame discussions around how the policy benefits Canadians or the country's healthcare needs, versus talking about what nurses need. Decision makers and politicians listen better when they hear advocacy for the public rather than for a vested interest group.

When Judith mentors "up and coming" nurses, she instills in them the "power of one." Her philosophy is that each nurse needs to understand how she or he can play a significant role in building partnerships and working with colleagues on shared agendas. For her, this is essential. The voice of many nursing groups is dismissed because they do not have the sophistication to build the lines of strong leadership. "It is important that all of us in nursing have a sense of our role and responsibility for the external world," she says. Judith credits her vast international network with assisting in pushing through key agendas. "I would like to see nurses in critical government positions, including ministers of finance."

> *Her philosophy is that each nurse needs to understand how she or he can play a significant role in building partnerships and working with colleagues on shared agendas.*

Throughout her nursing career and her life, Judith has kept true to her values. She found jobs and chose to live in certain countries based on whether she could align her personal value system with them. She juggled work, family, school, and research to overcome obstacles on the road to success. She took risks even if it meant "my head would end up on the chopping block." She believes it is important that nurses take credit for their successes.

In June 2004, Judith decided to leave the federal government to become president and chief executive officer of the Victorian Order of Nurses (VON) Canada. This organization is the largest nonprofit, charitable home care and community health organization in Canada. This highly regarded organization, founded in 1897, provides much-needed home care in communities across Canada. Once the Canadian leader in this role, VON Canada now competes with other healthcare providers that offer similar healthcare services in each province. With her strong background in governmental affairs, her high-profile reputation, and her international network, Judith is well-positioned for the job of leader at VON Canada. She provides the voice for strengthening public access to healthcare in Canada and advocates for policy directions that are needed. It is incredibly hard work, but the right thing to do. "When we get back to the shining glory

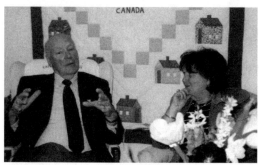

PRESIDENT OF THE REGISTERED NURSING ASSOCIATION OF ONTARIO.

that the organization used to be, Canada will be a stronger and better place," she says. With nurse leaders as determined as Judith to improve and keep watch over an entire country's healthcare system, the citizens of Canada are in good hands.

REFERENCE

RN with a cause. (1997). *Chatelaine*.

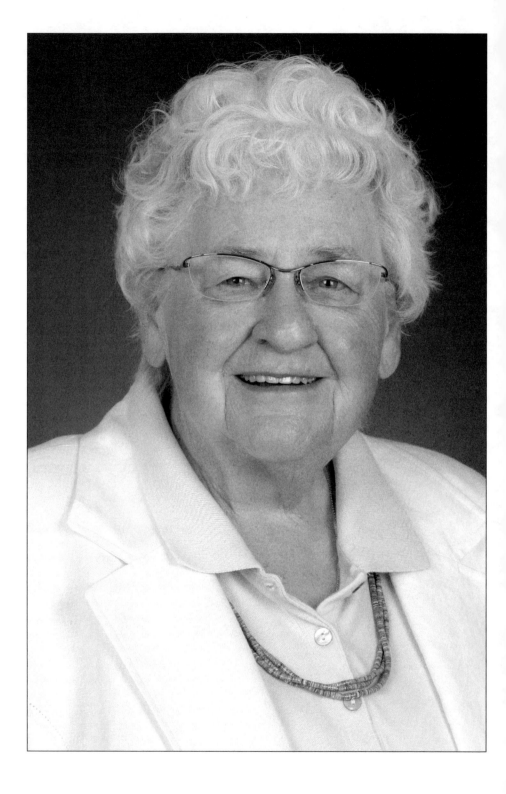

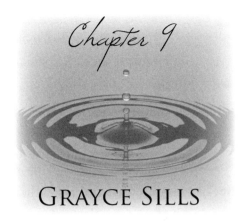

Chapter 9

GRAYCE SILLS

"The best lessons I learned came from the school of life."

—Grayce Sills

Grayce Sills, PhD, RN, FAAN, grew up in Bremen, Ohio, USA, a small town with roughly 1,100 people and 11 churches. Because of its small size, the community provided residents unique opportunities not available in large cities. It was a healthy environment. Children were raised by extended families and had the good fortune of being exposed to strong community influences. Bremen did not, however, allow for much privacy, and diversity was limited to the distinction between Catholic and Protestant, which took on the same mean-spiritedness that drives other forms of discrimination. Everyone knew each other's business and, according to Grayce, some knew more than you ever wanted them to know. This sense of togetherness and belonging to a community—both the positive and negative aspects—had a major impact on Grayce's life and influenced her research, leadership, and teaching. As Grayce says, "I found and continue to have an appreciation for the richness that diversity brings to our lives and have a concern and passion for social justice."

Grayce was the youngest of four children, each 2 years apart. She was orphaned at 2 1/2 after her mother died and her father, overwhelmed with the family responsibilities, subsequently abandoned the family to live and work in another community. She was raised by her grandparents and other relatives—later by the church pastor's wife—and went on to become a leader in psychiatric nursing and an advocate for psychiatric patients. It is no wonder the small-town values of family, community, and church were responsible for shaping her perspective on life. "The best lessons I learned came from the school of life," Grayce says.

THE EARLY YEARS

Grayce's mother died of septicemia. Her father, unable to handle the responsibilities of being a single parent to four children, left home for work in another community and returned only once or twice after that. He had tried to keep them all together for the first year, but he lost his job during the middle of the Great Depression and then just left town. This is where Grayce came to know the value of extended family and the community. The community pulled together as the problem solver. She and her three older siblings were raised mostly by her mother's family with the support of her father's relatives in Bremen. Grayce remembers the strong family and community ties that helped to make up for the absence of her mother and father.

As life would have it, at age 9 Grayce lost her grandmother, who had been a second mother to her. With her grandmother gone, Grayce leaned on the community and church for support. Almost everyone in town went to church. "People made it their business to monitor who went to church and who skipped," Grayce says. She attended the Presbyterian church, and the minister's wife became like a third mother to her. The minister's wife was also her high school English teacher, as well as Girl Scout leader and church choir director. It was this link to the choir that taught Grayce a keen lesson that she carries to this day: No matter how much you care about people, you have to be kind but unbiased when judging their talents. Grayce wanted to sing in the choir. The minister's wife, who clearly cared deeply for Grayce, never let her be a choir member. Grayce had numerous strengths, but singing was not among them. She later realized how wise a decision it was for her not to sing in the choir and what an important lesson it taught her.

During her teenage years, Grayce blossomed under the guidance of the pastor's wife, who shared intellectual gifts and cultivated in Grayce the desire to pursue higher education. No one in Grayce's family had been to college. Furthermore, she did not know anyone in the community who spoke of going away to college. The only individuals Grayce knew who were college-educated were her schoolteachers. Luckily, her lack of financial means did not prevent her from attending college, as people within the community stepped in to help with a

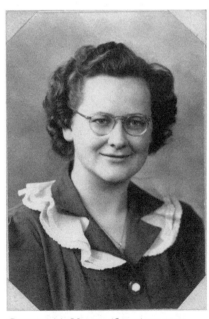

GRAYCE MCVEIGH (SILLS) IN HER HIGH SCHOOL GRADUATION PHOTO FROM MAY 1944.

scholarship. Even while making plans to attend college, Grayce had no idea what she should major in or what career she should pursue.With a $100 scholarship and not the slightest idea of what she was going to do, Grayce enrolled in Ohio University (OU) right out of high school. She laughs as she remembers how it must have seemed that she was "going to major in life," as she had no particular direction. During the 1940s, OU was a small liberal arts school with an emphasis on scholarship. At that time, much emphasis was placed on the liberal arts component. To assist in paying for her tuition, Grayce worked for the Presbyterian minister's family. She earned her room and board by doing the family cooking and cleaning and babysitting the couple's four adopted children.

By her sophomore year, her adviser asked her what she wanted to do with her life. Grayce knew she enjoyed working with people but did not want to be a social worker. Her adviser told her about the American Friends Service Committee, which was hosting a summer work camp at a

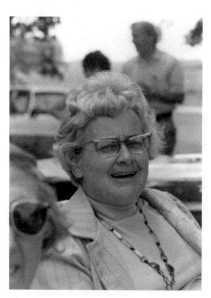

GRAYCE AT A FAMILY REUNION IN 1992.

mental hospital in New York. The United States was just coming out of WWII, and funds were being invested in training for some of the lower level positions in the New York state hospital. The summer camp paid $50 a month, along with room and board. The camp staff would provide training classes to prepare Grayce and the other students for working with mentally ill patients. "I thought this would be a great way to broaden my horizons and make a little money for myself," she says. She hoped to save enough money so she would not have to borrow from her grandfather for her remaining college tuition.

At age 20, she boarded the train from Ohio to New York, the first time she had taken such a significant trip. It was quite an adventure for her. Once there, Grayce met up with more than 100 other college students who were equally as energetic—and clueless as to what they were getting themselves into. The Rockland State Hospital was one of the largest psychiatric state institutions in the world. "It was a grim setting in days when patients were treated with electric shock treatments, mixed with the equally noxious paraldehyde," Grayce says.

The scene in the movie A Beautiful Mind *where insulin shock therapy was used is very close to what I saw on a regular basis.*

Grayce still shudders when she remembers the appalling conditions. Psychiatric patients were stripped of their dignity and treated with little or no respect. "The scene in the movie *A Beautiful Mind* where insulin shock therapy was used is very close to what I saw on a regular basis," she says.

At the time, physicians thought these treatments were beneficial, but they came to be a powerful lesson for Grayce. "It was an era of cold packs, full-sheet restraints, and electric shock therapy," she says. "We did not have the benefits offered today with the range of drugs and behavioral therapy." Grayce is still tormented by the horrific memories of these early treatments and vividly remembers the hopeless situations patients faced. Because of the aggressive treatments used in her early days as an aide, Grayce says she is "cautious about new drugs and their side effects, as well as new medical technology being used on extreme psychiatric problems."

Of more than 100 students who worked through the summer, only six decided to accept the offer to extend their stay over the entire year. The pay of those willing to stay on increased from $50 to $100 per month. Grayce felt this opportunity would provide her the needed income to go back to OU and finish her last 2 years.

It was during this extended year that Grayce became interested in psychiatric nursing. A head nurse named Betty Oliver seemed to work magic with patients and greatly influenced Grayce's decision to go into nursing. Even as a psychiatric aide, Grayce observed how Betty could walk into a room and within minutes bring comfort and calmness to her patients.

NURSING SCHOOL

After she decided to go into psychiatric nursing, Grayce enrolled in Rockland State Hospital's 3-year diploma program. While in nursing school, the students were paid $30 a month, along with room and board. "I knew I wanted to be a psychiatric nurse, but I was not too sure about the other areas of nursing," she says. "I still have the bumps and bruises from those 3 years!"

One nursing instructor during Grayce's operating room rotation was a role model of how *not* to teach students. This teacher would tell students they were either "funny bunnies" or "dumb bunnies." Grayce had the misfortune to be in the "dumb bunny" group. "I have often used this to emphasize the importance of being very careful to not label students," she says. In this particular case, the instructor told Grayce she was the "dumbest bunny of all." The teacher's disparaging comments made Grayce wonder if she belonged in nursing school and if she was smart enough to do the job.

One nursing instructor during Grayce's operating room rotation was a role model of how not to teach students.

Grayce and three other classmates supported each other during this challenging clinical rotation. To this day, no matter how much a student is struggling, "I am careful not to be sarcastic with them or label them," she says. The teacher's words had a powerfully negative effect on Grayce. The label given to her as a student made her question her aptitude and intelligence for many years to come.

The instructor told Grayce she was the "dumbest bunny of all." The teacher's disparaging comments made Grayce wonder if she belonged in nursing school and if she was smart enough to do the job.

In 1950, Grayce graduated from the Rockland State Hospital nursing program. She had completed 2 years at OU prior to nursing school. During the 1950s, her 5 years of combined education qualified her to teach in the diploma program at Rockland. She knew her educational path was not complete and wanted to finish her baccalaureate degree. Immediately after finishing Rockland's diploma program, Grayce was accepted into the baccalaureate completion program at Teacher's College in New York City. Mildred Montag, her adviser, told Grayce that since she had 3 years in a diploma program, 2 years at OU, and 2 years of psychiatric nursing experience, she should also be part of the new psychiatric nursing master's program.

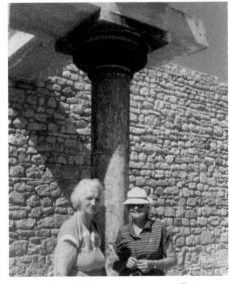

HILDEGARD PEPLAU, LEFT, AND GRAYCE SILLS IN KNOSSOS IN THE GREEK ISLES IN 1983.

Grayce had her first course with Hildegard Peplau, one of psychiatric nursing's foremost authorities. Grayce could not understand most of her concepts. Hildegard had developed an experiential mode of teaching based upon nurses' interactions and experiences with mental patients. She emphasized the therapeutic value of interpersonal relations between nurses and patients, as well as the role the environment played in changing behavior.

Grayce vividly remembers Hildegard talking about "high-level concepts of which I had no understanding. … I thought I was competent in nursing up until this point." The other students seemed to have read the research studies and literature, which Grayce had never heard of. "I was swimming in deep waters," she says. "With my sister ill, an excuse was there for me to leave midway through the second semester." Grayce was glad for the opportunity to be out of the course, because she did not understand Hildegard at all. "Dropping out of school felt very much like a failure to me," she says. Hildegard's approach was beyond what Grayce could initially comprehend, but the interpersonal approach to patient care left an impression.

FIRST LEADERSHIP POSITION IN NURSING

Grayce was needed by her sister and family back in Ohio, so she accepted a position at Dayton State Hospital as the associate director of nursing. There were four administrators and almost 700 aides and attendants. Her experience at Rockland State Hospital had taught Grace that the training provided for psychiatric aides and attendants was important. In Ohio, employees were hired to work on the units and given keys, with the hope they would learn from people who were already there. Obviously, the outcome was not always desirable and turnover of personnel was high.

The first program Grayce implemented was a training program. It was the first psychiatric aide training program in Ohio and soon became required curriculum in the state. Completion of the program was tied into the state pay scale, so employees eagerly participated.

The state hospital was designed according to the Kirkbride tradition, where the main building had ancillary wings extending out from a central corridor with men on one side and women on the other. Kirkbride's philosophy was that every patient should have access to an outside window. To accomplish that, long corridors with big windows in the sleeping rooms were required. However, the main rooms where patients spent the majority of their time were dark, while their bedrooms were painted white with natural sunlight shining through. "The thought was excellent, but the execution in this case was something else," Grayce says.

In 1956, Associate Director of Nursing Grayce Sills did not always have answers for her staff. In those cases, "I walked fast and looked like I was going someplace very important ... as if I were on the way to another meeting," she says. In reality, she was thinking, "Don't interrupt me, because I don't have any idea of how to handle some of the things you are going to ask me." She learned to do the job, all the while being acutely aware that she did not always have the answers. Instead, she found that being aware of available resources led her and her staff to answers or decisions.

Grayce always taught nursing students that during their career, they would be offered positions they did

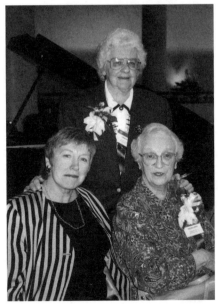

PAT MURPHY, LEFT, GRAYCE, CENTER, AND HILDEGARD PEPLAU, RIGHT, AT GRAYCE'S RETIREMENT SYMPOSIUM IN 1994.

not feel qualified for, but as long as they extended themselves to continue learning, they should embrace those challenges. "You tell yourself, 'I have to keep learning and developing more in this area.' Being willing to learn is how people improve themselves. It is sad to watch people take a leadership position and think they 'have arrived' when actually they are far from it," she says.

Over more than a decade, Hildegard Peplau spent summer months traveling to mental hospitals all over the United States to give 1- to 2-week workshops. She taught skills for interviewing patients, basic interpersonal skills, and psychiatric nursing concepts. She also gave hope to nurses by describing treatments that were helpful for patients. This was during the time frame when psychiatric care was moving from custodial to therapeutic care.

While Hildegard was working one summer in the neighboring state of Indiana, nursing consultants from Ohio attended her workshop. The consultants asked her to present her workshop in Ohio. Hildegard said she would be happy to come because Grayce Sills lived there, and she was one of the brightest people Hildegard had ever worked with.

"When I heard her comment, I thought, 'Wow,' I am not a dumb bunny after all,'" Grayce says. "It was Peplau who told me for the first time in my life that I was bright." Grayce often illustrates the power of positive affirmation by comparing Hildegard's comment to the former instructor's "dumb bunny" remark.

Hildegard asked Grayce to join her in teaching. From that point forward, her psychiatric nursing career blossomed. "We developed a relationship that spanned more than 30 years of collaboration and friendship," she says. It took a few years, however, before Grayce was ready to move on and accept Hildegard's offer.

Prior to meeting Hildegard, Grayce was an expert in descriptive psychiatry. During the late 1950s and 1960s, she was starting to learn about psychiatric diagnoses and how to plan a patient's care around that information. In the 1960s, she was influenced largely by Peplau's work and that of Sullivan and other interpersonal theorists. The 1960s were rich years for psychiatric nursing, when the profession was trying to develop the content out of the experience. The patient interview process provided the information to develop concepts and strategies for care. "Hildegard began to prompt me to go back to school and earn a master's degree," Grayce says.

While working at Dayton State Hospital, she completed her Bachelor of Science in Nursing degree at the University of Dayton. She also taught diploma students during their 3-month clinical rotation at the State Hospital. As administrator of the hospital, Grayce became acutely aware of a peculiar trend. After more then 100 diploma students completed their rotation experience, none of them applied to work at the state hospital. The conversion rate of clinical experience to applicant was zero. "We never got any of these students as employees, and I found that mystifying," she says. It would be natural to think that after 3 months of clinical experience, some students could be convinced to come back. Grayce said to the director of the nursing, "I want to be in a job where I teach students how to 'work' with patients, rather than 'do' to and for them." She really believed this would enrich the experience of the students, so they would want to apply for a job after graduation and pursue a career in psychiatric nursing.

Grayce took on the new position herself and was successful in creating interest among nursing students to the point where they actually applied for jobs at the hospital. Her new position expanded further to include professional development training among nursing staff at the hospital. She found it rewarding and was very happy in the new role, but when Hildegard Peplau came every summer for the training workshops, she urged Grayce to go back to school. Hildegard envisioned Grayce teaching graduate students in nursing. "I finally decided she was right," she says. "I did need to expand my own knowledge base of nursing."

Interestingly enough, her decision came at the same time Grayce met a psychiatrist at the hospital. They soon married. He was older, and they assumed they could not have children because of the age difference. As nature would have it, she became pregnant with a daughter soon after they were married. "She was the best thing that ever happened to me," Grayce says. She is now a proud grandmother of two.

Grayce left Dayton to attend graduate school at The Ohio State University, located about 1 hour from Dayton. She brought her daughter with her, but the marriage did not last the separation.

One of the first decisions facing Grayce when she arrived at Ohio State was whether to go into nursing or sociology. Two of her personal friends

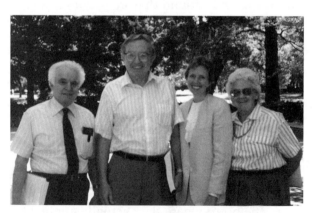

GRAYCE WITH OHIO STATE UNIVERSITY SOCIOLOGY DEPARTMENT FACULTY MEMBERS AND KAREN DAUGHERTY, AN OSU NURSING DOCTORAL GRADUATE, IN 1985. FROM LEFT TO RIGHT: SIMON DINITZ, AL CLARKE, KAREN DAUGHERTY, AND GRAYCE.

directed the graduate program in psychiatry at Ohio State. Her friends, who were from Cornell University and had in-depth psychoanalytic training, were at opposite ends of the theoretical spectrum from her. As much as they liked her personally, they advised her not to come into the nursing psychiatric graduate program. They encouraged her to attend the sociology program, which had a very interpersonal approach, because they knew it would be a closer fit to her interests.

In the sociology program, Grayce felt very much at home. "The people in the sociology department were as welcoming to me as you could imagine," she says. "I was from an outside field and was considered somewhat of a 'tourist.'" The sociology major had more men than women, and the faculty was chauvinistic to the few female students. Grayce, who was not viewed as a threat to the men, did not personally experience any of this chauvinism. The faculty knew that once she graduated, she would return to the nursing profession. Grayce observed this same chauvinistic treatment extended to the female doctoral faculty in sociology. "The men simply felt no woman could ever do field work in sociology, and they should stay back and manage the computers and the data in something of a secretarial function in research." It was a reflection of the time in history and a lack of sensitivity that bordered on arrogance.

Grayce enjoyed graduate school immensely. It was unusual in 1960 to be a single mother supporting a child, no less taking on the rigors of graduate school. Grayce successfully balanced her schooling and role as mother. Just before graduation, she was asked to apply to the doctoral program in nursing. During the 1960s, a federal program provided funding for unique partnerships among academic departments. For instance, at Case Western and several other academic institutions, students were dispersed in various majors: sociology, nursing, anatomy, or physiology. Each of the academic departments received a stipend just for accepting these students into their programs. "In order to get nurses through graduate education, the federal government provided funding from the nursing traineeship division," she says. Grayce was one of the first to break down the barrier of coming into the sociology doctoral program, which received no nursing funds. She earned a PhD in sociology.

While Grayce was working on her doctorate, the Vietnam War was raging, along with much political upheaval and anti-government sentiment among students. The climate surrounding this era was leaking onto the Ohio State campus. Grayce was one of six elected graduate students who requested a meeting with the university provost to discuss problems in the sociology department. In his reply, the provost said the department chair was doing his job very well, as far as he was concerned. The provost assured the students that the chair would take care of any problems in good time. About a week later, African-American students on campus took over the administration building, which brought out the Ohio National Guard and the Ohio State Highway Patrol.

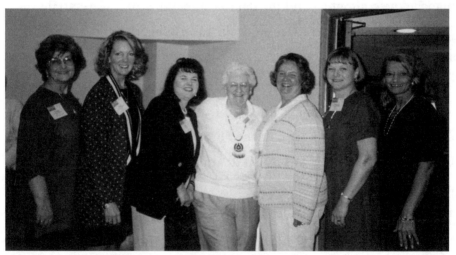

OHIO NURSE EDITORS AT THE COLORADO INANE MEETING. FROM LEFT TO RIGHT: LEAH CURTIN, KAY BALL, TINA MARELLI, GRAYCE, AND KATHY STONE. JOYCE FITZPATRICK IS ON THE FAR RIGHT. [WITH APOLOGIES, WE HAVE BEEN UNABLE TO IDENTIFY THE WOMAN SECOND FROM RIGHT.]

Grayce and her colleagues sent another letter to the provost stating, in essence, "Apparently there is only one way to be heard on this campus, and we still would like to have an appointment." The students quickly received a response granting a meeting with the provost. "I will never forget the march from our building to the administration building, which was surrounded by armed personnel," she says. The guards saw six students—5 shaggy-haired, bearded men and Grayce—approaching the administration building. When they focused on Grayce, who already had grey hair, the armed guards nodded and allowed them to pass. "We got into the elevator, and I told the men that I was their entrance ticket," she says.

Through that experience, Grayce discovered how it felt to be part of a subculture. More importantly, she learned how the university system worked and how to accomplish goals within that system. The incident illustrated the relationship among the provost, department chairs, and faculty. Grayce learned that leadership is a function, and it can be exerted from any level. "When it goes forward, the positional power is more potent, but if you have a dean or director who has positional power and knows how leadership can be a function, you have a powerful leader," she says. The experience helped Grayce gain a richer sense of social justice.

Between her master's work and doctoral program, Grayce taught for a year at The Ohio State University School of Nursing. She and her two colleagues from Cornell University had a plan for the psychiatric nursing program. The two colleagues would be retiring at a time that would coincide with Grayce finishing her doctorate, and she would take over the psychiatric nursing program. The plan worked out perfectly, except that when Grayce took over the program only one student had been recruited. She soon got a second part-time student and told everyone she had a 100% improvement in enrollment!

Grayce had noticed a similar situation in the psychiatric nursing program at Dayton State Hospital. Something was wrong when students did not migrate to psychiatric nursing practice. Since she was successful in turning around a similar situation once before, she believed she could do the same for this psychiatric program. "I knew I had to approach and work with these students differently," she says. The field of psychiatric nursing was just developing its theory and content beyond that of descriptive psychiatry. It was now extending beyond simply teaching nurses to carry out whatever the physician ordered.

Grayce worked at The Ohio State University the majority of her career in nursing. In the 1970s, nursing faculty members were discussing how to transition from a nursing school to a college. At Ohio State, the large units with deans were called colleges, while the smaller units under them were schools led by directors. The deans controlled the budget and access to the provost and helped develop policy for the institution. The schools were considered lower in the hierarchy, so information was slow to filter down to them. The budget also went from the school to the dean to the provost level. "We were a school in the College of Medicine that was an afterthought, for the most part," she says.

The School of Nursing had little voice in the operations of the university. Colleagues outside the school encouraged Grayce and other faculty to take action. They needed an initiative that would allow them college status. At first, the nursing faculty did not know where to start. The impetus they needed came when they realized that most university faculty members were on 9-month contracts, while the nursing faculty was paid the equivalent of 9-month wages but under 12-month contracts. Something was very wrong with that picture. "It was gender bias, but at the same time, we were not as academically qualified as the [college] faculty groups at that particular point," she says. The colleges had faculty who were prepared at the doctoral level or higher. The School of Nursing still had full-time faculty who held only a bachelor's degree. While this practice was on par with some other nursing programs and universities across the country, it did not make for a competitive edge within the Ohio State academic culture.

The first thing the nursing faculty focused on was the salary and equity issue. "We had to convince the faculty that here was an issue worth taking on," she says. Many of the nurses were married and had husbands who were the primary breadwinners, so they were less concerned about stirring the pot. In public universities, salaries are public information. Grayce and the leadership team used this information to create a level of discontent and dissatisfaction to motivate everyone to push for change.

Equalizing the salary discrepancy sounds logical and should have been obvious, but it took several years before any action was taken. "We presented our proposal to administrative people, the dean, and his college administration," she says. They were met with the initial response, "There is no money." Grayce and her team countered with the proposition that they would then accept their current pay but work only 9 months, as was common with the other faculty groups. That triggered a response and negotiations began. The nurses were finally being heard. Their intense discussions included threats of striking. "We decided collectively as faculty we would never go on strike, but that is how passionate we were about being heard," she says.

If more action was needed, the group decided that Grayce should go to the media. Grayce, who had her doctorate and tenure, could be the spokesperson since she had nothing to lose. However, the university administration did not push the group that far. The salary and equity were adjusted, but not without an admonition from the provost, who said that since nursing faculty members would be off in the summer, they could obtain the advanced degrees needed to pursue scholarship. Grayce could not argue that point, as it was true. The nursing faculty did use the time to pursue advanced degrees, and many enrolled in doctoral programs at Ohio State.

Now that the salary adjustments were complete, the issue of making the school a college needed to be addressed. Faculty members met with colleagues within the university in an effort to build a sense of consensus for their cause. They strategically used campus politics to garner support. The hospital and health science center were in the same area as the university, so the faculty built support among this group of colleagues. While some faculty focused on getting the proposal ready for submission, others focused on collaborative relationships. The faculty of the other colleges would vote on the proposal, so buy-in was essential. "We had them in our pocket, because they understood our aspirations and thought we were pursuing a good thing," Grayce says. The proposal passed and the School of Nursing officially became the College of Nursing.

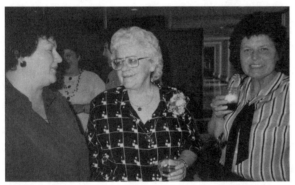

JOANNE STEVENSON, LEFT, GRAYCE, CENTER, AND MARY MACVICAR CELEBRATE THE CHANGE FROM SCHOOL OF NURSING TO COLLEGE OF NURSING AT OHIO STATE UNIVERSITY IN 1982.

The next discussion centered on who would become dean, as none of them had administrative experience. They asked the associate provost, who was familiar with nursing issues, if she would delay her retirement 1 year and provide leadership. She agreed and a formal search was conducted. The agreement specified that Grayce would be associate dean during that year, because the two worked together very well. After a year of searching for a new dean, the president offered Grayce the position. "I said, 'That is fine on a temporary basis, but I'm not going anywhere, so if we bring somebody else in we will be twice as strong.'" Grayce accepted an acting dean position until the search was complete. The first dean of The Ohio State University College of Nursing was Dr. Carole Anderson. Grayce held her position as associate dean for a year and interim dean for two years before stepping down to accept a department chair position. "We needed continued strength in our senior nursing leadership, so this allowed us to bring in new blood," she says. Sometimes Grayce wonders if she should have accepted the dean of nursing position, because it would have been an opportunity for her to grow as an administrator and leader.

Even with a career rich in academics, Grayce never forgot her patients and was committed to improving the quality of care. She was instrumental in advocating for community-based mental health services as well as stress-ing the importance of family and commu-nity involvement in patient care. "I have dedicated my career to integrating family and community care in the treatment of psychiatric patients," Grayce says. She spent her career trying to recreate that small-town support system for the vulner-able, less-fortunate psychiatric patient.

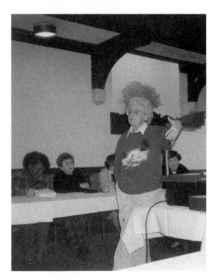

GRAYCE SILLS, INTERIM DEAN FOR OHIO STATE'S COLLEGE OF NURSING, AT OVERHEAD PROJECTOR DURING A FACULTY RETREAT IN 1983.

Grayce was on the governor's com-mittee for comprehensive mental health planning as a member of Franklin Coun-try's planning committee for outpatient and emergency services. Following her re-tirement from Ohio State, Grayce chaired

Ohio's study committee on mental health services and was a member and chair of the board of trustees for university hospitals.

Grayce left her legacy at The Ohio State University. From her perspective: "Every organization needs both perchers and nesters. The nesters have the painstaking task of establishing order and building a system, while the perchers, like me, come along and enrich it and fix it and often leave their debris behind." Grayce found herself in a position of leading the charge most of her career, which meant she did leave debris along the way. How-

Every organization needs both perchers and nesters.

ever, she accomplished most of what she set out to do. She became a faculty member in 1968 and stayed at Ohio State until her retirement in 1991.

PROFESSIONAL ASSOCIATION WORK

While in graduate school, Grayce became actively involved in promoting the development of the American Nurses Association (ANA). She passionately pushed nurses to join and get involved in ANA. She thought it would be great to have units or clinical areas within ANA for participation in nurses' specialty areas. During the mid-1960s, ANA was divided primarily into two areas of representation: bedside nurses and administrative nurses. After 7 or 8 years of trying to promote divided units within ANA, the group of psychiatric nurses found a home with the National League of Nursing and became the Interdivisional Council on Psychiatric Nursing. Grayce chaired the council in Ohio, her first leadership position unrelated to her employment.

The council disseminated information via providing opportunities for continuing education. It was after this time frame that ANA created divisions within the association; thus, the Interdivisional Council moved over to ANA.

One issue Grayce passionately promoted was the importance of diversity and human rights in professional practice. "I pressured the Ohio State Nurses Association to develop the first statewide committee on human rights," she says. The committee began to discuss what could be done at the state level to improve diversity within the profession. Discussions revolved around teaching people to work with differences and to understand and value diversity. During these years, "there were distinctions made between Black nursing groups and White nursing groups, which needed to be undone," she says.

At the 1970 ANA convention in Miami, Florida, a resolution was passed that allowed creation of the Commission on Human Rights at the national level of ANA. Grayce served on that first commission and then on the cabinet level for 12 years. "We helped the profession come to grips with diversity issues and its responsibility," she says.

In 1976, Grayce was elected to the Academy of Nursing and subsequently held two terms on its Governing Council. "We developed a position paper for the academy on the issues of diversity and human rights," she says. "They were exciting times and a turning point for ANA and the profession

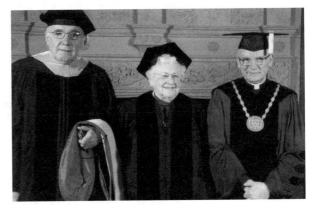

IN 2003, GRAYCE RECEIVED AN HONORARY DOCTOR OF SCIENCE DEGREE FROM FAIRFIELD UNIVERSITY. SHE IS PICTURED HERE WITH FR. JAMES BOWLER, S.J., LEFT, AND FR. ALOYSIUM KELLEY, S.J., PRESIDENT OF FAIRFIELD UNIVERSITY.

of nursing, as these were turbulent times." During this era, ANA's relationship with the National Student Nurses' Association improved, and a new level of cooperation developed. "It never led quite to where I had hoped, and this is an area of disappointment for me," she says. "I felt the student nurses should have been provided some form of membership within ANA as a bridge."

Grayce was an advocate for ANA offering credentialing to the various specialty areas of nursing, and it was not happening fast enough for her. "We waited and waited, but when there was no action taken in this area, a group of psychiatric nurse leaders published the standards with certification and founded the Society for Education and Research in Psychiatric Nursing," she says. The other nursing specialty areas had not developed their credentialing standards, and ANA was waiting for them to accomplish that. "Our area of psychiatric nursing needed certification in order to gain reimbursement from third-party payers and support our practice," she says.

One of Grayce's frustrations is that many times, nursing moves toward the lowest common denominator from the perspective of national associations and even within work settings. "You have to play to the highest common denominator," she says, "knowing you may not get there, but you need to keep striving." In Grayce's opinion, the importance of knowledge, data, and research was ignored during these years in favor of more emotionally compelling concerns. "This would not have been tolerated in medicine or law," she notes.

Grayce was reluctant to bring the certification outside ANA, but it was a priority at that time. "I have to remind myself that it is the American Nurses Association and not the American Nursing Association ... The organization focuses on nurses first, and I want it to focus on nursing first."

Intellectually, she understands ANA's focus on nurses, but emotionally she is more passionate about improving the profession of nursing.

Although she was a strong and loyal advocate for ANA, Grayce did not always see eye to eye with other association leaders. However, she stood up for her principles and made difficult choices. "Whether it may or may not look politically correct, one has to stand by what they believe to be the right thing," she says.

INTERNATIONAL PSYCHIATRIC NURSING

Grayce had an opportunity to work with the Psychiatric Nurses Association in Korea, Japan, Thailand, and Italy. "When I was president of the American Psychiatric Nurses Association, we had a vision to see what was going on in psychiatric nursing around the world," she says. This project accomplished little, but the work remains and could be picked up by the International Council of Nursing.

Grayce served as a consultant to programs in South Korea and was impressed at how practice changed as a result. Walking into the mental hospitals in Korea was like "stepping back to Dayton in the 1950s," she says. Grayce worked with Dr. Susie Kim to develop a national model of nurse-led community After Care. This model spread quickly and with good results throughout South Korea, where community resources, church, and families are effective bridges for

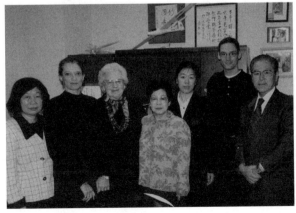

GRAYCE SILLS, THIRD FROM LEFT, VISITS FUKOKUA UNIVERSITY, JAPAN, IN 1997.

patients in mental hospitals. A large number of patients in the country are hospitalized, because there are no length-of-stay restrictions. As a result of the work done by South Korean psychiatric nurses, fewer patients are now hospitalized, and many more are successfully cared for in the community.

THE RETIRED NURSE

Grayce continues to work hard in her retirement years. She still serves as visiting professor at Ohio State and works on numerous projects within the state. She has seen many changes during her years in the nursing profession. "Nursing is no longer the field I entered," she says. "The knowledge available and yet to be discovered has expanded exponentially in my lifetime." Grayce believes research and evaluation are the tools in making information useful. If Grayce were to restructure nursing education, all nurses would hold graduate degrees.

Grayce Sills, professor emeritus at The Ohio State University, has received numerous honors, including three honorary degrees—the Honorary Doctor of Science from Indiana University, the Honorary Doctor of Science from Fairfield University, and the Honorary Doctor of Public Service from The Ohio State University, a rare honor for OSU to bestow such recognition on one of its own. In addition, Grayce has been named the Psychosocial Nurse of the Year from the American Psychiatric Nurses Association, has received the Teaching and

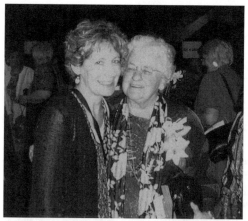

THE AMERICAN NURSES ASSOCIATION (ANA) AWARDED GRAYCE SILLS THE HILDEGARD PEPLAU AWARD IN 2002 FOR HER WORK IN PSYCHIATRIC NURSING. SHE IS PICTURED HERE WITH HER DAUGHTER, KATHLEEN M. SILLS.

Service Award from Ohio State's College of Medicine, and was awarded the Alumni Award for Distinguished Teaching, the university's highest honor for teaching. In 1995 she received Ohio State's Distinguished Service Award, and in 2000 she received the American Nurses Association's Hildegard Peplau Award for contributions to psychiatric nursing. She also was named a Living Legend by the American Academy of Nursing.

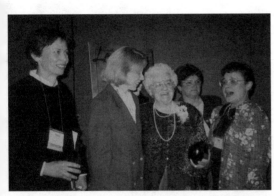

1999 AMERICAN ACADEMY OF NURSING (AAN) LIVING LEGENDS RECEPTION. FROM LEFT TO RIGHT: GAYLE PAGE, BERNADINE HEALEY, GRAYCE, BARBARA SMITH, AND FRAN HICKS.

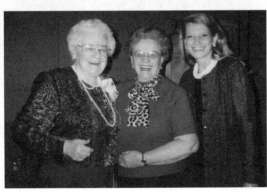

MADELEINE LEININGER, CENTER, AND JOYCE FITZPATRICK, RIGHT, HELP GRAYCE CELEBRATE HER LIVING LEGEND RECOGNITION AT THE ANNUAL AAN MEETING IN 1999.

Grayce dedicated her career to improving psychiatric care and treatment. She was a genius at taking elements from other disciplines and applying them to the nursing profession. Because of her graduate education in sociology, she brought a broader perspective to nursing. Grayce has left a legacy not only as an administrator at The Ohio State University, but also as a leader to psychiatric nurses across the country. When asked what she is most proud of, she laughs that besides her daughter and grandchildren, her role as an educator has been the most rewarding. "I do my best helping other people do their work," she says. That simple credo, which continues to fuel her relentless drive and ambition in a career that spans 55 years, is responsible for her latest honor, a doctorate of public service from The Ohio State University.

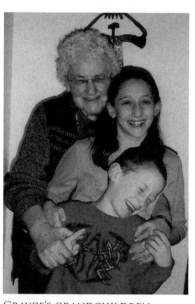

GRAYCE'S GRANDCHILDREN (GRANDSON SAGE IN FRONT; GRANDDAUGHTER TALIA IN THE MIDDLE), ALONG WITH HER DAUGHTER KATHLEEN, ARE HER PRIDE AND JOY. HERE THEY ARE PLAYING AROUND IN 2004.

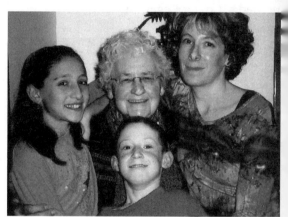

SURROUNDED BY HER FAMILY IN 2004. FROM LEFT TO RIGHT, GRANDDAUGHTER TALIA, GRAYCE, DAUGHTER KATHLEEN, AND GRANDSON SAGE IN FRONT.

Most recently, Grayce completed an 11-year tenure as editor of the American Psychiatric Nursing Association's journal, which she started in 1994 with her former student Nikki Polis, PhD, RN. Now Grayce is deploying the full force of her personality, professional acumen, and management expertise to coordinate an interdisciplinary health-training program funded

I do my best helping other people do their work.

by the Columbus Medical Foundation and the Ohio Department of Mental Health to integrate behavioral and physical healthcare services for needy populations. The pilot program has a two-fold mission: integrating the training of students in psychology, social work, nursing, psychiatry, marital and family counseling, and primary care; and bringing behavioral health services to the primary care setting. This project places students in nontraditional settings, including supportive housing sites for the homeless, youth corrections facilities, traditional substance abuse programs, and inpatient psychiatric facilities.

Grayce has no plans to quit shaking up a system that she feels has failed to adequately prepare the healthcare work force with the skills to meet the needs of a constantly changing clientele. Most importantly, Grayce hopes to break down barriers and encourage collaboration across the health sciences, something she has successfully done throughout her own career.

Grayce approaches most issues with humor and wit. "The ability to see incongruities in life, to notice the incredible mismatches between what is and what ought to be is to know joy," she says. "I have a deep appreciation for the paradoxical nature of the life we have on this planet. You have to be able to see what is fun in that."

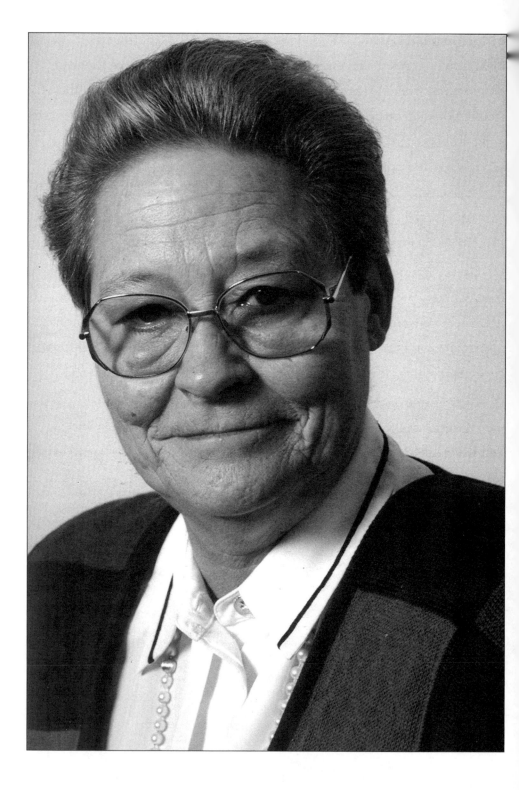

KIRSTEN STALLKNECHT

"I am a nurse, and that is what I am. My father was a ship's captain, and he became a managing director and someone started to call him a director. He said, 'I'm not a director, I'm a captain. All idiots can be directors, but not all idiots can be captains.' I have the same attitude" (Hilton, 2004, Honor after honor section, para. 5).

—Kirsten Stallknecht

Kirsten Stallknecht, RN, FAAN, has lived in Copenhagen, Denmark, her entire life. She has a rich international leadership background that she has used to improve nursing throughout Denmark and worldwide. As a young nurse leader in the 1960s, Kirsten wasted no time proving her effectiveness. At 29 years old, and with only 10 years of nursing experience under her belt, she was elected president of the Danish Nursing Organization (DNO), which had a membership exceeding 30,000 registered nurses. Other career highlights include organizing the first nurses' strike in Denmark; becoming president of the International Council of Nurses (ICN); and receiving the Commander of Dannebrog, the Order of Dannebrog, and the Knight of First Degree for outstanding services to the Danish health system and Danish nurses, all awarded by Queen Margrethe II of Denmark. These are stellar accomplishments for anyone, but especially significant for someone who never graduated from high school.

Kirsten was taught in childhood that whatever she started, she must see through to completion. She was not allowed to float from one interest to another. If she wanted to start dance lessons or music lessons, she had to see them through until she had accomplished a basic level of understanding and expertise. This belief system was a strong influence in her nursing leadership. "There were times in my career when things became so challenging the thought of quitting might have crossed my mind, had it not been for such a strong ingrained belief in finishing all that I undertook," Kirsten says.

It was this philosophy that carried her through the stretch of being a charge nurse in a hospital one day to winning a national election that would place her as head of the Danish Nursing Organization the next. Championing the winning campaign was only half the battle. In those early days, Kirsten was naïve about leadership. It was through "trial by fire" that she learned many lessons firsthand.

THE EARLY YEARS

Kirsten Stallknecht was born in 1937 to a mother who was 32 years old and had given up hope of being able to bear children. Her parents were thrilled with their unexpected new arrival. Her father had been in a prior marriage, so Kirsten had a half-brother who was 10 years older. As she was the only child from this marriage and born to a mother who had given up hope of having children, she describes herself as rather spoiled. In reality, with the effects of World War II and the economic depression, she was spoiled in love but not material items. Kirsten was raised in a very traditional, European-style home, where the father was the provider for the family and the mother stayed home to take care of the house and children. During the worst of the financial depression, Kirsten's mother would attempt to take in some part-time work, but her husband put a stop to it immediately.

> *"I was taught that we were not to buy new things. We were to make do with what we had already. It is still a philosophy that haunts me to this day."*

From 1939 to 1952, Kirsten's father was working as a sea captain on ice breakers during the very harsh Danish winters. He would be away for weeks at a time on his ship with the responsibility of ensuring the ice had been broken and paths were cleared to accommodate safe passage of vessels in and out of the harbors. During this period of time, the family relocated from the center of Copenhagen to the outskirts of town, where the effects of the war were milder.

There were not many "extras" during the war years. To get back and forth to school or to the grocery store, most families traveled by bicycle and did not even spend money on

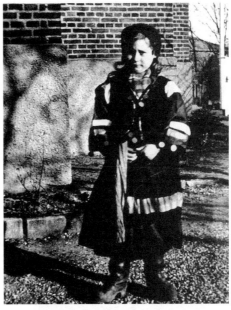

IN FEBRUARY 1943, KIRSTEN PREPARES TO COLLECT MONEY FOR THE POOR ON SHROVE MONDAY.

public transportation. Children were taught at an early age the importance of reusing and saving everything. The whole atmosphere of the country during this time was centered around making ends meet. Whatever it was, it could be used again and again. "You never threw anything out, whether it was scraps of food, material, or old clothes," Kirsten says. "I was taught that we were not to buy new things. We were to make do with what we had already. It is still a philosophy that haunts me to this day."

However, even during times when money was not plentiful, she was never deprived. "My mother was very artistic, and she had a terrific appreciation of culture," Kirsten says. She was sent to dance classes at age 4 and loved it. She attended the first grade in 1944. Because the school building was occupied by refugees from Germany, her classes were held in private homes, even though it was the public school system. It was not until 1946, when the German refugees left Denmark, that Kirsten attended classes on the actual school campus. Education was very important to her parents, but it is also mandatory in Denmark.

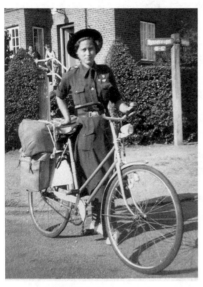

KIRSTEN STALLKNECHT READY FOR GIRL SCOUT CAMP IN 1952.

At age 7, Kirsten asked her mother if she could join the Girl Scouts. She enjoyed all the outings and experiences offered by the scouting group. By age 13, she was placed in charge of her troop. To this day, she credits the Girl Scouts with mentoring her for the transition into leadership. "It was my responsibility to arrange our hikes and make sure all safety measures were followed." She continued as troop leader until age 15 and found the experience invaluable.

Kirsten enjoyed and excelled in her classes through the ninth grade. At age 14, her life turned upside down. "I started high school and was so unhappy," Kirsten says. Her home life was unsettled. When her parents sold their house and moved to another part of Copenhagen, she lost all her schoolmates and friends, and these circumstances were reflected in Kirsten's school performance. Her parents noticed she was not doing well in school and her grades were suffering, but her father was convinced it was laziness. He pulled her out of school and put Kirsten in a housing school—a place where women learn to cook, clean, take care of children, and keep house. There were many of these schools located all over Europe, all well-attended. Kirsten enjoyed her new school because she was able to work with her hands and have an actual finished product. The term was less than 8 months; upon completion, she was ready to find employment.

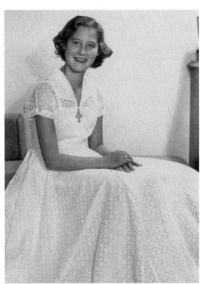

KIRSTEN ON HER CONFIRMATION DAY IN OCTOBER 1951.

In addition to her native language, she could understand German and speak English. Her parents wanted her to learn more languages, so they found her a job as an au pair in Switzerland. Off she went in 1954, at 17 years of age. She had never been out of Denmark before, and it was the first time she had been in the mountains. "I had never seen a mountain, so it was amazing to me," she says. Kirsten learned to enjoy her new position and gained an understanding of French and Italian. The job lasted about a year. At the end of the year, she returned home to Denmark with the dream of becoming a nurse. She was 18 years old and could not explain why she wanted to be a nurse, but that is what she wanted. Even her parents tried to impress other possibilities on her. In Kirsten's reminiscence, she feels that her reasons for wanting to be a nurse included the prospect of being independent from her home, living at the college, and getting the small salary.

NURSING SCHOOL

Kirsten loved being around people and was very social. The independence that nursing offered and the opportunity to work with others drew her into the profession. In the 1950s, those accepted into nursing school received a small salary (equivalent to approximately $10 a month), a uniform, and free housing. At age 18, she applied to a diploma program at University Hospital in Copenhagen. She was accepted into the nursing program without having earned her high school diploma, as was normally required. Her experience from abroad and her family background opened the door for her.

Nursing school was tough for Kirsten, but she knew she was in the right place. Most importantly, she felt independent. She was open to practice in all areas of nursing and did not want to specialize in any one area. In 1960, the year she graduated from nursing school, Kirsten met a medical student, and they fell deeply in love. They married in the spring of 1961, but it lasted only 4 years before she realized it was "the mistake of my life." They parted ways and divorced.

Her obvious eagerness for new experiences is shown by the fact she worked in four different wards—surgery, medical, otolaryngology, and neurosurgery—in her first 5 years as a professional nurse. One day the matron, or charge nurse, of the neurosurgical ward asked her what she was planning to do with the rest of her life. Kirsten's response was "enjoy myself." She liked her job and the workload was reasonable, so she was quite content with her career. Her matron told Kirsten she had great potential and should further develop herself in the profession by going back to school. This inspired Kirsten. Even though she was concerned about her qualifications—she lacked a high-school diploma and the Danish university requirements had recently been strengthened—she filled out the paperwork and attached a letter that reflected her desire for more education. She also shared the dilemma of her educational background. "I asked them to make an exception for me," she says. Once again, Kirsten had luck on her side, as an exception was granted and she was allowed to pursue further education in nursing leadership and education.

Denmark: Understanding the Healthcare System

To understand Kirsten, it is important to first understand a little of the background of her country. The Danish population is 5 million and, until recently, was very homogeneous. Denmark is divided into 14 counties that are responsible for the hospitals and 273 communities that are responsible for home care and social systems. Since the end of the 19th century, Denmark has been highly organized in the labor market and is generally regulated by collective agreements between trade unions and employer associations. "It creates a society where there are few very rich people and little poverty," Kirsten says.

> *"It creates a society where there are few very rich people and little poverty."*

Taxes in Denmark are high, but all schools from the beginning through university level are free to citizens. All medical support, hospitals, general practitioners, home care nursing services, public health nurses, and midwives are free. All people over 67 years are entitled to a state pension. Disability pensions also exist for those in need.

Modern nursing came to Copenhagen in the 1860s, when health authorities sent "responsible" women to London to hear and see what was going on in nursing. The purpose was to observe and learn what was being taught in the Nightingale schools and bring home the information, so it could be introduced in the Danish system. According to Kirsten, the general criteria for women to become nurses in the 1960s were:

- be an adult woman;
- have a good moral reputation;
- have good health;
- be willing to work long, hard hours;
- be orderly in work and behavior;
- be obedient to physicians and other authority figures; and
- be unmarried.

In Denmark, the title *nurse* is protected and can only be used by those who qualify for state registration after fulfilling the educational requirements. The registered nurse license is awarded by the state, based on the results of a state-controlled examination. There is only one educational route for entry into practice as a registered nurse, and specialties have to build on the basic registered nurse education. This system has allowed the Danish nurses protection of their registered nurse title and profession. "This has made life difficult, but it has also made life that much easier," says Kirsten. Patients in Denmark know what a nurse is and what the term *nurse* stands for, which is a privileged situation compared to many countries, including the United States, where the title is not defined by universal educational standards. In Denmark, however, a midwife is not a nurse and a nurse is not a midwife. Individuals can be both, but they have to have completed two separate educational tracks.

The membership rolls of the Danish Nursing Organization (DNO) include 95% of nurses in Denmark. The organization was founded in 1899 with a focused mission and purpose of organizing all nurses, developing professional education and standards for nursing, and improving the living and working conditions of nurses.

In modern society, it is important to have a "brand," an identifier of some sort that is recognizable as unique and different. The founders of DNO decided at their first board meeting in 1899 that members of DNO should wear a badge when working professionally and in uniform. They still wear the same badge today. For more than 100 years, it has been the sign that tells patients they have a registered nurse in front of them. The membership number of each nurse is printed on the back of the badge, and the badge must be returned to DNO if the nurse discontinues membership or passes away. Nurses value this insignia so much that the badges are respectfully returned when no longer being used.

STEPPING INTO NURSING LEADERSHIP

Once Kirsten was accepted in the university, it took her two semesters to finish her diploma (the equivalent of a bachelor's degree in the United States), and she graduated with the highest grade point average in her class. Upon graduation, she returned to Copenhagen and accepted a position as a ward sister or charge nurse in the university hospital, called Rigshospitalet, or simply "Riget," which is Danish for "national hospital."

Part of her agreement with the matron, in accepting the position, was that she be allowed to make some changes in how nursing care was provided. "I wanted to change the way we treated patients," Kirsten says.

The hospital unit was a research or science ward where patients from all over the country who were not responsive to basic treatment were sent.

Research studies were conducted on these patients, and new treatments and outcomes were documented. "We had to be very precise in our work to document any and all reliable results," Kirsten says. While attending the university, she had learned how team nursing had been implemented in U.S. hospitals, but the trend had not yet started in Denmark. Since all the Danish hospitals are public and do not have the same funding as private hospitals, team nursing could not be implemented 24 hours a day. It could, however, be applied during the day shift. She decided she would apply the best features of the idea to her system on a 32-patient ward. It was quite a shift in treatment and an innovative practice to be instituted by a 28-year-old nurse. (The changes may seem small in today's hospital settings, but at that time, the regimen for patients was very strict.) Previously, patients arriving at the hospital went first to a reception ward, where they had a bath and all their clothes were taken from them. They felt very much reduced to a number. Kirsten persuaded the chief medical officer that "her" patients did not have to follow this routine. They came straight to the ward, where they were given a bed and a small cabinet. They could keep their own clothes on except when they had to undergo treatment or special examinations. These patients often were very insecure after enduring long sicknesses without knowing what they had or how they could be cured. Keeping their trousers, as some male patients said, gave them a sense of being an individual.

Kirsten also changed how the nurses and doctors interacted. Nurses prepared what the individual doctor needed to communicate and investigate with the patient, but unless the patient could not speak due to illness, doctors could not count on a nurse just standing by as a servant. Nurses spent more time talking with patients and doing what the patients needed. Furthermore, Kirsten changed the old hierarchy among nurses, letting the younger nurses present material and support when the professor was on patient visits. Before these changes, only the ward sister usually had direct access to the professor. This created a relaxed atmosphere for both patients and nurses. Job satisfaction increased and, at the same time, patients expressed their appreciation. The little things made the biggest difference and gave patients a much better experience, even when they were seriously ill.

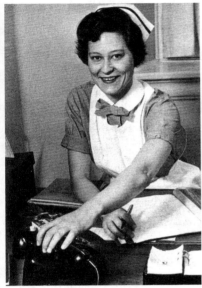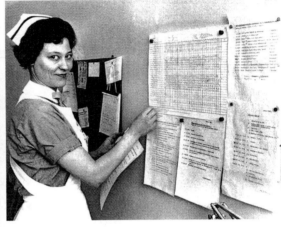

KIRSTEN IN HER ROLE AS ASSISTANT MATRON FOR RIGSHOSPITALET IN DENMARK IN 1967.

After the system had proven to be successful, the same model was adopted in other hospitals throughout Denmark.

At this point in Kirsten's young career, she did not stop at changing the area of patient care; she also addressed the relationship between physicians and nurses—specifically, how they interacted. Danish nurses have a long history of fighting for independence within hospital systems. Early in the 1900s, with nurses supporting the policy of "nurses lead the nursing staff," Denmark made the determination that nurses would be managed by the matron, or head nurse, based on the British model. This effectively kept management and leadership of nurses in the hands of nurses and away from physicians, which was not what the physicians preferred. Even after World War II, physicians continued to fight the independent attitude of Danish nurses, expecting nurses to serve as their personal assistants.

This expectation was prevalent throughout Denmark, including in the Riget. Kirsten, however, was determined to end that practice. "I stood up to the physicians who complained the nurses were not doing enough for them by informing them that nurses were not at the hospital to service physicians—nurses were at the hospital for the patients," she says. In this battle, she had the support of the chief medical officer. When physicians would report her and others on the nursing staff, the administration supported the nurses. Patients benefited the most from the change, as nurses had more time to spend attending to patient needs.

The leadership at her hospital created a wonderful, accepting environment conducive to change. She had been asked by many to write up all her changes and findings in the *Danish Nursing Journal*. At the time, it was the only nursing journal in the country. She published the article "Man tager en afdeling" (translated to mean "One Takes a Ward"), even though it was not a scientific study. In the article, she highlighted how people can make change from within the system if they approach the problem in the right manner and have the necessary support.

Once the article was published, nurses wanted to hear more about her changes, and Kirsten was asked to speak at meetings around the country. Suddenly, she was building a reputation and name for herself, without intending to. At the same time, some of the nurses in Copenhagen had approached her to run for election to the National Council of Nurses. She agreed and was elected in 1965, at age 28.

PRESIDENT OF THE DANISH NURSING ORGANIZATION

While Kirsten was serving in her role at the National Council of Nurses, the president of the DNO decided to retire. Kirsten was approached by a group of younger nurses who were seeking change within the organization. "There was a lot of unrest among the youngsters in the late 1960s, all over the world," she says. This rebellion for change during the 1960s was felt internationally in nursing, and Denmark was no exception.

"Being naïve is a good thing at times of great risk."

After much consideration, Kirsten decided to run for the presidency. She was receiving considerable support from various media sources. There were three candidates running for the presidency in a national nursing election voted on by all 33,000 members of DNO. She won the election. At the time, she knew very little about organizations or about economics, but she did understand nursing. Accepting this position was the riskiest move in her nursing career, which she did not realize at the time. "Being naïve is a good thing at times of great risk," she says.

On leave from the hospital, Kirsten started this full-time, paid position for DNO in May 1968. She was excited, but also scared of what she did not know. At times, it was overwhelming and intimidating. Calling upon her early childhood lessons of finishing what she started, she was always able to continue moving forward.

Her job responsibilities included addressing any issues related to the nursing profession and labor trade. "Since I did not have all the answers, I was extremely dependent on good advice from people who wanted to support me, but on the other hand, demanded that I do things myself," she says.

On the personal front, Kirsten met and married a Norwegian just after her election to the DNO presidency. It was 1968, and the marriage lasted only 2 years before she realized it was "a new mistake." They parted ways and divorced.

LESSONS FOR A NEW LEADER

As a new president, Kirsten had no experience being a spokesperson to the media, but she was now in the position of speaking on behalf of 33,000 nurses throughout Denmark. It was quite a learning experience for the 29-year-old. At times, she felt it was like jumping into the deep part of the ocean and just swimming to survive.

"I LEARNED BY DOING MY ENTIRE CAREER."

She made the mistake most new leaders make when stepping into a position of authority and power. "I wanted to change everything at the same time, and of course that does not work. It was like having a full plate and not knowing quite how to use a knife and fork. That was my situation," Kirsten says. She learned very quickly that it was impossible to tackle everything at once. As she moved forward with change, she made mistakes but learned from them and strategized more effective methods the next time around.

One of Kirsten's top priorities upon accepting office was further developing and strengthening shop stewards (the spokesperson and union representative) by providing education, so they could properly represent the association on workplace issues and at the same time, come back from the workplace setting with information about the concerns of bedside nurses.

YOU ARE NEVER FREE IF YOU ARE AT THE MERCY OF WEAK FINANCES." Her second major area of focus was to change the financial situation of the association. During these early years as a leader, Kirsten describes the financial situation of the association as "having a beautiful house without curtains, cabinets, or furniture. ... We had no money."

Kirsten starting managing every penny and was sure the staff thought she was too tight with the purse strings. She would not allow them to spend anything unless it was absolutely necessary. Of course, what the staff viewed as essential was not quite the same as what Kirsten considered necessary expenses. "We had lots of internal office arguments and board discussions early on, but I was absolutely sure that only by strengthening our economic position could we get the progress we demanded," she says.

At that time, the DNO board of directors was comprised of 42 members, including the president, and she was the youngest member. Being the youngest and in such a powerful leadership position had its challenges. Kirsten was fortunate to have gained the support of the majority upon taking office.

Since its first publication in 1901, the *Danish Nursing Journal* (*DNJ*) was the only professional nursing journal in Denmark until 1980. The journal is a DNO membership benefit and reaches nearly all nurses in the country. It was a wonderful communication tool for Kirsten to share her vision with the membership. The publication has helped give strength to DNO and security to its members. For years, the journal has made a profit for the organization. *DNJ* continues to be published every 2 weeks, but it faces the challenges that technology brings to the competitive market. Many other sources are readily available to nurses online. Although wonderful in their own way, online resources pull readers away from the *DNJ*.

"OUR STRUCTURE WAS NOT STRONG ENOUGH, SO WE WERE REALLY POWERLESS."

Kirsten never lost sight of her vision for strengthening the association. Because DNO was both for professional and trade union issues, the organization had to be able to step in and advocate for nurses. As a new leader, Kirsten prioritized moving the organization into a stronger position. "There were a lot of conflicts between people of the 'old school' and the new youngsters coming in and saying we will have to change everything," she says. The media was following DNO's progress very closely because, in Kirsten's own words, "I was an interesting animal, being so young, being a female in the trade union movement, and being so outspoken." The resulting stories were not always favorable. Being publicly chastised in the press is difficult for any leader, but especially so for a novice. She remembers feeling tremendous internal struggles early on in her leadership.

"I JUST THOUGHT IT WAS AWFUL TO MAKE ONE MISTAKE AND THE NURSE LOSES HER LICENSE."

Kirsten felt that nurses who struggled with a substance abuse issue should be treated with dignity and provided the option of professional counseling and treatment intervention. In Denmark during the 1970s, if a nurse was found guilty of abusing alcohol or drugs of any kind, his or her license was revoked. Kirsten witnessed nurses who had their livelihood taken away as a result of an alcohol or drug problem. She wanted first-time offenders to be provided treatment, with only a suspension of their license for a period of time. "I felt that giving that trust to a nurse, at that time, was a huge step for our nurses," she says. However, Kirsten did not pull off this change solely by her own efforts. Her mentor was Eli Magnussen, the chief governmental nurse and an international nurse leader. She helped to raise the additional funds needed to support the rehabilitation program, as well as additional funds to help nurses pay their bills while in treatment, as they were not able to draw a paycheck.

The rehabilitation program was a practical issue of great value to nurses, the administration of the hospitals, and the patients. "With the implementation of this intervention, our society did not lose a good worker who was struggling with personal issues," Kirsten says. The power of her mentor allowed Kirsten to believe that she could change the country's professional outlook on this issue. Doing so gave her the strength of confidence.

Even at the pace Kirsten was keeping, she had time to meet the real love of her life when she was about 40 years old. "I met him during my work as a trade union nurse, and we have been together over 25 years," Kirsten says. He had children from a prior marriage, so they had a full family.

Organizing Denmark's First Nursing Strike

Hospitals in Denmark are publicly owned by the counties, who are the main employers. Employers, of course, are not always willing to raise salaries for nurses or provide retirement plans in keeping with the economic times. Kirsten was seeking both salary increases and adequate retirement plans. The employers were trying to divide the power of nurses by telling them to find representation from several different unions. Some nurses were listening to the employers, but Kirsten was advocating the strength of solidarity. The home care industry was another force that challenged her every step. "We have a strong home care nursing system in Denmark, and that was the other big guy I was up against," she says. If Kirsten's efforts to increase wages were successful, they would be costly for all areas of healthcare.

It took Kirsten 5 years to turn around the DNO resources. "For the first time, we were making a profit," she says. "Now we were ready to go to the negotiating table to talk about nursing salaries." This was 1973, and the county employers were not willing to give up a penny more in salary to

> "Nurses were now given the highest pay raise of any public employee that year in the country, and it was a very powerful time for the profession."

the nurses. However, the nurses now had both the stamina and power to fight back. "After some unsuccessful negotiations, we gave them our strike warning," she says. "They did not believe us, so we followed up our threat and for the first time in history, the nurses of Denmark went on strike."

Kirsten again felt like she was swimming in the deep end of the ocean without a life preserver, as this experience could go either way for the nurses. She hardly slept, as the stress was taking its toll on her.

"You could not have a leader organizing a strike who did not care about patients, so we made sure that all emergencies could be handled," she says. No patients suffered, as there were provisions made throughout the strike. The right of nurses to strike is based on a general agreement between the employers and DNO. That agreement includes a clause that all essential care shall be delivered even during a strike. The number of essential staff for this situation is to be negotiated before the strike starts and to be presented to the government arbitrator appointed by law.

Once the strike was initiated, it took 6 weeks to achieve the desired resolution and the change in attitudes among the professionals themselves. "Nurses were now given the highest pay raise of any public employee that year in the country, and it was a very powerful time for the profession," Kirsten says. The nurses, who today are over 60 years old, remember the effects this particular strike had on the country, and it would be 20 years before the nurses in Denmark would go on strike again. "The nurses had the right to do it, as they were grossly underpaid and worked horrendously ong hours," she says. Interestingly enough, the nurses had the support of their patients—the Danish public.

The last strike for Danish nurses was in 1995, due to unfair wages. This time the government let the strike run for 25 days before Parliament intervened and secured the right to negotiations, based on a government-driven analysis of nurses' economic development from 1973 to 1995. Strike warnings have been given since, but the weapon has not been used. The most common reasons for both strikes were disagreement about salary increases and the status and compensation of nursing administrators when compared with other healthcare disciplines.

Pensions were as much of a concern to the DNO as salaries and working conditions. Many of the retired and elderly nurses had so little to live on that they suffered serious hardship and had to leave their apartment or housing when they became ill. Nurses of this generation were not allowed to be married and remain a nurse until the 1940s, so most had lived in flats or rooms owned by and connected to the hospital, the home care service, or wherever they worked. When they retired, they had to move out of these facilities, and their quality of life typically changed dramatically. Therefore, securing housing for nurses became an important issue. During the 1930s, a "nurses house" was built in Copenhagen. Since the 1960s, the nurses pension fund has invested heavily in properties for nurses all over the country.

Staffing ratios were never accepted as negotiable by any healthcare employer in Denmark. By combining negotiations related to the number of hours per shift, per day, and per week, along with the number of weekends free per month and length of pregnancy leave, some indirect influence has been possible on adjusting staffing ratios. All wards must have registered nurses responsible for the nursing service 24 hours a day, so the contractual stipulations keep the workplace conditions competitive.

After the 1940s, when nurses were allowed to marry, it became clear that something had to be done to protect pregnant nurses, whether or not they were married. Nurses are still engaged in general negotiations to secure better conditions during pregnancy and while mothering small children.

Danish nurses were the first Nordic nurses to organize themselves, but soon the rest of the Nordic countries followed suit. Norway, Sweden, Finland, and Iceland were all very active on the international scene in supporting nurses.

By the 1980s, with the professionalization of labor organizing, DNO became the only recognized organization for registered nurses with negotiating rights in relation to the country's labor laws.

The main ingredient of the strength of Danish nurses is that they have been unified in support of their profession for more than 100 years, from the most junior students to those in the highest positions of esteem and authority. The second major factor is that Danish nurses have managed to adjust their constitution and benefits offered to membership to meet new needs and accommodate the changing social order. No rule is inflexible, no decision is forever, and negotiation and compromise are ways of life.

A third factor is the dramatic change in the internal workings of DNO, its economic administrations, and the frequent use of non-nurse professionals to do its work and fulfill its responsibilities.

INTERNATIONAL NURSING

The DNO has been a member of the International Council of Nurses (ICN) since 1909. Kirsten attended her first ICN Congress in Montreal in 1969, at which time the newly elected ICN president introduced her to the Nordic Nurses Federation (NNF), which is comprised of a conglomerate of ive Nordic nurses associations. As Kirsten networked within the NNF, she continued attending the international conferences for nursing. In 1971, he attended the Council of National Representatives and then went again when it was held in Mexico in 1973. She learned more and more from her international colleagues and brought the best of it back to Denmark. The CN has been strong and influential in the development of nursing policies of the DNO.

Kirsten asserts in some of her writings that one of the traits unique to Denmark is that the Danish have always depended on cooperation with other countries to get inspiration, to trade goods, and to obtain raw material to produce goods. "Our culture is therefore very much influenced by other countries, but at the same time is very Danish," Kirsten says. Denmark is such a small country that the people do not need to use their resources to create new processes and systems, but they do need to learn and take from the best of what other countries have found effective. This concept has influenced Kirsten's approach to leadership and change. Instead of approaching situations thinking she has all the answers, she listens first to what ideas others have to offer and applies the best to her own situation.

"Many of our top nursing leaders attended school at Teacher's College in the United States or went to study in Britain before they became leaders in Denmark," Kirsten says. "What one needs to realize is that one can see the great ideas in practice,

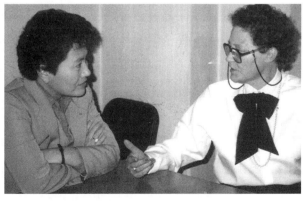

KIRSTEN, THEN PRESIDENT OF THE DANISH NURSES ORGANIZATION, WITH DR. HIROKO MINAMI IN JAPAN IN 1985.

but our country has to take and pick what can best fit into our general system of healthcare. … We cannot just adopt whatever comes out next."

However, in Eastern Europe and other smaller countries, one of the biggest problems has been the lack of relevant literature in their own language. A lot of well-meaning people have brought advanced nursing literature printed in English that only a few nurses had access to, even fewer were able to read, and still fewer understood.

In 1981, during an international nursing congress in Los Angeles, Kirsten was asked by a group of her peers if she would consider running for an ICN board position. She ran for election in Europe and was elected to serve as a board member during the years of 1981-1985. She was assigned to be chairman of the Social and Economic Committee because of her strong background and reputation in labor relations throughout Europe. Kirsten chaired this committee while continuing her full-time job as DNO president.

In 1985, following her first term as board member, Kirsten was elected second vice president of ICN. She was proud of the international board position, because it showed "how a leader from a small country, without the highest educational credentials, can be recognized for their work and contribution to the profession." From 1997 to 2001, Kirsten served as president of the International Council of Nurses. She thoroughly enjoyed this position. Because she had left her full-time job at DNO, she could take time to follow more closely what was going on in the nursing profession at the international level. It was very interesting for Kirsten to observe firsthand the conditions many nurses worked under, and she came to admire her profession even more as she recognized the obstacles they had to cope with on a daily basis.

During her ICN presidency, she also realized that around the world, nursing culture has similarities that are independent of national policies and social, religious, and cultural differences. These similarities enable nurses worldwide to exchange professional news, even when they do not speak the same language. It sets the stage for tremendous trust in the profession and the potential of nurses, given the possibilities to further the health and well-being of people.

One of the highlights from her years of service to international nursing was during the 100th anniversary of ICN in the Royal Albert Hall in London. "The Royal Albert Hall is really special in English culture, and that is where the nurses of the world were gathered to celebrate the 100th anniversary of international nursing. ... It was spectacular," she says.

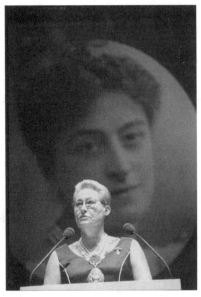

KIRSTEN GIVES HER PRESIDENTIAL SPEECH, SUNDAY, 27 JUNE 1999, IN LONDON'S ALBERT HALL.

INTERNATIONAL TRAVEL

Other highlights of Kirsten's nursing career include her travels to other countries to view their nursing practice firsthand. In the late 1970s, as a member of the Nordic nursing group, she traveled to Moscow to help organize a nursing conference on workplace conditions. The Nordic nurses were allowed to visit some of the hospitals and clinics in Russia. It was very different from nursing in the Western part of the world.

During the 1970s, nurses working in the Eastern bloc were seen as assistants to physicians and not independent professionals. They did not have access to new, international knowledge about nursing and were not aware of ICN. Kirsten was amazed to find they did not even have access to basic ethical guidelines. This trip opened the gate to forming an ongoing relationship with nurses from the Eastern bloc, as nurses in small delegations were able to come to Denmark and other Nordic countries to learn more about nursing practice in the West. Over the years, Kirsten has traveled back to the former USSR countries and has been to all the Eastern and Central European countries.

In 1979, the U.S. Department of Labor invited Kirsten to visit the United States. Although it was not her first visit, this trip was special for her, as she was invited to travel the country for a full month and visit hospitals, schools, clinics, and long-term care facilities. She arrived in Washington, DC, and went to Louisiana, New Mexico, Arizona, California, Washington state, Kansas, and Massachusetts.

In addition, Kirsten traveled to both China and Japan as an invited member of the Chinese-Danish Friendship Association. In the 1980s, she stayed in China 10 days while touring hospitals, schools, farming communities, and so on. She also went to Japan and received tours of one of the major private universities that had been influenced by Danish philosophers. Through her leadership at DNO, she also hosted exchange trips for Japanese nursing students to come to Denmark and other European countries. A group of Japanese nursing students came every year, and she in turn would go back to Japan. A strong bond formed between DNO and the Japanese Nurses Association.

"The Japanese Nurses Association is a very large union, but they do not have negotiating rights as we know them in Europe," Kirsten says. "It is not their tradition, as they are women." The Japanese nurses may not have negotiating rights as other countries have, but the nurses have learned to leverage what they do have to their advantage. "They are so smart, and they have the knowledge of how their system works, so they are effective in being heard."

All this international nursing experience has given Kirsten a broad perspective on healthcare systems worldwide. There are portions of systems in many countries that stand out as excellent, but no one system would work for all countries. In the United States, patients who can afford healthcare services have access to excellent technology, research, pharmacological interventions, and highly educated medical personnel. The downside is that not all citizens have equal access to these services, as the best services are generally the most expensive. These services are available only to those who either have good insurance or private financial means. This system of providing healthcare would not work in the poorer countries of the world.

Canada and many countries in Europe have heavy taxation, but in return they provide coverage of all healthcare and educational services. The technology and research available may not be the latest, but it is quite good, and patients are not discriminated against based on income level. Individuals who struggle to make ends meet are assured care by physicians and hospitals in the same manner as wealthy individuals, since the government pays the reimbursement out of tax monies.

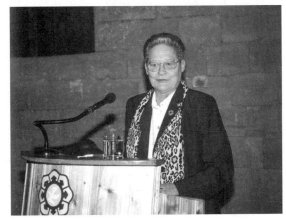

KIRSTEN, ICN PRESIDENT, IN CYPRESS, 1999.

Hospital care in Denmark is free to its citizens because of the taxation structure. It is a different attitude of care, as it is the Danish philosophy that everything should be done for everybody in need. In other countries, the philosophy is everything shall be done if you can pay for it. One of the challenges of socialized medicine is longer wait times for surgeries and technical procedures. As Kirsten says, "In Denmark we try to keep the wait list no longer than 2 months for scheduled procedures, while cancer patients always have the privilege of being taken first." Countries that have socialized healthcare systems also have private hospitals available to patients with private insurance.

International consultants must be aware of the culture, economics, social dynamics, and political issues related to healthcare in other countries. There is an international nursing shortage, but most countries do not experience the dire situation that Africa experiences. When Kirsten traveled throughout Africa, she saw conditions where there was only one nurse available to care for several villages within a 100-mile radius. Most countries do not experience this critical level of nursing shortage.

THE RETIRED NURSE LEADER

"I always said nursing can lead to anything one wants out of a career," Kirsten says. She worked as president of the Danish Nurses Organization for 28 years and was never bored. She was on overload most days, and her secret as an international nurse leader is never lacking the courage to take on new risks. In addition, Kirsten's leadership went beyond nursing. "I was involved not only in my profession, but kept very busy working on issues outside of nursing as well," she says. Kirsten was commissioned by the government to work on issues not related to nursing. In 1992, her last job for the government was serving as chair of Wonderful Copenhagen, the tourist association of the capital of Denmark. "It gave me a much broader area to function within, both for the benefit of DNO and for society," she says. Today, Kirsten still keeps busy working on a voluntary basis for the government.

> *She learned to measure success in small increments or steps. The path of reaching her goal was more important than the speed of getting to the finish line.*

As Kirsten reflects on her years in nursing and leadership, she remembers growing up during a generation in which women did not pursue careers. "I was an exception to be a strong female leader who helped to influence our healthcare system and nursing profession," she says. It has been 10 years since Kirsten officially retired from DNO, and she continues to consult on nursing issues and speak throughout the country. "It takes a lot of energy and time to be an effective leader, so I don't work full time, but I do work on smaller projects."

One of the leadership lessons Kirsten learned is to have a little more patience with people. "I was never patient when I was young. I wanted to change everything at the same time," she says. Along her journey Kirsten learned patience, one step at a time. She would set her goals, but realized change could not happen overnight. She learned to measure success in small increments or steps. The path of reaching her goal was more important than the speed of getting to the finish line.

In 1990, Kirsten received a national honor bestowed by Denmark's queen. "It is not commonplace to receive an honor from the Queen, no less someone who has a strong labor union background ... so I was honored when the employer and the ministries recommended that the Queen consider me for my first honor, which is called the Knight of Denmark," she says. Kirsten's father was alive to witness her awarded honor. "My father, who had been so worried when I was young, and who took me to the special school of housekeeping ... he was so proud of me ... it was the biggest day in both our lives." Years later, Kirsten was awarded an even higher honor that no other nurse in Denmark has been awarded: a special Commander's Cross by the Queen. The award recognizes all her service to nursing and healthcare in Denmark and internationally. She was nominated by many of the same employers and nurses she had represented during her years of service. It was upon leaving her service with the ICN that she was given this honor.

In 2004, Kirsten was invited to the United States to receive the International Distinguished Leadership Award, an honor bestowed by the Commission on Graduates of Foreign Nursing Schools. "I was very touched by this because I had been harsh on the Americans for what I viewed as their lack of sensitivity in many issues, but I have always liked the Americans. ... I just never thought anybody in the States would bestow me with an honor," she says.

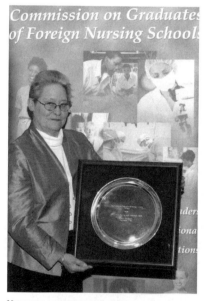

KIRSTEN RECEIVED THE INTERNATIONAL DISTINGUISHED LEADERSHIP AWARD IN 2004. THIS IS AN HONOR BESTOWED BY THE COMMISSION ON GRADUATES OF FOREIGN NURSING SCHOOLS.

With all the choices young adults have these days in making a career choice, Kirsten still believes nursing is one of the best choices. "I want to encourage young people in nursing to trust in their own capability to develop nursing, because we have a tendency in nursing to feel sorry for ourselves, victimizing ourselves. ... It is outdated thinking. ... It is about saying, 'I can do this and I make a difference in my patients' lives.' "

Since nursing is a profession that is needed by every human being, nursing is a powerful choice. "We should be proud about being in a position where others cannot function without us," Kirsten says.

REFERENCE

Hilton, L. (2004, November 30). Leader, teacher, mentor. *Nursing Spectrum*. Retrieved October 18, 2006, from http://www.nursingspectrum. com/InternationalNursing/News/Articles/LeaderTeacherMentor.htm

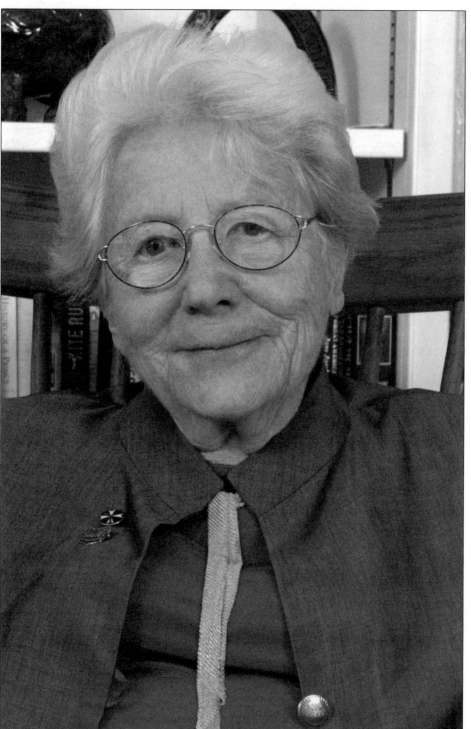

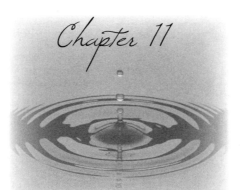

FLORENCE SCHORSKE WALD

"Nursing's role is to save the future of healthcare!"
—Florence Wald

Death and dying strike a chord of fear and anguish in most people. In the 1960s, the diagnosis of cancer boded death, pain, suffering, and separation.

In Latin, the word hospice means to host a guest or stranger; Florence Wald, RN, MN, MS, FAAN, centered her work on hosting a pain-free, dignified life while facilitating the dying process. She started by founding the first hospice in America in 1974. The concept has since proliferated to more than 3,300 hospice programs that have served millions of patients and families. Florence believes the holistic hospice philosophy and mission are the "essence of nursing," and from the beginning of her career, she sought to instill this philosophy in her nursing practice. Florence's pioneering efforts changed the heart of society to accept and engage in an end-of-life process that she describes as "appropriate, understanding, and natural."

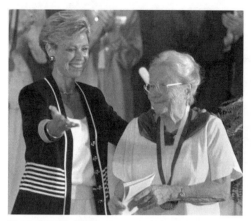

FLORENCE'S 1998 INDUCTION INTO THE
NATIONAL WOMEN'S HALL OF FAME.

The impact of Florence's work is so profound that in 1998 she was inducted into the National Women's Hall of Fame, which honors American women for significant contributions to society. This honor puts her in such legendary company as Eleanor Roosevelt, Helen Keller, Susan B. Anthony, Harriet Tubman, Sandra Day O'Connor, and Florence's idol, Lillian Wald. Her leadership journey has not been without its ups and downs, including being unceremoniously "fired" 18 months after opening the doors of the first American hospice program in Branford, CT.

Florence has contributed to the nursing profession as a researcher, staff nurse, and faculty member at Rutgers and Yale universities. She was dean at Yale University School of Nursing for nearly a decade, and she has been an international leader for end-of-life care. At age 81, she was named a principal investigator for a feasability study evaluating the need for hospice in Connecticut State Correctional facilities. Influenced by family values, timing, colleagues, serendipity, and risk-taking, Florence has never been put off by challenges, and no task has ever appeared too large for her to accomplish. When she observes the enormous medical challenges today, including inconsistent quality, untenable cost, and too little health maintenance, Florence unabashedly declares that "nursing's role is to save the future of healthcare!"

EARLY INFLUENCES

The Schorske children were second-generation Americans, but their values and culture were heavily influenced by their German heritage. Theodore

Schorske and Gertrude Goldschmidt grew up in New York City (NYC), where each was acutely aware of the challenges presented to immigrants at the beginning of the 20th century, including housing discrimination, unfair labor practices, and disparity of health and education benefits. Before Theodore and Gertrude married, they were supporters of the NYC settlements, including the famous Henry Street settlement, founded by Lillian Wald to assist immigrants in acclimating to a democratic society that was not always egalitarian, particularly to those who did not speak the language.

On April 6, 1917, the United States entered World War I. Thirteen days later, Florence was born into a German family in a divided world. The Schorskes felt like social outcasts in America, regardless of the fact it was the country of their birth. Gertrude Schorske would tell of the neighbor who declared, "Well, there is my little enemy," as she glared at Florence's 2-year-old brother in the carriage. At that time, Florence's father was vice president for Deutsche Spaar Bank in New York City. The ethnic pressure was so pervasive that the bank was renamed Central Savings Bank to Americanize it. Before the war, the Schorske family spoke German at home so the children would be bilingual, but fear of isolation turned them to English speaking.

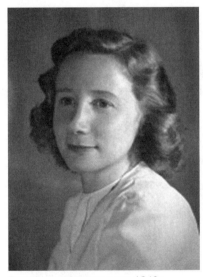

FLORENCE IN THE MID 1940S.

On April 6, 1917, the United States entered World War I. Thirteen days later, Florence was born into a German family in a divided world.

Florence's parents were well-read and self-educated, but neither had a college degree. Extensive self-study and soul-searching left her parents in the position of being devout pacifists, which made the war and its effects more distressing. As members of the Socialist party, they "leaned to the left" and became known for their political beliefs. The dinner conversations were rich with discussion of current events, culture, politics, and philosophy. When Mr. and Mrs. Schorske traveled, the children went with them as a part of their "worldly education." All encounters, negative or positive, were viewed by the Schorskes as opportunities to learn something new as family.

In 1929, the family traveled to Germany and experienced the culture and beauty of their forbearer's homeland before the devastation of Hitler and

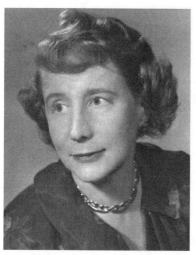

THIS 1958 PHOTO WAS PUB-
LISHED IN *THE NEW YORK TIMES*
TO ANNOUNCE FLORENCE'S
APPOINTMENT AS ACTING DEAN OF
THE YALE SCHOOL OF NURSING.
ULTIMATELY, THIS PHOTO LED TO
HER MARRIAGE TO HENRY WALD.

World War II. In 1932, Florence and her mother returned to visit family in Berlin and found an entirely different Germany. The Nazis were promoting anti-Semitic activities and organizing pro-Hitler rallies. Florence remembers the terror of being literally trapped in the middle of one of these rallies and surrounded by "shouting, jostling Nazis calling us auslander [foreigner]." The country seemed to teem with unexpected outbursts of hate and violence. This validated what the Schorskes had been reading in the U.S. papers and led them to help Jewish families immigrate to America.

THE DESIRE TO BE A NURSE

Florence's early influences of cultural isolation and ethnic discrimination influenced her thinking of what a nurse could be. She understood that exteral stress can create tremendous undetected internal distress. As a result, Florence came to believe that healthcare extends beyond the disease and must include the internal distress of the patient and family that is associated with the illness. This, too, came from her lived experiences.

Florence came to believe that healthcare extends beyond the disease and must include the internal distress of the patient and family that is associated with the illness.

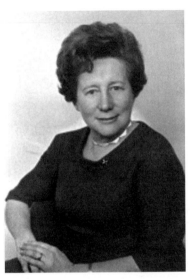

FLORENCE, TAKEN IN 1968.

As a young child, she suffered numerous bouts of pneumonia. In 1926, when Florence was 7, the Schorske family traveled to Florida to facilitate Florence's recovery from a bout of life-threatening pneumonia. On the return trip home, they stopped in Washington, DC, where she was then diagnosed with scarlet fever. This meant weeks of isolation in Garfield Hospital, which Florence described as being trapped in a "vintage Civil War hospital." This was the first time Florence had been separated from her family, and it was a challenge for everyone. Her private nurse, Eunice Biller, from Richmond, Virginia, was as concerned about Florence's spiritual being as her physical being. Florence still remembers the comfort and caregiving presence that Miss Biller gave to her. This spiritual support involved music therapy, play therapy, and communication techniques that made Florence "feel like a person, not a patient with a contagious disease."

From this time forward, Florence was committed to becoming a nurse. At age 17, when preparing for college, she discovered that her father's "old-fashioned beliefs" did not see college as necessary for women. Conversely, her mother had always wanted to attend college and believed that Florence should be allowed to follow her dreams. Her older brother, Carl, sided with Florence and their mother; he believed that education was important and gender was irrelevant. Carl had been the family scholar, attending Columbia University as an undergraduate and Harvard University for his graduate education. Carl, who incorporated the family passion for politics and culture into his studies, would go on to win the 1981 Pulitzer Prize for general nonfiction as author of *Fin-de-Siecle Vienna: Politics and Culture*. He has had academic appointments at Wesleyan University, the University of California at Berkeley, and Princeton University.

> *Annie believed that nursing's purpose was to respond to the patient as a human being, which directly aligned with Florence's vision.*

When it was obvious that Mr. Schorske was outnumbered three to one, he agreed to allow Florence to attend Barnard College and live at home. Florence had another idea—Mount Holyoke College—which meant she would live hours away in South Hadley, MA. Her father was not happy, but Florence won the battle and began a new and independent life.

Florence received a bachelor of arts degree in physiology and sociology from Mount Holyoke College in 1938 and immediately enrolled in the 30-month nursing program at Yale University. At that time, Yale University School of Nursing was for college graduates only who earned a master's degree in nursing; many students came from Mount Holyoke College. Annie Goodrich, founder of the Yale University School of Nursing, had consulted with Mount Holyoke faculty in designing the nursing curriculum. Annie believed that nursing's purpose was to respond to the patient as a human being, which directly aligned with Florence's vision. Yale University School of Nursing, however, was also influenced by the medical model, with a primary focus on the disease, *not* on the patient. This disease orientation was result of the rapidly growing knowledge in medical science that was over-shadowing everything else at the time. Florence was dismayed that nursing was lost in the treatment of the disease, and she questioned if she had made a major career mistake.

After graduation, Florence accepted a staff nurse position at Children's Hospital in Boston before she went on to work at the Henry Street Settlement in NYC—the very patient-focused organization that she had heard of as a child. Unfortunately, timing being what it was, Florence arrived at Henry Street just as the Visiting Nurse Service separated from the rest of the settlement to become the Visiting Nurse Service of New York. When it was part of the Henry Street Settlement, the Visiting Nurse Service was nurse-driven and patient-focused. However, after the reorganization in 1944, the Visiting Nurse Service of New York was based on a physician-driven model. Florence found physicians were unprepared to accept the nurse vision and collaboration. She remained with the Visiting Nurse Service of New York for 2 years (1941-43) but left dissatisfied. For Florence, the art of nursing was still being lost to the science of medicine, and patients were not being viewed as humans or individuals.

Leadership Lesson Learned

"One's image of what one does in the nursing profession may not fit with what is going on in the industry at a particular time."

The real question a leader must ask is, "How are you planning to correct your professional course when the environment no longer matches your original vision?"

Florence had not anticipated these two professional dead ends, as both Yale University School of Nursing and the Visiting Nurse Service were influenced by the medical model. She left the nursing profession for 8 years (1944-52). She resorted to psychoanalysis to sort things out. World War II was raging, and it was a difficult emotional time. She wondered if her pacifist beliefs fit the circumstances of the times.

In early 1944, Florence did the unthinkable in her pacifist family and enlisted in the Army. She felt an obligation to help the military men and women who were fighting the atrocities of Hitler. Ironically, Florence was assigned to a small maternity ward at the United States Military Academy at West Point. Eighteen months later, the war ended, and so did her military service.

Not all beliefs, she had come to understand, fit all circumstances.

Florence's decision to join the military, which went against the grain of what she had so firmly believed before, revealed to her that she was capable of seeing things differently when the situation called for it. Not all beliefs, she had come to understand, fit all circumstances.

Her first collaboration was with the United States Army Signal Corps to evaluate physiological changes when subjects were exposed to extreme climates. Florence recalls that the research questions were interesting, but the methods were poorly designed. Nonetheless, very good outcomes came from the experience—she discovered the importance of clinical research. During her 8-year sabbatical from nursing, Florence became a clinical research assistant at Columbia-Presbyterian Hospital on a surgical metabolism unit. The surgery department research team was developing new laboratory techniques to measure blood volume, assess electrolytes, and explore intervention in vascular and heart surgery. Additionally, the team evaluated which blood vessels and transplanted tissues best tolerated surgical intervention, identified surgical interventions most appropriate in liver failure patients, and even explored the feasibility of repairing an aortic aneurysm—pioneering research at the time. Secondly, it was here that she met her husband-to-be, Henry Wald, one of Florence's research subjects who was in officer's candidate school.

Florence and Henry dated 3 years before he proposed marriage to her in 1948. Henry had completed his military service and had graduated from the Cooper Union for the Advancement of Science and Art in NYC with a degree in engineering. Because Florence's father was dying, her mother had breast cancer, and her professional path was uncertain, she put Henry's proposal aside until serendipity reunited them many years later.

This glimmer of a paradigm shift in acute care practice convinced Florence to consider a return to nursing and hospital care.

By 1952, her psychoanalysis and research experiences had piqued her interest in how children fare when separated from parents and how people react during episodes of high stress. Florence became interested in the work of John Bowlby, Anna Freud, Dorothy Burlingham, and others who reported on the effects of war on children in England. Because of a nursing shortage during the war, a hospital in Newcastle, England, had utilized parents as providers of care for hospitalized children. Out of this workforce crisis came a new vision of family participation in pediatric care, and the reports from patients, families, staff nurses, and physicians were very favorable. As a result, this hospital changed its policies to expand parent visitation and integrate families into the pediatric patient's care. This glimmer of a paradigm shift in acute care practice convinced Florence to consider a return to nursing and hospital care.

Florence joined the staff at Babies & Children's Hospital of New York at Columbia Presbyterian Hospital late in 1952. She collaborated with the unit head nurse in convincing the physicians to "allow parents to feed their children and settle them in for the night." Florence finally believed she was making a difference. Now, focused on the spiritual and psychological aspects of nursing, she decided to pursue a second master of science from Yale—this time in psychiatric nursing.

At last, her career seemed back on track. She lamented the 12 "misguided, nonproductive, and professionally useless years" [1941-52]. Today, she wonders what might have happened if she had gotten on track sooner, but she firmly believes that "things can't be ordered into place," but instead they must "fall into place."

TAKING A NEW DIRECTION

Upon completing her psychiatric nursing master's degree from Yale University in 1956, Florence was invited to join the Rutgers University faculty. This opportunity was particularly appealing, because Rutgers was beginning a master's program in psychiatric nursing. More importantly, she would have the privilege of working with Hildegard Peplau. For Florence, she was finally in the right spot, at the right time.

Hilda Peplau was a visionary nurse leader who was enhancing communication and creating the scientific foundation of the patient-nurse relationship. She was at the peak of her career and was known as a "mover and shaker" at the National Institute of Mental Health. Florence became her assistant. She describes Hilda as "most original and most able to help psychiatric patients."

Florence found Hilda to be "highly respected by colleagues and students, although some found her overwhelming and obdurate. ... Hilda was briliant, and she knew that she was brilliant." Florence also believed that the opportunity to work with this kind of brilliance—with the gifted pioneer in patient care and teaching that was Hilda—was a once in a lifetime experience.

In addition to her own conceptual thinking and methods of approach, Hilda also introduced students to other nurse educators in the field, such as Dorothy Marinas at New York University, Ruth Gilbert at Columbia Teachers College, Helen Mannock at Boston College, and Gwen Tudor Will at Chestnut Lodge. Through this exposure to some of the brightest minds in the profession, Hilda opened Florence's eyes to the social science approach to systematic study of nursing.

Leadership Lesson Learned

"Learning should not be limited to the ideas of one. ... Diversity of thought is an essential element to professional expansion—one's own ego should not become a barrier when preparing the next generation of thought leaders."

Hilda was not fully appreciated in her time, Florence says. People didn't always understand what she was attempting to accomplish because "Hilda had a deeper grasp of issues." According to Florence, Hilda would "coax students down a path they were fearful to take." Fortunately, Florence followed Hilda's lead.

Florence left Rutgers University in June of 1957, but this decision left her feeling conflicted. She had much left to learn from Hilda, she believed, but another door was opening. The dean of Yale University School of Nursing, Elizabeth Bixler, had asked Florence to return to Yale and help at a critical time. Yale President A. Whitney Griswold had proposed closing its school of nursing in the major shift to move the university to an "ivory tower" and exclude disciplines of practice. Numerous irate alumni and faculty members convinced Griswold to rethink his decision, with the condition that the future of the nursing school depended on curriculum enhancement and strong leadership. Florence knew Yale's culture and had been part of in developing the master's curriculum at Rutgers.

Initially, Florence was hired to be an instructor of psychiatric nursing. By the end of the summer, she was asked to take over as the director of the psychiatric program when Marion Russell, then director, sent a telegram announcing she wouldn't be returning for the fall semester. These changes were early signs of things to come for Florence and Yale.

In short order, Florence discovered that most of the faculty, and the dean herself, retreated behind closed doors. A small group of faculty members who were already teaching advanced nursing willingly discussed a new curriculum, while the remainder were either making other career plans or watching from the wings. Dean Bixler made it clear that the school's future was in the hands of the next generation of leaders. The situation appeared more fragile than Florence had originally realized.

A few of the faculty began to meet with the intent of creating order out of chaos. Out of these early meetings, Florence became impressed with one particularly "vigorous" faculty member—Ida Orlando. Ida was conducting research on how to help students develop relationships with patients. She was an "energetic, tough character from Brooklyn" who was proud of her Italian heritage. Ida was critical of psychiatric nurses who utilized complex approaches such as Freudian, Sullivanian, and Reichian methods. She believed that patient communication and relationships needed to be simplistic. Ida proposed good listening skills and validation of assumptions with the patient by asking, "So are you saying …?" Ida believed that it was the responsibility of nurses to advocate for patients' needs. Ida's approach was a back-to-basics methodology, and Florence thought it made great sense. See-

After agreeing to the interim deanship, Florence discovered a surprising gift—Virginia Henderson.

ing the talent in Ida and others slowly begin to emerge, Florence became hopeful that they could create a vision the president would support.

In December 1956, with the dean's permission, Florence, Lucy Conaut, and Martha Pitel went to President Griswold to discuss a new curriculum. A growing faculty group agreed to prepare a brief outline of the new curriculum for his review. The group, now including Ernestine Wiedenbach and M. Elizabeth Tennant, prepared a one-page curriculum proposal. This was drafted and then accepted by the president. The document was the roadmap for the School of Nursing for advanced education in midwifery, psychiatric nursing, and public health, with systematic study of practice. In early 1958, President Griswold offered Florence the interim deanship.

Florence knew that accepting the interim leadership position was risky, but she had a vision of what the program could be, and enough confidence in the people who were committed to work with her, that she took the position. It turned out to be worth the risk.

After agreeing to the interim deanship, Florence discovered a surprising gift—Virginia Henderson. In 1953, Virginia had left Teacher's College. Under the auspices of Yale University, Virginia held a research appointment to co-author a book with Leo W. Simmons titled *Nursing Research: A Survey and Assessment,* which would be published in 1964. Florence recalls that Virginia's research appointment had a small salary, but she needed a place to work. As luck would have it, the office next to Florence's was empty.

Florence describes Virginia as "brilliant, with a broad scope of knowledge and experience ... visionary, articulate, and strategically very wise." She

Doors were open now, unlike before, and the dialogue was brisk and productive.

was a leader, Florence quickly understood, who didn't need a title to be effective. Serendipity had created the meeting, but a deep mutual respect formed a remarkable friendship.

In 1959, Florence officially became the fourth dean of Yale University's School of Nursing. She immediately began to integrate with other schools at the university—including sociology, anthropology, and psychology—to broaden the content and methodology within the school of nursing. The sociology department nominated Robert Leonard, a new faculty member, for a dual appointment with the School of Nursing. He became instrumental in creating methods of research to study practice. When working with master's-level students, Leonard encouraged and assisted them in publishing their findings. He wanted nursing students to publish in nursing journals and to be first author. He extolled the importance of publishing, and through his commitment to nursing students launched many nurse researchers, including such luminaries as Ada Sue Hinshaw, Donna Diers, Rhetaugh Dumas, and Angela Barron McBride.

Things were finally coming together at Yale, and Florence credits Ida Orlando's ideas, Ernestine Wiedenback's practice, Virginia Henderson's vision, and Robert Leonard's methods with providing the building blocks for the new curriculum. Synergy was occurring within the faculty team, and everyone seemed to contribute to the progress. Doors were open now, unlike before, and the dialogue was brisk and productive. Florence is adamant that change of *any* magnitude does not happen as a result of one person. She is emphatic that her leadership just "ornamented, strengthened, and widened" how others operationalized the vision.

Florence recalls one major regret during her deanship—her handling of external pressure to change the leadership in the psychiatric program. Ida Orlando was director of the psychiatric program, and she was being challenged about the simplicity of her analysis of nursing practice. As Florence puts it, Ida was "in the wrong time for unacceptable ideas." Ida was strong-willed and self-confident.

Nursing theory builders were emerging, but Ida believed the theorists' thinking was counterproductive and could compromise patient welfare. She equated theory building to adding layers, and she was committed to removing layers. Florence admits that Ida "had a singular view and was obdurate." The Yale School of Nursing psychiatric program received significant funding from the National Institute of Mental Health (NIMH), and the NIMH review board didn't approve of Ida's simplistic format. For 3 years, the NIMH asked Florence to remove Ida from the leadership role. Florence resisted because she believed in Ida. Her observations had led Florence to believe that "all of that proliferation of ideas about theoretical approaches to process was terribly misguiding to nurses." Florence adds, "Frankly, I have yet to hear students say they felt theory was a help rather than a hindrance." Unfortunately, the pressures continued. Dissatisfied with Florence's lack of action, the NIMH threatened to discontinue support for the psychiatric nursing fellowships and financial responsibilities for the psychiatric program. The message was clear: It was Ida or the NIMH. Florence didn't have the finances to replace the potential NIMH losses, so she asked Ida to step aside. Florence has not forgotten or forgiven herself for the decision she felt forced to make. She is also disappointed that those kinds of pressures can be imposed on a leader and an institution.

According to Florence, leaders must be open to the conversations around the controversy. Ida was set in stone with her ideas and allowed no hint of a compromise to enter her discussions. Florence observes that "listening is as important as moving forward and feeling the need to impart an idea." Ida lost a good concept to a flawed process. Florence has learned from Rashi Fein, of the Harvard University School of Public Health, that "society will only accept what it is ready for, and you must temper your ideas with what can be moved forward at that time." Additionally, Florence had 3 years' notice of a collision of internal and external ideas. It is the leader's responsibility, she emphasizes, to recognize the resistance or conflict. Had Florence taken a more active role in creating compromise on both sides of the controversy, would the outcome have been better?

Florence also had a major personal triumph as a result of being named dean—after 10 years she reconnected with Henry Wald. As Henry was sitting in a coffee shop, the man next to him had a newspaper open to an article and picture announcing Florence's deanship. Henry had been married for nearly a decade and, with two children (Shari and Joel), had recently lost his wife in a car accident. He couldn't believe he had found Florence for the second time in his life. In 1959, Florence, at 40, and Henry, at 35, met again and soon married. Florence was delighted to also have found two wonderful children, who were 6 and 8 at the

Prior to patient-rights discussions, cancer care involved secrecy, with cancer diagnoses often being kept from patients.

time, to complete a family. Today, Shari Wald Vogler is a registered nurse who intends to one day open a hospice, and Joel is a communications consultant.

THE EPIPHANY: HOSPICE CARE IN AMERICA

The 1960s in the United States is well-recognized as the era of civil rights.

It was a period when society was assessing the boundaries around human rights, which then precipitated the discussion of patient rights. Private matters such as healthcare treatment were becoming issues of public discussion. It was a time of protest and change.

Prior to patient-rights discussions, cancer care involved secrecy, with cancer diagnoses often being kept from patients. Patients were commonly placated and told something akin to, "We had to remove a breast because we found a few bad cells, but this doesn't mean you have cancer." Physicians did not want to take away hope, and they thought they were doing the right thing. This was American culture at the time, and faculty and students in nursing practice at Yale New Haven Medical Center were urged by physicians not to answer patient and

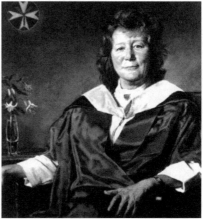

OIL ON CANVAS AT YALE SCHOOL OF NURSING

FLORENCE WALD WAS THE FOURTH DEAN OF THE YALE SCHOOL OF NURSING. SHE BECAME ACTING DEAN IN 1958. IN 1959 SHE WAS APPOINTED FULL DEAN, A POSITION SHE RETAINED UNTIL 1967 WHEN SHE STEPPED DOWN TO PURSUE HOSPICE WORK.

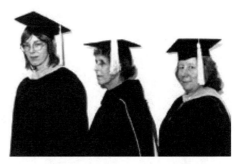

YALE UNIVERSITY SCHOOL OF NURSING DEANS DIERS, ARNSTEIN, AND WALD, SEPTEMBER 1972.

family questions about their progress and their discontents. Social scientists call that system of communication *closed awareness.*

The curative model was then pursued at all costs, even if the patient's condition was worsening. A palliative model didn't exist. Dying pain-free and with dignity was seldom an option in the early 1960s. However, an awakening to the total suffering of dying patients and their families was taking place in the United Kingdom under the leadership of Cicely Saunders. She was a nurse, a social worker, and a physician who studied pain relief in all its manifestations and created a hospice setting where physical comfort, respect, and spiritual and psychological support were there for those who were facing death.

> *Cicely was the first to coin the phrase "total pain" to represent the physical, social, psychological, spiritual, and emotional aspects of end-of-life care.*

In 1963, as plans for St. Christopher's Hospice in the UK were advancing, Cicely came to the United States in search of others with similar interests in palliative care. Bernard Lytton, a Yale urologist who had met Cicely in London, invited her to Yale to speak to medical students about her ideas. Virginia Henderson, who had read Cicely's first publication, attended the lecture and was spellbound by the photographs of patients and their families shown before and after their suffering was addressed. Virginia told Florence of the standing ovation Cicely had received from the students and described what she had heard as "the essence of nursing."

At Virginia's urging,

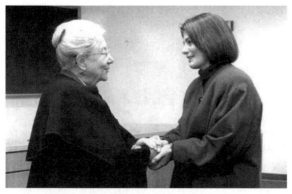

FLORENCE GREETS THE NEWLY NAMED DEAN, DEAN CATHERINE GILLISS, APRIL 1998.

Florence asked Cicely to speak at the School of Nursing on the following day. Florence describes the experience as a "professional epiphany." Cicely was the first to coin the phrase "total pain" to represent the physical, social, psychological, spiritual, and emotional aspects of end-of-life care. The nursing school audience members connected with the discussion on "total pain" through the presentation of color slides showing patients and their families before and after the patients' needs were addressed. Cicely spoke of family involvement, financial considerations, and how care was complex and essential to the patient as a human being, rather than as the host of a disease. She emphasized the value of an interdisciplinary team of nurses, physicians, social workers, and clergy to accommodate diverse patient and family issues.

Cicely articulated in one lecture what Florence had been seeking for her entire career.

Cicely had concluded that the medical care system did not serve these patients well. She had already designed an environment for this special population and was raising funds for St. Christopher's Hospice in southeast London, which would open in 1967.

Florence was particularly moved by Cicely's grasp of what was in the patient's heart and mind. "It was the epitome of nursing," Florence says. Cicely articulated in one lecture what Florence had been seeking for her entire career. She walked away from the discussion knowing that hospice care was here to stay. Three years later, Florence invited Cicely back for 6 weeks as a Yale University School of Nursing visiting professor. Cicely was involved in clinical rounds of the various hospital services including pediatrics, medicine, surgery, and psychiatry to understand the culture of the organization. At the end of her stay, Cicely gave a speech to a packed auditorium titled "The Moment of Truth," which described patients' needs and rights when dying. Cicely also held a workshop that attracted the few people she knew who were working in the field of death and dying, including Elisabeth Kübler-Ross, Colin Murray Parkes, Ray Duff, the Rev. Gregory Reeves, the Rev. Edward Dobihal, and social scientist Leo Simmons, among others, to exchange ideas and make professional connections.

In the years that followed, American culture was reshaped by social scientists and practitioners developing the knowledge base on death and dying. Society was beginning to talk about death, and some physicians were able to understand the distinction between quality and quantity of life. Finally, Florence's ideas were in synergy with the future direction of patient care, and she was in a position to lead hospice care in America. Florence maintained close contact with Cicely, and her hospice knowledge and experience nourished Florence's thinking.

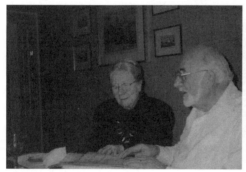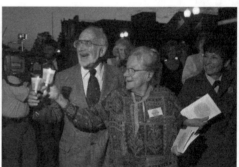

FLORENCE AND HENRY WALD AT HOME, LEFT, AND AT A 1998 CANDLELIGHT VIGIL.

NEXT STAGES

By 1965, Florence came to the realization that it was time to consider leaving the deanship at Yale, but she wanted to do so gracefully. Her heart was already invested in creating hospice care. In 1968, Margaret Arnstein became the fifth dean of Yale University School of Nursing, and Florence assumed a research associate position, which provided her an academic connection and resources for research efforts.

The role transition gave Florence time to see St. Christopher's Hospice in London firsthand. Florence stayed for a month, and she worked in every part of the organization—from bedside care to administration. Florence was preparing herself for hospice in America. Henry Wald was so energized by the work at St. Christopher's that upon their return home, he sold his partnership in his engineering company, Wald and Zigas, and started on a health facility planning degree at Columbia University's School of Architecture so he could contribute to planning the Connecticut hospice. He wrote the hospice feasibility report as his thesis.

> "How can we create an institution in this country such as hospice? We are trapped by the buildings and the technology. How can we get out?"

Florence remembers the day she stood at the front of the Yale-New Haven Hospital and thought, "How can we create an institution in this country such as hospice? We are trapped by the buildings and the technology. How can we get out?" She had seen the possibilities in England, and the outcomes were compelling. She saw the potential of hospice care as clearly as she saw the obstacles to it.

On her way to lunch that day, she encountered three people: Dr. Ray Duff, author of *Sickness and Society*; the Rev. Edward Dobihal, director of religious ministry at Yale-New Haven Hospital; and Dr. Morris Wessel, a family-centered pediatrician. Florence invited them all to join her for lunch. She spent the entire lunch talking about her hospice experience and exploring the possibilities of hospice care at Yale-New Haven Hospital. Collectively, the four-member group decided to meet regularly to work on the project. The group obtained a small grant to conduct a study (1969-71) they called "A Nurse's Study of the Care of Dying Patients and Their Families."

Rather than observing how nurses and doctors were caring for those who were dying, as had Ray Duff and August Hollingshead in previous work, the researchers—Florence and Katherine Klaus, RN—gave the care themselves to discover what they could accomplish, how it helped, and what the obstacles were by keeping diaries of the patients' care. The research team also searched for resources in the community.

Barriers to pain relief were rigid. Morphine intervention was shunned even when all hope was gone. As patients' conditions deteriorated, medical caregivers avoided the patients and their families. However, hospital staff nurses were relieved and grateful for the nursing care Florence and Katherine gave. The nurses wished they had time to provide that kind of care as well.

Hospital staff nurses were aware of the patients as human beings, but not enough to relate to them as anything other than as a diagnostic and curative problem. Care of the family was not perceived to be part of their role. Involving the family was a monumental task because this meant "breaking the code of silence, which had been decades in the making," Florence says. The process was moving healthcare from disease management to symptom management, and the barriers were enculturated in years of practice.

During the study, 22 dying patients were cared for. It was quickly evident that the greater New Haven community did not serve dying patients or their families appropriately or well. Cicely Saunders had been in touch by letter and personal visits during those years. In a visit on 21 November 1970, she stated her conviction that Florence and her colleagues were ready to plan for hospice services. Cicely urged the team to begin with home care service first, while an inpatient unit was being planned.

Hospice Inc. was established as a not-for-profit, tax-exempt institution. Those who were part of the caregiving team became the incorporators, including the Rev. Robert Canney, the Rev. Edward Dobihal, the Rev. Fred Auman, Katherine Klaus, Ira Goldenberg, Morris Wessel, Florence Wald, and Henry Wald.

Cicely Saunders continued to maintain regular contact as an observer and adviser. The planning stage was organized in areas of the necessary tasks—patient care, building and site location, personnel, finances, research, and community and professional relations. The relationship of the tasks was integrated into a time line. Once the planning process was determined, volunteers from the community joined the staff in carrying out the work. Soon volunteers were more plentiful than the tasks at hand.

Project funding was a priority. Private foundations worked in collaboration with each other once a budget was estimated. The van Ameringen Foundation, The Commonwealth Fund, and The Ittleson Foundation (initially) contributed to planning, home care, and building, respectively. Local community contributions followed. Housing for the enterprise was provided by local institutions.

The beginnings of the hospice home care came 3 years later. Sylvia Lack, a London physician who had been on staff at St. Christopher's Hospice, headed up the home care program. She had been recommended by Cicely Saunders and brought invaluable experience to the New Haven Hospice program. Meanwhile, plans for the building and site were drawn up for board approval by a task force headed by Virginia Henderson and Henry Wald.

Lo-Yi Chan was selected as the architect and given the charge to create an environment that would make patients and visitors comfortable and at ease, as well as to keep the hospice part of the community. The 48-bed building was divided into two parts to make it a reasonable size, with spacing for both togetherness and privacy. Easy access to the outside, including for bed-bound patients, was incorporated into the design. Ultimately, the building would open in 1980.

While planning and home care moved forward as projected, state licensure and a certificate of need lagged. The federal agencies for planning were unstable. Regional medical programs created under the administration of U.S. President Lyndon Johnson had recently been replaced by state health agencies under President Richard Nixon's term of office. An aging Connecticut state health commissioner, Franklin Foote, who was about to retire, was uncertain how to assist in the birth of a new, unique health service such as hospice.

No one on the board of directors or the planning staff had the background to guide the process, nor did other community agencies or health care administrators at Yale find successful solutions. However, an expert who had helped the city of New Haven in government relations for urban renewal was hired as a consultant. Dennis Rezendes was successful in obtaining a certificate of need.

> *When Florence was on vacation, Dennis informed them that if he were to continue, they must ask her to resign.*

UNDERSTAND THE DYNAMICS OF ORGANIZATIONAL GROWTH

As the planning progressed, Florence noted a fracture forming between the home care staff and the soon-to-be inpatient staff. Dennis had no experience in clinical care, but that did not matter at the time, because Florence was to lead this portion. Dennis, educated in the Wharton School of Business, had a corporate administrative style that was inappropriate to

Florence's democratic, collaborative, decision-making notions. Home care staff preferred his classic style of taking charge rather than her consensus-building style. Dennis also knew the ways of ascendancy. He had been appointed by the board as administrator. When Florence was on vacation, Dennis informed them that if he were to continue, they must ask her to resign. When Florence refused to offer her resignation, the board ended her appointment.

Florence was devastated. Her dream had been taken from her. She had already seen the denouement, and she consulted with Seymour Saruson, a Yale University organizational psychologist, to make sense of the situation. Seymour had studied new kinds of organizations that were expanding and changing. His work demonstrated that, regardless of the kind of organization, when the "original innovators bring on other people to expand the idea, discord develops, and the second group essentially kills off the first group." He compared this organizational behavior to what happens in the theater. The author writes a play. The play can't reach the audience without a director, who applies a slightly different interpretation of the original work. The play comes to life through the actor, who has the capability to modify the director's perspective. The growth of ideas, from different perspectives, can result in a successful interpretation or in a "destructive internal force," with the original message blurred in the translation.

Florence admits that this chain of events was a result of a "strategic blind spot." She didn't envision the first U.S. hospice as a role model for the rest of the nation. She simply wanted to adapt St. Christopher's hospice model to Greater New Haven. Dennis had a national vision and a dynasty mentality. When he developed the National Hospice Organization and held the first meeting in 1975, he had estimated that 200 people would attend, but nearly 1,000 arrived. Additionally, Florence did not think in terms of organizational complexities, including policy and the dynamics of controlling rapid growth. When the board was formed in 1971, she considered taking on the role of president, but chose not to be considered. She was concerned that a woman and a nurse would not command the necessary respect. Florence had the ability to lead a large organization, as was demonstrated through her deanship at Yale University School of Nursing. Today, Florence would advise nurses to "step up and assume leadership roles that appear to be a stretch," and to not allow gender or professional hierarchies to be measures of capability.

Florence continued to actively disseminate the hospice model of care in America through national and international channels. She has been part of many end-of-life care discussions and has a keen interest in hospice services across the country. The hospice literature and leadership credit Florence with being the American founder of the hospice movement, but she sees its ownership as much more diverse. She may have lost an important leadership battle when the board ended her assignment, but she won the war that created a paradigm shift for end-of-life care in America. Today, there are more than 3,300 hospice programs in the nation, and millions of patients and families have benefited from her courage in taking the first step and from those others who formed a wider base.

On the other hand, Dennis may have won the battle but lost the war. Upon assuming leadership, Dennis almost immediately changed the name of the organization to the Connecticut Hospice Inc. and hired Rosemary Johnson Hurzeler as an assistant. Ironically, within 1 year of opening the building, Rosemary had "forced Dennis out." Twenty years later, Rosemary left the original hospice building and sold it for $1 to

Fleet was a good Buddhist scholar who had made some bad choices that resulted in a 25-year prison sentence for drug trafficking.

in order of nuns who suffered physical disabilities, and it was subsequently renamed the "Monastery of the Glorious Cross." Rosemary reclaimed a corporate building on a beautiful site as the new location for Connecticut Hospice. After that, the vision ebbs and flows.

CONDUCTING RESEARCH IN HER 80s

In 1994, Florence received a grant from the Center on Crime, Communities, and Culture to study adaptation of hospice care to prisoners in the Connecticut State Department of Corrections. The study incorporated six prison infirmaries serving Connecticut's 23 prisons to explore health management practices of terminally ill patients in prison custody.

Florence first learned of the concept of hospice care for prisoners from her daughter, Shari, a member of the same Tibetan Buddhist group as Fleet Maull. Fleet was a good Buddhist scholar who had made some bad choices that resulted in a 25-year prison sentence for drug trafficking. While serving his sentence at Springfield Federal Penitentiary in Missouri, Fleet was shaken as he witnessed inmates die with minimal care. He and other inmates had the compassion and commitment to end-of-life care but lacked the formal skills. The prison chaplain and the prison warden engaged the local Springfield, hospice program to train the prisoners as volunteers.

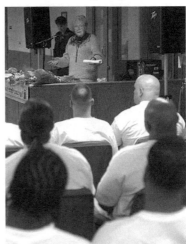

FIRST GRADUATING CLASS OF HOSPICE VOLUNTEERS (2002) AT CONNECTICUT'S MACDOUGAL-WALKER CORRECTIONAL FACILITY.

In 1987, Fleet established the first U.S. prison hospice with the help of a Buddhist group. In 1991, he disseminated the prison hospice concept by establishing the National Prison Hospice Association, and Florence, along with Elisabeth Kübler-Ross, became a member of the advisory board.

In 1997, Florence and Nealy Zimmermann approached A. Siobhan Thompson, MPH, to help write a grant and design a feasibility study on the needs and resources for hospice care in Connecticut correctional facilities. Nealy was president of the Connecticut chapter of the National Prison Hospice Association, and Siobhan was directing a research study on HIV infection rates among the all-female prison population of the Janet S. York Correctional Institute.

"Today, the hospice program has earned a place in the correctional community, but it wasn't an easy road to pave. When we introduced the idea of inmate volunteer caregivers, only about half the correctional staff supported the idea, and their support was with caution," Siobhan says. However, as of January 2007, a decade after the feasibility study, the seventh class of hospice inmate volunteers was graduated; 120 incarcerated men and women in Connecticut's correctional system are now trained to help deliver hospice care.

"Even in a prison setting, caregiving can transform sadness in the bleakest of circumstances into satisfaction and even great happiness, when people actually love what they do," Siobhan says.

The prison hospice experience has provided Florence with a broader scope of understanding of caregiver transformation while caring for the terminally ill. For inmate caregivers, the role was described as "evoking a sense of respect, understanding, and forgiveness for those who are finding final moments of peace." Florence is still in touch with the prison hospice program, and she describes the experience as a "rich setting to work with the disadvantaged and those who are marginalized."

WORDS OF WISDOM

Florence openly declares that she is not sure exactly what a leader is. She has difficulty defining the word "leader." "There are so many different tracks, and it is a very changeable state—much like an amoeba," says Florence on the topic of leadership. She believes that leadership strength requires knowing oneself and capitalizing on special competencies as a leader. According to Florence, Donna Diers, dean emeritus of Yale University School of Nursing, is a "gifted writer who possesses a remarkable style and interest in using words properly, so her leadership as a writer may be the natural and driving strength behind her leadership as a dean." She states that not everyone can be good at everything, but it is important to identify and maximize innate talents.

True to her leadership lessons, Florence also reminds emerging leaders that leadership is not a title. "The right title allows you to join the circle, but it is not the true influence." Florence points out that Virginia Henderson didn't have a leadership title at Yale University, but she was a great leader who influenced the lives of many with her gifts of writing and teaching. The Yale School of Nursing and hospice moved forward because of her contributions. Title or no title, it is important to acknowledge and recognize those leadership influences that are moving the art and science of nursing—they are seen as the pillars holding up the vision.

When Florence discusses the individual recognition she has received for her hospice work, she becomes visibly unsettled. She wants the world to know that the awards really belong to the group that pioneered the hospice effort with her. "No one person accomplished this, and it is almost embarrassing to be singled out." Florence does take pride that the nursing profession has received due praise for

"The right title allows you to join the circle, but it is not the true influence."

the hospice movement, because this is the "essence of nursing—nurses practicing nursing to its fullest potential."

"As assisted suicide is practiced today, the family can't be a part of the process and that puts the onus on the patient." Florence takes the controversial stand that ending suffering in terminal illnesses via euthanasia is an acceptable alternative. She believes that patients and family should have the choice after the options and consequences are completely considered and discussed. According to Florence, the term "assisted suicide" is an inappropriate concept, because it puts the patient in an isolated position and that puts the onus on the patient." The word suicide is so "unacceptable" in most cultures—except Japanese—that society predictably reacts negatively.

When reflecting on the current state of healthcare delivery, Florence believes that nurses can be saviors of an unhealthy medical care system. She has believed for many years that medicine has been glorified and made imperative. Society has an unrealistic image of what medicine can do. She believes prevention is the essential role and should be universal and ubiquitous. She further suggests that "nursing divest itself as the assistant to medicine." Nursing, she believes, is branching out and identifying problems and solutions from a humanistic and holistic perspective. Nurses will flourish as healthcare moves into the next century, notes Florence, and the hierarchy in medical care will begin to diminish.

> *Florence believes that nurses will be the saviors of an unhealthy medical care system.*

SUMMARY

Hospice has become synonymous with goodness and compassion. Receiving hospice services has been described as "finding the light after being in a dark tunnel." One family member interviewed described hospice nurses as "angels on earth who have the gift of turning the destructive storm into a rainbow." Hospice has become a service that family, physicians, nurses, social workers, and case managers depend on to ease the "total pain" of dying. Florence Wald, among a band of pioneers, made this come about in the United States.

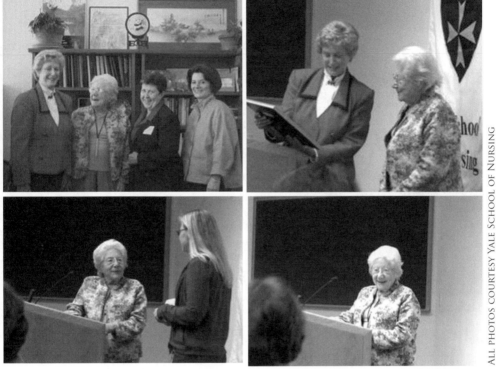

TOP LEFT: THEN CONNECTICUT LT. GOVERNOR JODI RELL (NOW GOVERNOR RELL), FLORENCE, LINDA SPOONSTER-SCHWARTZ (CONNECTICUT'S COMMISSIONER FOR VETERANS AFFAIRS), AND DEAN CATHERINE GILLISS. TOP RIGHT: JODI RELL PRESENTS FLORENCE WITH THE CONNECTICUT TREASURE AWARD.

Florence continues to leave a legacy of patient- and family-centered care that has elevated nursing practice and clinical autonomy to new and unexpected levels. She believes that the mentor influences in her life—Hildegard Peplau, Virginia Henderson, and Cicely Saunders—provided her the platform for developing her ideas in a scholarly manner and the cour-

> *The profound nature of her work has certainly allowed others the privilege to get their lives in order and pass in peace with the dignity they and their families deserve.*

age to act on them. As she reflects on her life, Florence is grateful for all the lessons learned, because each encounter prepared her for the next task and ultimately to "change the face of dying."

In July 2005, Cicely Saunders died from breast cancer. Florence knows that Cicely had lived her dream and made a difference.

So has Florence. Today, she "is in good heart." Hospice is firmly entrenched in healthcare and society. Her final goal is to organize her papers so the hospice journey will be accurately recorded but, she says with a grin, "I hope I live long enough to leave my desk in order!"

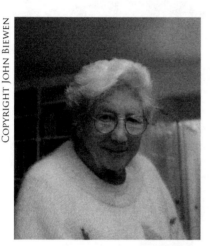

FLORENCE IN HER HOME, 2005.

The profound nature of her work has certainly allowed others the privilege to get their lives in order and pass in peace with the dignity they and their families deserve.

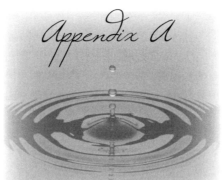

Appendix A

LEADERSHIP CHALLENGES

Instructors and students: These leadership challenges are provided to inspire you to challenge your own leadership skills in relation to the lessons learned throughout the book. Use them within a course or simply to reflect on how you might react to the same situations these leaders experienced.

CHAPTER 1 – RICHARD CARMONA

1. Leadership is often an exercise in perseverance. Rich Carmona identifies his ability to fail and "just keep getting up" as a key ingredient in his ultimate success. Reflect back on a time when you may have given up on a project or an aspiration. Did you give up too early? What could you have done differently to change the outcome? Did your failure to "just keep getting up" again affect your career? As a leader, imagine yourself in a situation in which you are looking to motivate someone to get up one more time. What would you say to inspire an individual to make a second or third effort?

2. Our leadership style and ability are influenced by our life experiences. Describe how your life experiences have contributed to your leadership style and abilities. Identify a person or circumstance that has prompted you to see yourself in a different way. Have you influenced the leadership styles or abilities of others? If so, in whom and in what ways?

3. Rich spoke of being a new leader and facing complacency in the workplace. How would you approach complacency in an organization that claimed to be dedicated to excellence? What would help you to identify the hidden agendas that threatened to interfere with your leadership goals?

4. Describe a project or mission you were assigned that seemed impossible to complete. What were the barriers that caused you the most trouble? How did you overcome these barriers? Who did you enlist to help you overcome the obstacles? In what ways did you earn leadership credibility during this time of challenge?

CHAPTER 2 – MARY ELIZABETH CARNEGIE

1. Elizabeth was determined to make a difference for African-American nurses in this country. She saw very quickly the discrimination that was occurring and felt it should not be tolerated. She stood up for what she believed in and made a difference for all African-American nurses. This is her legacy to the nursing profession. What "wrongs" still exist in the nursing profession? How can you help turn these around for other nurses?

2. Elizabeth was an African-American woman who stood up for herself at a time when it was not always welcomed or accepted. She was professional in her demeanor, but firm in her position of equality. In numerous instances, Elizabeth could have lost her job or professional role for speaking up, but she did not. Have you ever been in a situation with so much of your professional career at stake? How did you handle yourself? What did you learn from the situation?

3. Elizabeth made a name for herself as a great nurse leader, but never forgot her roots. Today, her legacy continues through scholarships for African-American student nurses. What legacy do you plan on leaving the profession?

CHAPTER 3 – LEAH CURTIN

1. Leah Curtin spoke about "drawing a line in the sand." She reminded us of our responsibility to defend that line in the sand. [Drawing a line in the sand means to establish limits to what is acceptable to you.] Should a leader avoid drawing lines in the sand? What justifies drawing lines in the sand? What local and national healthcare issues are you aware of for which national or international nurse leaders have drawn lines in the sand? Describe the professional risks and benefits of taking a leadership role in these issues.

2. Leah believes that the "real nurses" are the nurses who practice at the bedside. How do nurse leaders manage the dilemma of moving farther away from the bedside with each leadership promotion? Is it possible to be a "real nurse" and hold the title of a nurse administrator? In your opinion, what is the definition of a nurse leader?

3. Courage and candor would aptly describe Leah's leadership journey. Leah had no problem pointing out the obvious and asking the difficult questions that begged to be addressed. Can you describe a clinical circumstance when no one asked the important and obvious patient care question? If so, describe such a situation. How does your organization manage ethical dilemmas? Would you have the courage to "do the right thing" if you believed your job was on the line? What kind of systems should organizations have in place to support healthcare providers in challenging the status quo?

4. Leah spent decades writing about the politics, power, and possibilities of the nursing profession. She demonstrated the "power of the pen" for most of her career. Identify two areas of professional interest (identified through your experience or observations) that beg to be published and write the first paragraph for each topic. Read one of Leah's editorials from *Nursing Management*—pick one, any one will do—and describe her style of writing, risk-taking choices, and leadership messages in the article.

Chapter 4 – Imogene King

1. Imogene learned one of her early leadership lessons from her father, who taught her to be open in her communication and respectful to others when choosing her words. Have you ever witnessed a leader "lose her cool" or react inappropriately for the circumstance? What impression did that leave with you? How might she have respectfully handled the same situation? Has this ever happened to you as a leader? If so, describe the situation, your response, and how you would do it over if given the chance.

2. Imogene saw the importance of leaders asking questions in order to make necessary change. During her first professional association meeting, she sat quietly. Later, she asked her mentor why no nurses had challenged the speaker's statements during the meeting. Imogene became very involved in her nursing associations as a mechanism to change the profession and bring a voice to nurses. Are you involved in your state nurses association? If not, how are you effecting public policy change for the profession? What are some ways you can get involved in effecting change for the nursing profession?

3. Imogene is renowned for her work on the Goal Attainment Theory. She stresses the primary importance of nurses setting goals with their patients versus planning the care without patient involvement. Do you take the time on a regular basis to work through goal setting with patients, or do you (or the physicians) make the decisions on what goals your patients should achieve?

Chapter 5 – Ruth Lubic

1. As demonstrated in Ruth Lubic's chapter, timing can be everything to a leader. As a leader stepping into a new position, have you ever walked into an organizational "mess" that was left over and took the heat for it? How did it make you feel? How did you resolve the issue?

2. One critical lesson Ruth learned was actively listening to her patients and their unique health history versus what the textbooks say should occur in the normal setting. During your career, has a patient ever provided a history different from what the textbooks taught? Which source did you believe initially? How did you handle the discrepancy?

3. Throughout Ruth's career, she has been in positions where she had to battle the political forces of "physicians versus nurses." How would you rate the professional level of communication with physicians throughout your career? In hindsight, as you reflect upon any confrontational or negative conversations with physicians, how would you handle that same interaction today? What would you teach a new nurse to do in a similar situation?

CHAPTER 6 – MARGARET MCCLURE

1. Maggie McClure was a leader in a hurry. She developed three distinct leadership roles that contributed to the profession of nursing: nurse researcher, professional organization leader, and nurse executive. Select one of these roles and describe the leadership attributes Maggie displayed in creating success. How did Maggie lead during adversity in the given role?

2. Maggie spoke of the "tail wagging the dog" when describing the dilemma of 12-hour shifts. Should hospitals revisit 8-hour shifts? If so, how would you as a nurse leader go about instituting this change? Describe a time that you were compelled to make an unpopular practice change because it was better for the patient. How did you create buy-in from the team?

3. The Magnet study was uncharted waters for the nursing profession. The researchers behind the study analyzed the workforce shortage from a different perspective—"why do nurses stay," instead of "why do nurses leave" their work environments? Identify an area of healthcare that would benefit from a different perspective of query. Describe your thoughts about nurse vacancy and turnover rates as the strongest predictor of Magnet work environments. As the nurse workforce shortage intensifies, do these indicators hold the same value? If not why?

4. Maggie reminds nurses of the power physicians have in creating healthcare policy that may directly impact nursing practice. As a nurse leader, what other alliances should we emphasize and build as we set our agendas to improve patient and nurse outcomes? What leadership role does nursing play in creating the interdisciplinary team?

Chapter 7 – Marla Salmon

1. According to Marla Salmon, the world is run by those who show up. What does this mean to nurses and the nursing profession? How do we show up for our patients and their outcomes? How do we best prepare ourselves for "showing up" prepared and capable of positively influencing the outcomes? Can you think of a time when you or nursing as a profession missed an opportunity to make a difference in healthcare? Describe the situation and hypothesize on how seizing the opportunities may have made a difference to the overall outcomes.

2. Marla's mother wisely reminded her family that, "You can't go somewhere without leaving somewhere." Have you determined where you need to go with your career? What talents have you yet to develop to go "somewhere"? What is holding you back from making the journey?

3. Describe a circumstance that defined or codified your leadership. What compelled you to speak up for something that wasn't right or take charge in a leadership vacuum? Did you feel differently about yourself immediately after the event or circumstance? Did others notice and support your leadership initiative? If not, what would you do to support someone in a similar position with you in the senior leadership role?

4. Marla is a risk taker who believes in the "why not" philosophy of life. What must you know as a leader to embrace the "why not" of individual choices? What is your personal leadership style? How does it help you achieve success? How does it contribute to "failures"?

CHAPTER 8 – JUDITH SHAMIAN

1. Judith had to learn the valuable lesson of accepting constant change early in her life. She lived in three different countries and had to learn new traditions and new ways to communicate. This level of continuous change taught her survival skills that she used to navigate through some rough waters in life. Change and ambiguity can be two of the most difficult obstacles for a leader and her or his team. How do you personally handle change and the thought of not knowing what your organization's next move might be? Have you worked in settings that seemed to function chaotically most of the time? How did you survive the environment? As a result, what professional advice would you give someone who is in a similar situation?

2. Judith grew up as a child facing much adversity due to circumstances beyond her control. She used this internal strength to her advantage later in her professional career and became a risk taker in healthcare by setting standards others tried to follow. As an executive nurse, Judith was setting golden standards in nurse staffing that were too costly for other hospital systems to follow. She was not always popular for being a trendsetter, but she was doing what she believed to be right for the profession. She was a fighter from an early age and remained true to herself. As a leader, are there times you or a superior has gone against the popular belief and made a stronger decision as a result? What did this experience teach you about leadership?

CHAPTER 9 – GRAYCE SILLS

1. Grayce learned as a young girl that critical feedback can be painful but necessary to move forward and be successful. These conversations are referred to as "crucial conversations." As a leader, have you ever had to have a crucial conversation with an employee to make a corrective action or share with someone their areas for improvement? How did you handle this conversation? In hindsight, could you have handled the conversation

more professionally? How do you think the employee felt by the end of the conversation?

2. Grayce was a visionary before her time. When she first recognized how psychiatric patients were treated in the late 1940s and early 1950s, it left an impression she never forgot. She knew psychiatric patients deserved to be treated with dignity. Her life's work centered on providing good standards of practice for psychiatric patients. What nursing experience left such an impression on you that it changed your life's work? Was it an experience from nursing school or later as a professional nurse? Is it this experience that helped you to choose a nursing specialty area of practice?

3. Grayce had a nursing instructor who "labeled" students and grouped them in unflattering ways. Grayce was put in the "dumb bunny" category. Besides the embarrassment, this caused deeper harm as Grayce came to accept her coined name as the truth and believe she was not as bright as the others in her class. This is obviously an example of poor instruction. Have you ever mentored a new nursing student who struggled with concepts or practices you thought were obvious or easy? If so, did you react to the student in a supportive way and work with him or her to encourage learning? Were you as patient and caring as you should have been or were you rushed into fixing the situation yourself?

CHAPTER 10 – KIRSTEN STALLKNECHT

1. At age 28, Kirsten "wanted to change the way we treated patients." Kirsten had studied the U.S. model of effective team nursing, so she set up a similar "test" system in her hospital unit. One leadership lesson Kirsten learned from international nursing is to take the best ideas and incorporate them into practice, as appropriate to that environment. What works 100% in the United States may not work exactly the same in Denmark; however, parts of the same concepts can be applied. What great health care concepts or processes have you seen in one system and tried to recreate in another system? Could you use the entire model, or did you have to modify the idea to "fit" your new organization?

2. Kirsten Stallknecht leaped into her riskiest leadership role as president of the Danish Nurses Organization, without really knowing what she was getting herself into. In hindsight, she admits she was naivé, but is clear that had she known the extent of the job she might have forgone the opportunity. Have you ever experienced a leap into a new leadership role that in hindsight you underestimated? What did you do to gain the necessary skills for the job? Did you consider stepping down from the position when you realized the full scope?

CHAPTER 11 – FLORENCE WALD

1. Along with a leadership title comes the responsibility of performing in the role. Florence Wald points out that a title allows one to "join the circle," but this is not the "true influence." Offer some suggestions of what may contribute to true influence. Identify three individuals in your life who demonstrate true influence. What are the characteristics or abilities that allow these people to demonstrate true influence?

2. Florence was devastated when an individual she recruited engineered her departure from the hospice facility that had been her dream. What proactive methods could a leader engage in to avoid "strategic blind spots"? Can you think of a time when a hidden agenda halted a worthy project or eliminated a good leader? Describe the circumstances and how you would have handled the situation differently.

3. Florence would ask, "How are you planning to correct *your* professional course when the environment no longer matches your original vision?" As a leader, it is your responsibility to change. What suggestions do you have about correcting your professional course when your vision is out of synch with the organizational culture or the direction of the profession or industry? What constitutes a professional challenge versus a professional mismatch? How would you know the difference? What would be your leadership choices in each circumstance?

4. Florence indicated that leaders must be open to conversations around controversy. How would you as a leader create positive outcomes around controversial conversations? Provide an example when a controversial conversation produced an unwanted outcome. In retrospect, evaluate what you could have done differently as a leader to avoid this outcome.

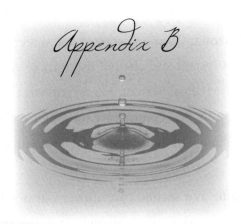

RICHARD HENRY CARMONA, RN, MD, MPH, FACS

Born to a poor family in New York City, Richard H. Carmona experienced homelessness, hunger, and health disparities during his youth. The experiences greatly sensitized him to the relationships among culture, health, education, and economic status and shaped his future.

After dropping out of high school, Carmona enlisted in the U.S. Army in 1967. While serving, he earned his General Equivalency Diploma and went on to become a combat-decorated Special Forces Vietnam veteran. After leaving active duty, he was able to attend Bronx Community College of the City University of New York through an open enrollment program for veterans. He earned an Associate of Arts degree and then attended the University of California, San Francisco, where he received a Bachelor of Science degree (1977) and medical degree (1979). At the University of California Medical School, Carmona was awarded the prestigious gold-headed cane as the top graduate.

Originally trained in general and vascular surgery after medical school, Carmona completed a National Institutes of Health-sponsored fellowship in trauma, burns, and critical care. He is a fellow of the American College of Surgeons. Recruited jointly by the Tucson (Arizona) Medical Center and the University of Arizona, Carmona started and directed Arizona's first regional trauma care system and chaired the State of Arizona Southern Regional Emergency Medical System. He served as a professor of surgery, public health, and family and community medicine at the University of Arizona and as the Pima County Sheriff's Department surgeon and deputy sheriff.

Public health came as a second career after Carmona went back to graduate school while working to complete a master's degree in public health. His interest stemmed from the realization that most of his work as a physician was for reasons that were preventable.

In 2002, Carmona was unanimously confirmed by the Senate to become the 17th surgeon general of the United States. President George W. Bush chose Carmona for the post because of his extensive experience in public health, clinical sciences, healthcare management, and preparedness and his commitment to prevention as an effective means to improve public health and reduce healthcare costs while improving the quality and quantity of life.

As surgeon general, Carmona had a very diverse portfolio of responsibility that included prevention, preparedness, health disparities, health literacy, global health, and health diplomacy. He also issued many landmark surgeon general communications during his tenure, including a definitive statement regarding the danger of secondhand smoke.

Carmona has published extensively and received numerous awards, decorations, and local and national recognition for his achievements. A strong supporter of community service, he has served on community and national boards and provided leadership to many diverse organizations.

After completing his 4-year term as surgeon general in 2006, Carmona was named to the position of vice chairman for Canyon Ranch, a health and wellness company. He also serves as chief executive officer of the company's Health Division and oversees health strategy and policy for all Canyon Ranch businesses. He is president of the nonprofit Canyon Ranch Institute and the recipient of the first distinguished professorship in public health at the University of Arizona's Mel and Enid Zuckerman College of Public Health.

M. Elizabeth Carnegie, DPA, RN, FAAN

M. Elizabeth Carnegie has made significant contributions to the development of nursing as a profession, science, and discipline. She has been a role model for teachers, scholars, academic administrators, and organizational leaders, particularly within the African American community. Carnegie was the first Black nurse elected to the board of the Florida Nurses Association and dedicated her career to breaking down the racial barriers for Blacks in nursing.

Carnegie received her nursing education through a diploma program at the Lincoln School for Nurses, a Bachelor of Arts degree from West Virginia State College, a Master of Arts degree from Syracuse University, and a Doctor of Public Administration degree from New York University.

Carnegie was employed at the American Journal of Nursing Company (AJN) from 1953-1978 and is editor emerita of *Nursing Research*. She has written, edited, and contributed chapters to nearly 20 books and is author of all three editions of the award-winning *The Path We Tread: Blacks in Nursing Worldwide, 1854-1994*.

Carnegie initiated the baccalaureate nursing program at the historically Black Hampton University in Virginia, where the archives are named in her honor. A past president of the American Academy of Nursing (1978-1979) and chair of the American Nurses Association's Minority Fellowship Program Advisory Committee (1988-1999), she served as dean and professor of the School of Nursing at Florida A & M University (1945-1953). From 1991-1995, she served on the Sigma Theta Tau International board of directors.

Since retiring from the Journal Company in 1978, Carnegie has served as an independent consultant for scientific writing and as distinguished visiting professor for the schools of nursing at Hampton University; University of North Carolina at Greensboro; Pennsylvania State University in University Park; University of Massachusetts at Amherst; University of Michigan, Ann Arbor; Indiana University, Indianapolis; and Commonwealth University of Virginia, Richmond. She has also occupied endowed chairs at Adelphi University, New York; Memphis State University, Tennessee; and Prairie View University, Houston, Texas.

Carnegie has received eight honorary doctorates and countless awards, including the Estelle Osborne Award from New York University; induction into Columbia University's Teachers College Hall of Fame; the American Nurses Association Mary Mahoney Award; the George Arens Pioneer Medal from her alma mater, Syracuse University; the President's Award from Sigma Theta Tau International; and the Living Legend Award from the Association of Black Nurse Faculty in Higher Education. Also, she was inducted into the American Nurses Association Hall of Fame in 2000 and the Florida Nurses Association Hall of Fame in 2001.

Leah Curtin, RN, MS, MA, FAAN

Leah Curtin is a clinical professor of nursing at the University of Cincinnati College of Nursing and Health and was editor in chief of *Nursing Management* for 20 years. She also is managing partner of Metier Consultants, editor in chief of *The Journal of Clinical Systems Management,* and director of Cross Country Education's Nurse Manager Boot Camp. She has co-directed *The Health Care Leadership Forum* since 1998 with Franklyn Shaffer, EdD, RN, FAAN. A graduate of the Good Samaritan Hospital School of Nursing and the University of Cincinnati, Curtin earned a master's degree in health planning and health administration from the university and a Master of Arts in philosophy with a major in ethics from the Athenaeum of Ohio. In 1982, she was elected a fellow of the American Academy of Nursing for her work in ethics, and in 1990 she was awarded an honorary doctorate from the State University of New York for the impact her editorials have had on the development of nursing and healthcare in the United States. In 2002, The Medical College of Ohio awarded her a second honorary doctorate for her humanitarian services.

In 1996, Curtin was scholar-in-residence at Ballarat University in Victoria, Australia. She also was a visiting scholar at the University of Oklahoma, Brigham Young University, and University of Eastern Kentucky. She is the first virtual faculty member of the University of Colorado School of Nursing. In 1998, Curtin was invited to Copenhagen, where she testified before Denmark's Ministry of Health on the impact that restructuring in U.S. hospitals has had on the safety of patient care. In 2001, and again in 2002, she was a distinguished lecturer for the Hong Kong Hospital Authority, Hong Kong, China. She has been listed in *Who's Who in America* since 1991 and in *Who's Who in the World* since 1992. She is the author of more than 286 articles and 400 editorials as well as eight books written for professionals. She also wrote the book *Sunflowers in the Sand: Children's Stories of War,* for a general audience. Researched in the Balkans, most notably Croatia and Bosnia Herzegovina, this book was endorsed by people as diverse as the executive director of UNICEF, the Roman Catholic bishop of Cleveland, and comedian Jerry Lewis. The book included a foreword written by Tony Danza and received a positive review in *The New York Times Sunday Book Review*. All proceeds from the sale of *Sunflowers* is sent to The Croatian Children's Fund for the care and treatment of children damaged by war.

Imogene King, EdD, MSN, RN, FAAN

Imogene King is universally recognized as a pioneer of nursing theory development and theory-based nursing practice. As one of the original nurse theorists, King has had an enduring impact on nursing education, practice, and research while serving as a consummate, active leader in professional nursing. Internationally known for her *Theory of Goal Attainment*, King has worked with nurses in Canada, Germany, Japan, Sweden, Denmark, and most recently, China, to shape professional nursing practice, scholarship, and education. Her theory has relevance and value in increasing diverse and outcome-oriented systems for the delivery of nursing and healthcare. Her nursing paradigm is an important model for healthcare in the 21st century and beyond.

King's legacy of service spans nearly 6 decades. Her numerous contributions to the American Nurses Association (ANA) include the first ANA Committee, in 1965, to plan clinical conferences. More recently, she served as the southeastern representative to the ANA Code of Ethics Task Force. King was the 1996 recipient of ANA's Jessie M. Scott Award for demonstrating the interdependent relationships among nursing education, nursing practice, and nursing administration. She has served in elected and appointed positions as a voice for the profession at international, national, and state levels and is known for asking relevant, critical questions that command evidence-based decision-making for the future of nursing and health-are. King has consistently demonstrated her willingness to mentor nurses and students across all roles and settings. Most importantly, King serves as a role model in demonstrating the importance of one's professional responsibility to actively contribute to the advancement of the nursing profession. As a result, she has personally influenced the life, community, and profession of nurses and nursing. King received her diploma in nursing from St. John's Hospital in St. Louis, Missouri, her Bachelor of Science in Nursing and Master of Science in Nursing from St. Louis University, and her EdD from Teachers College, Columbia University. King has won numerous honors and awards. She was inducted into the ANA Hall of Fame and the Florida Nurses Association Hall of Fame, and in November 2005, she was named a Living Legend by the American Academy of Nursing.

Ruth Watson Lubic, CNM, EdD, FAAN, FACNM

A diploma graduate of the Hospital of the University of Pennsylvania, Ruth Watson Lubic also received a bachelor's and master's degree in nursing from Teachers College, Columbia University, followed soon thereafter by a certificate of nurse-midwifery awarded by the Maternity Center Association (MCA)/The State University, New York (SUNY) Health Sciences Center in Brooklyn. Broadening her scope, she earned a doctorate in education (EdD) from Columbia in applied anthropology.

From 1970 to 1995, Lubic was general director of the MCA, a venerable organization founded in 1918 by socially prominent women and operated continuously by professional women of great distinction, including Frances Perkins. When Franklin Roosevelt appointed Perkins secretary of labor in 1933, she was the first woman named to a U.S. Cabinet post. MCA's focus is the health and welfare of childbearing families. Here, Ruth put her unusual education and personal philosophy to full use during her

25-year tenure as chief executive officer (CEO). While maintaining her Upper West Side residence in Manhattan with her husband, she currently serves as president and CEO of the District of Columbia Birth Center and is founder and president emeritus of the District of Columbia Developing Families Center in Washington, DC. She is also an adjunct professor at the New York University Division of Nursing and the Georgetown University School of Nursing. From 1995-1997, she was an expert consultant for Philip R. Lee, MD, assistant secretary for health in the United States Department of Health & Human Services.

Lubic's vision led to the establishment of the first freestanding childbearing center (CbC) in the United States. The CbC served as a model for more than 150 centers in this country, operating from the MCA townhouse in Manhattan (1975-1996) before being transferred to St. Vincent's Medical Center as the Elizabeth Seton Childbearing Center. Instrumental in the growth of this movement was the National Association of Childbearing Centers (NACC), of which Lubic was a co-founder and first president. Because of her knowledge and skills as a public speaker, she has consulted widely in the United States and with organizations in Japan, Australasia, and several European countries. Birth centers on the CbC model have been established in Australia, Sweden, and Germany. Her insights have led Ruth to redefine the stereotype of the low-income mother as consistently high-risk. Thus, MCA established its second freestanding birth center in 1988 in the depressed inner city area of the southwest Bronx. Apart from achieving remarkable medical statistics, the social and familial impact of MCA has been extraordinary. Turned over to a community health center in 1992, it continues to operate successfully.

Lubic's work has had much recognition for its numerous achievements in public health. In 1971, she was elected to the Institute of Medicine of the National Academy of Sciences. Subsequently, she was elected to fellowship in the American Academy of Nursing, the American College of Nurse-Midwives, the New York Academy of Medicine, the Association for the Advancement of Science, and the Society of Applied Anthropology. She was a member of the first official American medical delegation to the People's Republic of China in 1973. In October 1983, she was designated by *Ladies Home Journal* as one of "America's 100 Most Important Women." Honorary doctorates were awarded by the University of Pennsylvania and four other institutions. She is particularly pleased with the Rockefeller Public Service Award that was presented to her by Princeton University, her son's alma mater.

MARGARET L. MCCLURE, RN, EDD, FAAN

Margaret L. McClure is a professor at New York University, where she holds appointments in both the School of Medicine and College of Nursing. For almost 20 years, she was the chief nursing officer at NYU Medical Center, where she also served as the chief operating officer and hospital administrator.

A prolific writer and lecturer, McClure is internationally recognized as a nursing leader. Her best-known contribution to the literature is the study "Magnet Hospitals: Attraction and Retention of Professional Nurses," which she co-authored under the auspices of the American Academy of Nursing. More recently, she completed *Magnet Hospitals Revisited*, a compilation of the work that has been done to date regarding this subject.

A graduate of the Lankenau Hospital School of Nursing in Philadelphia, McClure received her baccalaureate degree from Moravian College in Bethlehem, Pennsylvania, and her master's and doctoral degrees from Teachers College, Columbia University.

McClure is a member of Sigma Theta Tau International and a past president of the American Academy of Nursing and the American Organization of Nurse Executives. She is the recipient of numerous awards, including an Honorary Doctor of Humane Letters degree from Seton Hall University and an Honorary Doctor of Laws degree from Moravian College. She retired from the United States Army Reserves with the rank of colonel.

MARLA E. SALMON, SCD, RN, FAAN

In 1999, Marla Salmon became dean of the Nell Hodgson Woodruff School of Nursing of Emory University, where she is also professor in both nursing and public health. In addition to her work in academic and clinical nursing, Salmon has held senior leadership positions in professional and national government service. Her career focus has been on national and international health policy, administration, public health, and workforce development.

As former Division of Nursing director and chief nurse of the U.S. Department of Health and Human Services, Salmon led key federal programs aimed at shaping the nation's nursing workforce. She continued this work when she chaired the National Advisory Committee on Nursing Education and Practice, and on an international level, while serving as former chair of the Global Advisory Group on Nursing and Midwifery of the World Health Organization.

Salmon has been called upon to play significant advisory roles nationally and internationally, including membership on the White House Task Force on Health Care Reform and the American Nurses Credentialing Center Magnet Think Tank. More recently, she served on several committees for the Institute of Medicine of the National Academies, including the Committee on the Options for Overseas Placement of U.S. Health Professionals and the Nursing Panel Committee on Monitoring the Changing

Needs for Biomedical and Behavioral Research Personnel Study. She has served as a consultant to the World Health Organization and has worked extensively with government and corporate partners in the Caribbean region and elsewhere.

Salmon serves on a number of professional boards, including membership on the Nursing Advisory Council of the Joint Commission on Accreditation of Healthcare Organizations, the board of directors for the National Council on Healthcare Leadership (NCHL), and the board of trustees of the Robert Wood Johnson Foundation, including former membership on its National Advisory Committee for the Executive Nurse Fellows Program. She has published extensively and is a member of several editorial boards, including *Journal of Nursing Scholarship* and *Nursing and Health Policy Review*.

Salmon has received prestigious awards and recognitions, including membership in the Institute of Medicine and the American Academy of Nursing. Her federal leadership led to her receipt of the President's Meritorious Executive Award and both the U.S. Public Health Service's Chief Nurse Award and Special Recognition awards. Salmon has received the American Nurses Association Community Health Nurse of the Year Award and was recognized by the National Black Nurses' Foundation for her role in enhancing the ethnic and racial diversity of the nation's nursing workforce.

Salmon received her Doctor of Science from The Johns Hopkins University School of Hygiene and Public Health, holds degrees in nursing and political science from the University of Portland, is a Fulbright scholar, and is the recipient of honorary degrees from the University of Portland and the University of Nebraska Medical Center. Salmon is a fellow with the W.K. Kellogg National Fellowship Program and the Hubert H. Humphrey Institute of Public Affairs.

JUDITH SHAMIAN, RN, PHD

Judith Shamian is president and CEO of VON Canada (Victorian Order of Nurses for Canada). She was chosen to head VON Canada effective June 2004. From 1999 to 2004, Shamian was executive director, Office of Nursing Policy, Health Policy & Communications Branch, Health Canada. She was appointed to lead the new national Office of Nursing Policy when it was created in 1999.

In her role as executive director, Shamian participated in a variety of national committees and working groups, and provided advice and support to the policy work of Health Canada. She represented Health Canada at the federal, provincial, and territorial Advisory Committee on Health Human Resources and the policy-setting Canadian Nursing Advisory Committee, both of which make policy recommendations to ministers of health on health human resources issues.

Shamian serves on numerous national and international committees concerned with health services and systems knowledge policy development and nursing.

Shamian is also professor, Faculty of Nursing, at the University of Toronto, and a member of the Nursing & Health Services Research Unit, maintaining an active research portfolio as a principal investigator, co-investigator and decision-maker. Her work has focused in the areas of leadership, health system outcomes, healthy workplaces, and healthy workforce issues, such as turnover of nurses. As co-investigator, she led the Ontario arm of the study in the International Hospital Outcomes Consortium, headed by Linda Aiken. Widely published internationally and in great demand as a speaker and consultant, Shamian has traveled to every Canadian province and territory, as well as throughout the Americas, Eastern Europe,

China, Israel, Africa, the Caribbean, Australia, New Zealand, and other regions of the world.

Shamian is past president and life member of the Registered Nurses Association of Ontario. Before joining Health Canada in 1999, she served for 10 years as vice president at Mount Sinai Hospital in Toronto. In that position, she developed and led the World Health Organization Collaborating Center for Nursing at Mount Sinai, the first such center based in a hospital setting.

Shamian's career in Canada began with her education in nursing at Shaare Zedek Hospital in Israel. She attended Concordia University in Montreal for her bachelor's degree and New York University, United States, for her graduate degree in public health with an emphasis in international health education. She earned her PhD in nursing from Case Western Reserve University in Cleveland, Ohio. Shamian has numerous awards, including the Jubilee medal, which was awarded during the 50th anniversary of Queen Elizabeth II. This award is bestowed on Canadians who have made significant contributions to their country. In 2005, Shamian received an Honorary Doctor of Laws from the University of Lethbridge, Alberta, and another in 2006, from Ryerson University in Toronto, Ontario.

GRAYCE SILLS, PHD, RN, FAAN

Grayce Sills, PhD, RN, FAAN, is professor emeritus at The Ohio State University (OSU) College of Nursing. She joined the faculty in 1964 as an assistant professor. She has served as director of graduate programs and interim dean. Sills was a leader in shaping Ohio State's College of Nursing, including the development of the master's and doctoral programs and acquisition of college status (the college previously was the School of Nursing in the College of Medicine).

She is an internationally recognized scholar and a gifted, inspirational, and compassionate pioneer in the field of psychiatric mental health nursing. Sills is a member of the American Nurses Association and American Psychiatric Nursing Association. She was the founding co-editor of the *Journal of the American Psychiatric Nurses Association* and served as editor until 2005. Her commitment and skill as a teacher earned her a Teaching and Service Award from OSU's College of Medicine and the Alumni Award for Distinguished Teaching. She was named a Living Legend by the American Academy of Nursing and received the Distinguished Practitioner Award from the National Academy of Practice, the Psychosocial Nurse of the Year Award from the American Psychiatric Nurses Association, and the Professional of the Year Award from the Ohio Association for the Mentally Ill. Sills holds a BSN from the University of Dayton, and an MS and PhD from OSU. She received an Honorary Doctor of Science degree from Indiana University, an Honorary Doctor of Science from Fairfield University, and an Honorary Doctor of Public Service from Ohio State University. She has held visiting professorships at the University of New Mexico, Rutgers University, Oregon Health & Science University, Case Western Reserve University, and Indiana University. A fellow of the American Academy of Nursing, Sills was an elected member of AAN's Governing Council and a trustee and chair of The Ohio State University hospital board (1985-2000). In addition, she is past president of the American Nurses Foundation.

KIRSTEN STALLKNECHT, RN, FAAN

Kirsten Stallknecht served 28 years as president of the Danish Nurses Organization. She retired in 1996, but was then elected president of the International Council of Nurses in 1997 and served in that position until 2001. During her career, she has been involved with nursing both nationally and internationally. During the last several years, Stallknecht has been involved with the World Health Organization (WHO) in developing international strategies for nursing and midwifery as a member of the Global Advisory Group of Nursing and Midwifery. Stallknecht has received the following honorary royal titles from Denmark's Queen: Commander of Dannebrog (2001), Order of Dannebrog-Knight of 1st Degree (1996), and Order of Dannebrog (1990). In addition, she received the Christensen's award (1995) and CGFNS International Distinguished Leadership Award.

Stallknecht believes that the most pressing concern today is lack of support for the advancement of nursing to serve the increasing needs of the population worldwide. As the world grows smaller, it is imperative that nurses communicate internationally, because health has no borders and illnesses "fly" from country to country all around the world. Stallknecht further believes that nurses can learn much from each other about how to solve problems as social, political, and economic trends shift. It is important, as well, that individual nurse leaders feel that they are not left alone with their problems and, together, they can overcome great challenges.

Stallknecht received her diploma in nursing from University Hospital in Copenhagen, Denmark, and her diploma in nursing education and management from the School of Advanced Nursing, Aarhus University. In addition, she has traveled extensively on behalf of the profession to such countries as the former USSR, China, USA, Canada, Japan, and the Nordic countries.

FLORENCE SCHORSKE WALD, RN, MN, MS, FAAN

A pioneer of the hospice movement in the United States, Florence S. Wald envisioned the need to maximize the quality of life for the terminally ill. Following a trip to England in the late 1960s to assess the care delivered at Saint Christopher's Hospice near London, Wald returned to the United

States and implemented a feasibility study to determine the need for a hospice in Connecticut. Since that time, her exemplary work with the dying has influenced the further development of hospice care.

Born Florence Sophie Schorske on 19 April 1917 in New York City, she was the younger of two children and attended school in Scarsdale, New York, where the family moved when she was a small child. She graduated from Mount Holyoke College with a Bachelor of Arts degree in 1938 and, in 1941, she received a master's degree in nursing from Yale University School of Nursing. In 1959, she married Henry Wald, whom she credits with being a constant, supportive force in her life.

Wald began her nursing career as a staff nurse with the New York Visiting Nurse Service. Ensuing positions included 6 years as a research assistant in the Surgical Metabolism Unit of the College of Physicians and Surgeons in New York and 2 years as an instructor at Rutgers University School of Nursing in New Jersey. In 1957, she was employed as assistant professor of psychiatric nursing at Yale University School of Nursing and in 1959, she was appointed dean and associate professor, a position she retained for 9 years. From 1969 to 1970, Wald continued at Yale as a research associate and from 1970 to 1980 served as clinical associate professor. At the same time, she was a member of the board and an integral part of the planning staff of Hospice Incorporated in Branford, Connecticut, the first hospice in the United States. Recognizing that the terminally ill have unique needs, Wald developed a hospice model that provides holistic and humanistic care for the dying person and requires appropriate understanding of the concepts of death and dying among nurses giving care in the hospice environment.

Wald has published widely and earned many distinctions, including a Founders Award from the National Hospice Association, a Distinguished

Woman of Connecticut Award from the governor of Connecticut, fellowship in the American Academy of Nursing, and three honorary doctoral degrees. In addition, the Connecticut Nurses Association established the Florence S. Wald Award for Outstanding Contributions to Nursing Practice in her honor.

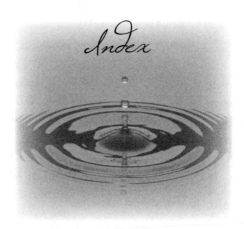

Index

B

C

D

E

J

K

N

O

P

U

V

W

Y–Z